The Biosynthesis of Vitamins
and Related Compounds

To

R. A. MORTON

The Biosynthesis of Vitamins and Related Compounds

by

T. W. GOODWIN

Department of Agricultural Biochemistry
University College of Wales, Aberystwyth, Wales

1963

ACADEMIC PRESS
London and New York

ACADEMIC PRESS INC. (LONDON) LTD.
BERKELEY SQUARE HOUSE
BERKELEY SQUARE
LONDON, W. 1

U.S. Edition published by
ACADEMIC PRESS INC.
111 FIFTH AVENUE
NEW YORK 3, NEW YORK

Library of Congress Catalog Card Number: 63—14041

PRINTED IN HUNGARY

INTRODUCTION

In the advancement of the scientific study of animal nutrition, which followed the classical studies of Eijkman, Funk and Hopkins at the end of the last century and during the first decade of this century, the significance of the vitamin concept clearly emerged. Since then vitamin research has passed through a number of phases. In the first phase a combination of brilliant classical organic chemistry with most painstaking applications of the newly developed techniques of bioassay led to the spectacular developments of the thirties when the structures of some 11 vitamins were elucidated. Since 1940 only two new vitamins, folic acid and vitamin B_{12}, have been described in detail. Although the elucidation of the structures of these compounds again represented a brilliant contribution of organic chemists to biochemistry, the 1940–1960 era represents the heyday of the second phase of vitamin research — the metabolic phase. During this period the fundamental significance of many of the water-soluble vitamins in nutrition was elucidated when it was found that they functioned as co-factors, or coenzymes, for specific enzymes. Further, more detailed investigations with purified systems frequently revealed that the vitamins as isolated in the early days were themselves rarely co-factors *per se*. Derivatives such as pyrophosphates (thiamine pyrophosphate), or nucleotides (nicotinamide adenine dinucleotide) or even more complex structures (coenzyme A) were found to be the true functional units. It is only during the last 2–3 years that the coenzyme form of vitamin B_{12} has been discovered, and there are still many fundamental problems to be solved in this area, especially in describing the coenzyme functions of the fat-soluble vitamins; in spite of this, however, during the past 5–10 years a third phase in vitamin biochemistry has been gradually developing — the biosynthetic phase. The rapid developments in our knowledge of the mechanism of anabolic processes in the main regions of metabolism (fats, carbohydrates, proteins) during the past ten years, combined with the development of new and powerful experimental techniques have allowed meaningful investigations to be carried out on the problem of the biosynthetic pathways leading to the formation of vitamins.

Investigations in this field are rapidly increasing both in number and in sophistication; the aim of this monograph is therefore to correlate for the first time the information currently available on the biosynthesis of vitamins and to present an overall picture of the present position within a framework of modern biochemical thought. In a few cases little information is available, and what is available is fragmentary; it will give satisfaction if these indications of the gaps in our knowledge stimulate appropriate investigations designed to make good the deficiencies.

Although the approach to each vitamin must vary to some extent, the general plan of every chapter dealing with water-soluble vitamins is the same. Firstly investigations on the biosynthesis of the basic vitamin structure are described; these by their very nature are usually confined to micro-organisms and higher plants, but it must be remembered that mammals can synthesize nicotinic acid from tryptophan, and rats can make L-ascorbic acid from D-glucose (it is phenomena such as these which make it difficult to produce a strict definition of a vitamin). In order not to make the treatment too narrow the approach in the first section of each chapter is widened, where appropriate, to include a discussion of the biosynthesis of compounds which are the source of the immediate precursors of the vitamins under consideration; for example, in considering pantothenic acid synthesis, the important problem of the formation of valine, the amino acid from which pantoic acid is synthesized, is fully discussed; similarly, the pathway of tryptophan biosynthesis is considered in the section dealing with the biosynthesis of nicotinic acid. This should help to place the many problems of vitamin biosynthesis in perspective in relation to other metabolic processes, and should also make the book valuable as a text for senior undergraduate students of biochemistry as well as a monograph for investigators directly concerned with vitamin research. In the second main section of each chapter the "activation" of vitamins — their conversion into coenzymes — is discussed; these reactions occur in animals as well as in plants and micro-organisms and all aspects of this problem are considered. The "metabolic lesions" which have occurred during the inexorable evolutionary processes and which make animals dependent on external sources of vitamins are dealt with in a final section.

In the chapters dealing with fat-soluble vitamins an additional problem arises because of the existence of provitamins. Certain carotenoids with the appropriate structure (e.g. β-carotene) can be converted into vitamin A by animals, and 7-dehydrocholesterol in the skin of animals can be converted *in situ* into vitamin D_3 (cholecalciferol) by insolation. In order to put the discussion of these processes on a wider basis, the biosynthetic pathways leading to sterols and carotenoids are considered in detail.

The trivial names of enzymes are generally used in the text, but the specific name, as recommended by the Commission on enzymes of the International Union of Biochemistry, is given in square brackets the first time an enzyme is mentioned. The recommendation of the Commission that "enzymatic" replace "enzymic" has been accepted — although somewhat unwillingly.

The literature has been covered to the end of 1962; but in some cases early 1963 references have also been included. This has only been possible because of the willing co-operation of the publishers.

In general only well-authenticated abbreviations are used; when uncommon abbreviations are used, they are fully defined the first time they appear. NAD^+ and $NADP^+$ are used to represent the oxidized form of nicotinamide adenine dinucleotide and nicotinamide dinucleotide diphosphate, respectively; the reduced forms are represented by NADH and NADPH; when neither the oxidized nor reduced forms are specifically concerned then the symbols NAD and NADP are used.

My thanks are due to Dr. B. H. Davies and Dr. E. I. Mercer who not only read the manuscript and made many valuable suggestions but also read the galley and page proofs; to Dr. D.R. Threlfall who read the galley and page proofs and prepared the subject index; to Miss J.T. Peel for typing the manuscript, and to my daughter Clare for helping to check the references.

Aberystwyth
August, 1963

T. W. GOODWIN

CONTENTS

CHAPTER 1

THIAMINE AND RELATED COMPOUNDS

1. INTRODUCTION

In a now classical series of experiments, C. Funk (1911) described the isolation of a fraction from rice polishings which cured beri-beri, and coined the term "vitamine" for substances which would cure such deficiency diseases. The terminal "e" was dropped in the early 1920's when it was realized that not all such compounds were amines. The material which cured beri-beri was originally termed vitamin B but, following on the demonstration by Emmet and Luros in 1920 that at least two biologically active compounds were present in rice polishings, the compound which was more labile to heat and which cured beri-beri was named vitamin B_1 by the British Accessory Food Factors Committee; this nomenclature is now universally accepted. The trivial name "aneurine" was suggested by Jansen, who first isolated the crystalline material, and it was used for a considerable time throughout Europe; however, it was not acceptable in the United States because of its therapeutic implications. "Aneurine" was eventually replaced by "thiamine" and this is now internationally accepted.

* R = the pyrimidine residue of thiamine; ⓟ = orthophosphate residue.

1

Crystalline thiamine was first obtained from rice polishings in 1926 by Jansen and Donath, but although it was subsequently crystallized from various other sources (e.g. yeast) by various investigators (see Robinson, 1951), it was not until 1934 that R. R. Williams and his colleagues worked out a much more efficient isolation procedure which allowed sufficient material to be accumulated for full chemical study. The investigations which led to the elucidation of the structure (I) of thiamine have been described in detail by Williams himself (1938).

Phosphate Esters of Thiamine

The functional form of thiamine, which acts as the coenzyme for the yeast enzyme carboxylase carrying out reaction 1, was shown

$$CH_3COCOOH \rightarrow CH_3CHO + CO_2 \qquad (1)$$

by Lohmann and Schuster (1937) to be thiamine pyrophosphate (TDP) (II). TDP is now known also to be the coenzyme for pyruvic dehydrogenase, α-oxoglutarate dehydrogenase and transketolase (Westenbrink, 1958). Under mildly alkaline conditions the reaction between TPP and oxo acids proceeds in the absence of enzymes (Mizuhara and Handler, 1954; Yatco-Manzo et al., 1959), and the discovery that, in experiments with model thiazole compounds, the deuterium of D_2O rapidly exchanged with the hydrogen on C-2 of the thiazole ring led to the formulation of a mechanism of thiamine participation in the decarboxylation of α-oxo acids which involved hydroxyalkyl derivatives (Breslow, 1957, 1958). "Active pyruvate" has been identified as α-lactyl-2-thiamine pyrophosphate (Holzer and Beaucamp, 1961); on decarboxylation this yields "active acetaldehyde" (III) which is acted on by yeast carboxylase (Krampitz et al., 1958; Holzer and Beaucamp, 1961) and wheat germ carboxylase (Carlson and Brown, 1961) with the production of acetoin. In the presence of an oxidizing agent, acetoin-forming systems produce acetate from hydroxyethyl thiamine (Krampitz et al., 1961). It has also recently been shown that hydroxyethylthiamine makes up 60—75% and 25% of the total thiamine in Escherichia coli and bakers' yeast, respectively (Carlson and Brown, 1961) and that it appears during the germination of maize seedlings although it is absent from the ungerminated seeds (Johnson and Goodwin, 1963). Thiamine monophosphate (TMP) and thiamine triphosphate (TTP) have been detected in liver (Rossi-Fanelli et al., 1952; Rindi and de Giuseppe, 1961); the function of TTP is not yet known, but, as discussed later-TMP is an intermediate in the biosynthesis of thiamine. As with many other vitamins there is no indication that free thiamine, that is the non-phosphorylated form, occurs to any appreciable extent in biological tissues.

II. BIOSYNTHESIS

A. *General*

(i) *Micro-organisms*

Apart from being universally required by animals, thiamine is also an essential growth factor for many micro-organisms and investigations into this problem yielded the first clues to the way in which the thiamine molecule is built up. The now classical work of W. H. Schopfer and of W. J. Robbins and their colleagues on the mould *Phycomyces blakesleeanus* showed that it required thiamine for growth and that this requirement could also be met by a mixture of the thiazole [4-methyl-5-(β-hydroxyethyl)thiazole, "thiamine thiazole" (IV)] and pyrimidine [2-methyl-6-amino-5-hydroxymethyl-pyrimidine, "pyramine" (V)] components of the molecule (Schopfer and Jung, 1937; Robbins and Kavanagh, 1937).

(IV)   (V)

Following on these observations, many fungi were examined with respect to their thiamine requirement. The results have been discussed in detail by Schopfer (1943) and here it is sufficient to record a representative set of data in Table 1; these results demonstrate that fungi can be separated into five categories according to whether they require (1) preformed thiamine, (2) both fragments preformed, (3) only the pyrimidine fragment preformed, (4) only the thiazole fragment preformed, or (5) no preformed thiamine or either fragment.

These observations have been extended to bacteria the great majority of which can synthesize thiamine; however, a few, for example, *Lactobacillus fermentii* (Sarrett and Cheldelin, 1944) and *Flavobacterium aquatile* (Weeks and Beck, 1960) require it preformed. Others can synthesize one component, for example *Brucella* spp. (thiazole) (Koser and Wright, 1942) and certain *Mycobacterium* spp.

TABLE 1. Requirements of Some Fungi for Thiamine and its Pyrimidine and Thiazole Fragments

Preformed thiamine	Both pyrimidine and thiazole components	Thiazole component only	Pyrimidine component only	Neither constituent components nor thiamine
Ceratostomella fimbriata	Absidia ramosa	Boletus luteus	Cenococcum grandiforme	Neurospora crassa
Ceratostomella penicillata	Amanita pantherina	Boletus piperatus	Ceratostomella coeruleum	Polytomella obtucum
Chalaropsis thielavioides	Boletus granulatus	Endomyces magnusii	Ceratostomella piceae	Polytomella uvella
Cortinarius glaucopus	Boletus variegatus	Mucor ramannianus	Ceratostomella quercus	Rhodotorula aurea
Phytophthora cinnamomi	Marasmius perforans	Stereum frustulosum	Ceratostomella stenoceras	Torula hansen
Phytophthra erythroseptica	Parasitella simplex		Dermatium nigrum	
Phytophthora infestans	Paxillus prunulus		Endomyces vernalis	
Tilletia tritici	Phycomyces		Mitrula pusilla	
Torula cremoris	Phycomyces blakesleeanus		Phythiomorpha gonapodioides	
Torula kefyr	Phycomyces nitens		Phytophthora fagopyri	
Trichophyton discoides	Piricularia oryzae		Phythium butleri	
	Polyporus versicolor		Phythium polycladon	
	Saccharomyces cerevisiae		Pilaira anomala	
	Tilletia horrida		Polyporus adustus	
	Tricholoma albobruneum		Rhodotorula flava	
	Tricophyton album		Rhodotorula mucilaginosa	
			Rhodotorula rubra	
			Schizophyllum commune	
			Sclerotium delphinii	
			Sclerotium rolfsii	
			Sphaerulina trifolii	
			Torula rosea	
			Torula sanguinea	

(pyrimidine) (Lutz, 1948), whilst others require both components but do have the ability to combine them to form thiamine (e.g. *Rhizopus suinis*) (Schopfer, 1943).

(ii) *Higher plants*

Isolated root tissues of the majority of plants require thiamine as a growth factor (Went *et al.*, 1938). Exceptions are maize (McClary, 1940), fleshy sections of carrot root (Nobécourt, 1940) but not seedling carrot root (Bonner, 1940), lucerne *(Medicago sativa)* and the white clover *Trifolium repens* (Bonner, 1938). Root cultures of some varieties of tomato require only the preformed thiazole component whilst others require both components (Robbins and Bartley, 1937). Pea roots have the same requirements (Bonner and Buchman, 1938), whilst flax roots, on the other hand, require only the thiazole residue (Bonner, 1940).

B. *Mechanism of Condensation of Pyrimidine and Thiazole Fragments*

In spite of the clear indications afforded by the nutritional studies discussed in the previous section that the final stage of thiamine biosynthesis involved the condensation of the pyrimidine and thiazole residues, the first direct demonstration of this awaited the development of isotope studies, and it was not until 1959 that Korte and his colleagues (Korte and Weitkamp, 1959; Korte *et al.*, 1959) showed that [2-^{14}C]-4-methyl-5-(β-hydroxyethyl)thiazole (IV) and [^{14}C]-2-methyl-6-amino-5-aminomethylpyrimidine (VI) are both incorporated into thiamine in all micro-organisms examined irrespective of the class (Table 1) into which they fell. It is doubtful whether (VI) is incorporated intact into thiamine as such; indeed recent

(VI)   (VII)

enzymatic studies with yeast extracts have demonstrated the conversion of (VI) into (V) before incorporation into thiamine (Camiener and Brown, 1960). [2-^{14}C]-4-Methylthiazole (VII) is not incorporated into thiamine (Korte *et al.*, 1959).

Harris and Yavit (1957) found that the condensation of (IV) and (V) to form thiamine, catalysed by crude extracts of bakers' yeast, required ATP, but that the ATP requirement was abolished if 2-methyl-6-amino-5-phosphorylmethylpyrimidine (Py-P) was substituted for (V). However, using purer enzyme preparations Leder (1959a) showed that ATP was still required even in the presence of Py-P, and that the first product of the reaction was thiamine monophosphate. These observations eventually led to the elucidation of the mechanism of the reaction (sequences 2–6) by a number of investigators almost simultaneously (Leder, 1959b; Camiener and Brown, 1959, 1960; Nose *et al.*, 1959, 1961; Suzuoki and Kobata, 1960).

$$\text{2-Methyl-6-amino-5-hydroxymethylpyrimidine} + \text{ATP} \xrightarrow{\text{Mg}^{2+}} \text{2-methyl-6-amino-5-phoshorylmethylpyrimidine (Py-P)} + \text{ADP} \qquad (2)$$

$$\text{Py-P} + \text{ATP} \xrightarrow{\text{Mg}^{2+}} \text{Py-P-P} + \text{ADP} \qquad (3)$$

$$\text{4-Methyl-5(}\beta\text{-hydroxyethyl)thiazole} + \text{ATP} \xrightarrow{\text{Mg}^{2+}} \text{4-methyl-5(}\beta\text{-phosphorylethyl)thiazole (Th-P)} + \text{ADP} \qquad (4)$$

$$\text{Py-P-P} + \text{Th-P} \xrightleftharpoons{\text{Mg}^{2+}} \text{Thiamine monophosphate} + \text{P-P} \qquad (5)$$

$$\text{Thiamine monophosphate} + \text{H}_2\text{O} \longrightarrow \text{Thiamine} + \text{P} \qquad (6)$$

The separation of the synthesis of Py-P-P into two stages (2 and 3) has been indicated by the following observations of Lewin and Brown (1961): (a) during the reaction Py-P always appears first; (b) a purified enzyme converts Py-P into Py-P-P without the intermediate formation of the free pyrimidine; (c) the activity of a Py-P-P-forming enzyme can be destroyed without affecting reaction (2), and (d) UTP, GTP and CTP can replace ATP in reaction (2), but not in reaction (3). A similar conclusion has been reached by Kawasaki *et al.* (1960) and Kawasaki and Fujita (1961).

Although the details of reaction (4) are not completely settled, it probably takes place as indicated because thiazole pyrophosphate has never been detected during the reaction.

The enzyme carrying out reaction (5), *thiamine monophosphate synthetase (thiamine phosphate phosphorylase)* is specific for the two substrates indicated. It has been purified 500-fold from yeast and exhibits a pH optimum at 9·2. The Michaelis constants for the pyrimidine and thiazole substrates are $1·0 \times 10^{-6}$M and $7·0 \times 10^{-6}$M respectively; pyrophosphate (8×10^{-6}M) inhibits the reaction non-competitively (Leder, 1961).

In 1959 Eberhart and Tatum described a number of thiamine-requiring *Neurospora crassa* mutants which will also respond to a mixture of the pyrimidine and thiazole residues of thiamine. A gene *thi-10* was also described which reduces the ability of one of the mutants *(thi-1)* to condense the two residues. Now that the biochemistry of the condensation has been worked out, it would be interesting to investigate the locus of action of *thi-10*.

C. *Formation of the Pyrimidine Residue*

The pyrimidine component (V) of thiamine differs from the pyrimidines found in RNA and DNA in one important respect — there is a methyl substituent at C-2. The hydroxymethyl substituent at C-5 can also be considered unique in the present context because such a substituent is only found in certain special DNA molecules such as bacteriophage T_2 (see Goodwin, 1960). As some micro-organisms require the pyrimidine residue of thiamine preformed, and as they must certainly be able to synthesize their nucleic acid pyrimidines, it is clear that the requirement for the thiamine pyrimidine (V) is the result of either: (a) its pathway of synthesis being different from the conventional pathway (Fig. 1); or (b) the inability of the organism to insert the required substituent at C-2 and/or C-5; or (c) the inability of the organism to remove ribose 5-phosphate from, for example, uridine 5-phosphate, because, as indicated in Fig. 1, pyrimidines are synthesized at the nucleoside 5-phosphate level whilst, as stated in the previous section, the free pyrimidine is the obligatory substrate for thiamine biosynthesis.

The problem of the synthesis of the pyrimidine residue of thiamine is now ripe for direct biochemical attack but at the time of writing very little work has been reported. A thiamine-less strain of *Esch. coli* which will grow on a mixture of the pyrimidine and thiazole residues of thiamine will also grow when the thiazole portion is replaced by a mixture of thymine and uracil (Nakayama, 1956). Pine and Guthrie (1959) found that *Bact. subtilis* (ATCC 6051) incorporates [^{14}C]formate specifically into the pyrimidine fragment of thiamine. As formate is not a component of the ring system of pyrimidines, it was concluded that it was present in the C-2 methyl and/or the C-5 hydroxymethyl carbons and was incorporated by means of a conventional 1-C transfer; this view is supported by the observation that the incorporation is reduced in the presence of amethopterin which specifically inhibits 1-C transfer. Somewhat similar results have been observed with [^{14}C]formate incorporation into thiamine in bakers' yeast (David and Estramareix, 1960; Goodwin and Howells, 1961) although in the experiments of Goodwin and Howells some activity was also found in the thiazole residue. The label from [^{14}C-methyl]methionine is also incorporated into the pyrimidine residue of thiamine in bakers' yeast but not as effectively as into the thiazole residue (Howells, 1962). According to David and Estramareix (1961) the label is not incorporated into the carbon attached to C-5 of the pyrimidine residue. If this report is confirmed

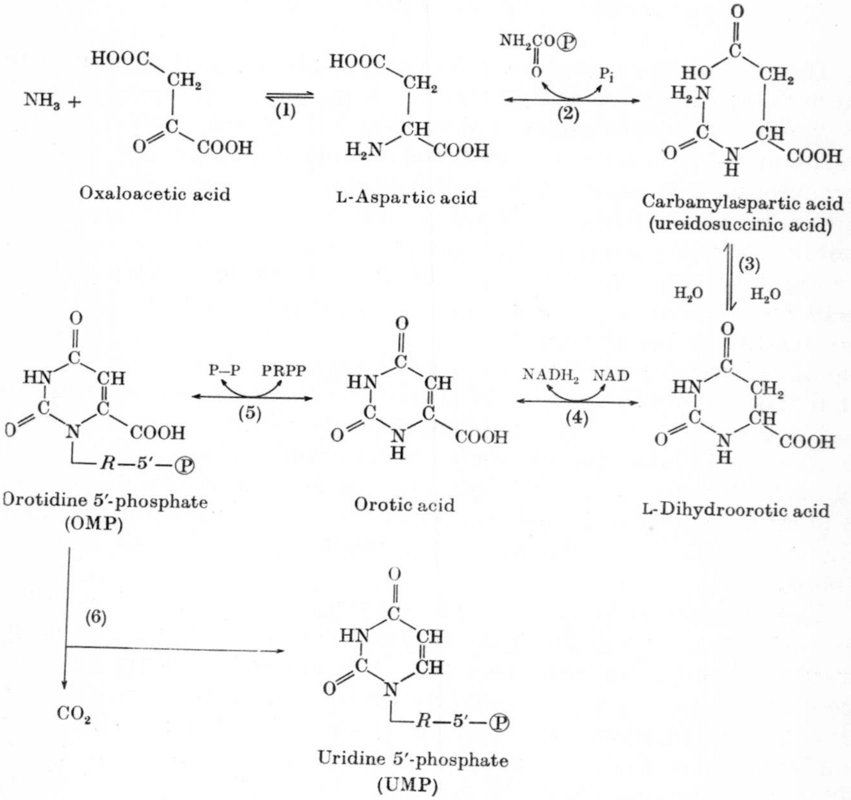

FIG. 1. The Pathway of Pyrimidine Biosynthesis.

then it is possible that the pyrimidine residue arises from β-methyl-aspartate and not aspartate (Fig. 1). This would yield a methyl substituent at C-5 which would not have arisen from a 1-C unit because β-methylaspartate is formed from glutamate under the influence of *glutamate isomerase* (Barker, 1961). Some support for this view comes from the report that tritiated β-methylaspartate is incorporated into thiamine by *Esch. coli* (Woolley and Koehelik, 1961).

Nutritional experiments indicated that isolated pea roots do not possess even a limited synthetic ability with regard to the synthesis of the pyrimidine residue; the absence of a 1-C substituent from C-5 or an NH_2 group from C-6 completely eliminated the growth promoting activity of the residue (Bonner and Bonner, 1948).

It has already been stated that 2-methyl-6-amino-5-aminomethylpyrimidine (VI) is converted into 2-methyl-6-amino-5-hydroxymethylpyrimidine (V) before incorporation into thiamine, and the same is true for 2-methyl-6-amino-5-methoxypyrimidine (Camiener and Brown, 1960); presumably a similar reaction occurs with (VI) in the yeast *Rhodotorula rubra* (Schopfer, 1938) and also in a thiamine-requiring strain of the bacterium *Esch. coli*, which can grow in the presence of (VI) and the thiazole residue of thiamine (Nakayama, 1956, 1957). 2-Methyl-6-amino-5-formylpyrimidine was also active in the *Esch. coli* strain (Nakayama, 1956, 1957), whilst 2-methyl--6-amino-5-cyanopyrimidine was inactive in both *R. rubra* (Schopfer, 1938) and *Esch. coli* (Nakayama, 1956, 1957). [4-^{14}C]-2-Methyl-6--amino-4-hydroxypyrimidine and 2,5-dimethyl-6-amino-4-hydroxypyrimidine are incorporated into thiamine only in micro-organisms which require the pyrimidine residue preformed.

D. *Formation of the Thiazole Residue*

Very little is known concerning the mechanism of the formation of the thiazole ring of thiamine. The claim (Bonner and Buchman, 1938) that isolated pea roots will condense thioformamide with acetopropanol according to reaction (7) has not been confirmed in either pea roots (Louis, 1951) or in the micro-organisms *Phycomyces* and *Neurospora* (Tatum and Bell, 1946). Furthermore, [^{35}S]-γ-mercapto-γ-acetopropyl acetate is not incorporated into thiamine by micro-organisms (Korte *et al.*, 1961). Harington and Moggridge (1940) postulated that thiazole arose from a-amino-β-(4-

$$\tag{7}$$

methylthiazole-5-)propionic acid (VIII) which in turn could be formed from methionine by the addition of acetaldehyde and NH_2 group (reaction 8). Some support for this view is that the L form of (VIII) is converted to some extent into the thiazole residue by yeast (Harington and Moggridge, 1940) and by isolated pea roots (Bonner and Buchman, 1938; Robbins, 1940) but not by

$$
\underset{S}{\overset{N}{\big|}}\!\!\!-\!\!CH_3
$$
$$CH_2CH(NH_2)COOH$$

(VIII)

$$\text{``}NH_2\text{''} + \underset{H_3C}{\overset{H}{\underset{S}{\big|}}}\overset{O=C-CH_3}{} + H_3C\underset{S}{\diagdown}CH_2CH_2CH(NH_2)COOH \longrightarrow \underset{S}{\overset{N}{\big|}}\!\!-\!CH_3 \; CH_2CH(NH_2)COOH \quad (8)$$

Phycomyces blakesleeanus [Bonner, quoted by Buchman and Richardson (1939)] or by *Staphylococcus aureus* [Knight, quoted by Harington and Moggridge (1939)]. Reaction (8) would require that the methyl group on C-4 should arise not from a 1-C transfer but that the methyl of methionine should appear at C-2; this conclusion is supported by the observation that [^{14}C]formate is insignificantly incorporated into the thiazole residue of thiamine by *B. subtilis* and bakers' yeast whilst [^{14}C-methyl]methionine is more effectively incorporated (Howells, 1962). Furthermore, [^{35}S]methionine is more readily introduced into the thiazole residue of thiamine in bakers' yeast than is [^{35}S]cysteine, and unlabelled methionine dilutes out the incorporation of $^{35}SO_4{}^{2-}$ into thiamine to a greater extent than does cysteine or homocysteine (Hitchcock and Walker, 1961).

The variations in the thiazole residue which can be tolerated by isolated pea roots are not great (Table 2): - compounds with the following substituents in place of —CH$_2$CH$_2$OH at C-5 are active: —CH$_2$CHOHCH$_3$, —CH$_2$CH$_2$CH$_2$OH and, as already indicated (p. 5), —CH$_2$CHNH$_2$COOH; replacement of —CH$_2$CH$_2$OH by —H, —CHOHCH$_3$, or —COOH results in an inactive molecule (Bonner and Bonner, 1948). Table 2 also indicates that no variation in substitution in C-5 of the thiazole residue can be tolerated in the intact thiamine molecule by pea roots.

On the other hand, Nakayama (1956, 1957) reported that thiamine auxotrophs of *Esch. coli* (26–43) and *N. crassa* (18558A), which can utilize the thiazole residue of thiamine, also respond to a limited extent to 4-methylthiazole (VII). Furthermore both mutants can be maintained in the absence of the thiazole residue by either cysteine, or 4-thiazolidine carboxylic acid (IX), but not by homocysteine, methionine or methanol. Because considerable amounts of thiamine

TABLE 2. Effect of Varying Substituents in Position 5 of the Thiazole Residue of the Thiamine Molecule on its Activity as a Growth Factor for Isolated Pea Roots (Bonner and Bonner, 1948).

In intact molecule		In thiazole fragment	
Substituent	Activity	Substituent	Activity
CH_2CH_2OH*	+	CH_2CH_2OH*	+
$CHOHCH_3$	—	$CHOHCH_3$	—
$CH_2CHOHCH_3$	—	$CH_2CHOHCH_3$	+
$CH_2CH_2CH_2OH$	—	$CH_2CH_2CH_2OH$	+
$CHNH_2COOH$	—	$CHNH_2COOH$	+
		$COOH$	—

and the thiazole residue of thiamine accumulated in cultures of these mutants when they were incubated with either cysteine or 4-thiazolidine carboxylic acid, reaction (9) was suggested as the route for biosynthesis. However, this scheme involves 4-methylthiazole as a key intermediate; as just stated, this is not an outstandingly effective intermediate in these mutants and, as indicated above, it is completely ineffective in isolated pea roots. Furthermore, (a) as stated on p. 5, [2-^{14}C]-4-methylthiazole is not incorporated into thiamine in a number of micro-organisms (Korte *et al.*, 1959), and (b) in isotope competition experiments, the incorporation of $^{35}SO_4^{2-}$ into thiamine by yeast is very effectively diluted out by the intact thiazole residue, whilst 4-methylthiazole had only insignificant activity (Hitchcock and Walker, 1961).

Plaut (1961) has recently suggested a third possible route for the synthesis of the thiazole residue of thiamine. It will be recalled that the thiazolidine ring of penicillin arises from condensation of cysteine and valine (reaction 10) (see Goodwin, 1960); analogously, cysteine could condense with, for example, glutamic acid to form a thiazolidine precursor of the thiazole residue of thiamine (reaction 11)

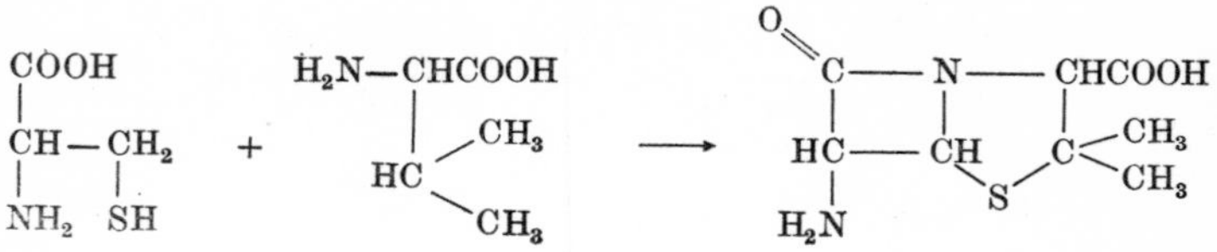

$$
\begin{array}{ccc}
\underset{\substack{|\\ \mathrm{CH-CH_2}\\ |\quad\;|\\ \mathrm{NH_2\;\; SH}}}{\mathrm{COOH}}
& + &
\underset{\substack{|\\ \mathrm{HC} \diagdown \mathrm{CH_3}\\ \mathrm{CH_3}}}{\underset{|}{\mathrm{H_2N-CHCOOH}}}
\end{array}
\longrightarrow
\qquad (10)
$$

$$
\mathrm{HOOCCHNH_2CH_2} \underset{\mathrm{SH_2}}{|} \quad + \quad \underset{\substack{|\\ \mathrm{CH_2.CH_2COOH}}}{\mathrm{H_2NCH.COOH}} \quad \dashrightarrow
$$

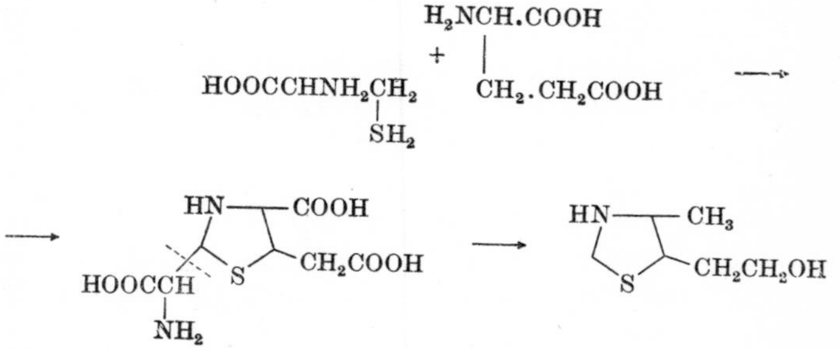

$$
\longrightarrow \qquad\qquad \longrightarrow \qquad\qquad (11)
$$

III. GENERAL FACTORS CONTROLLING THIAMINE FORMATION

A. *Higher Plants*

(i) *Vegetative tissues*

Bonner (1942) demonstrated in a number of ways that the leaf is responsible for thiamine synthesis in the tomato plant. For example, (1) transport of thiamine to roots occurs only in plants with intact leaves, and (2) girdling* of the petioles results in accumulation of the vitamin on the laminar side of the girdle. Maximal synthesis and transport occur in mature leaves. Although young, rapidly expanding leaves are capable of synthesis, little or no translocation occurs to or from these sites at this time.

Maximal concentrations of thiamine are found in the shoot apex and youngest leaves in tomatoes (Bonner, 1942), maize (corn) (Burkholder and McVeigh, 1940), peas (von Rytz, 1939), cotton (Sukhorukov and Filippov, 1940) and many woody plants (Burkholder and Snow, 1942). The reasons for these high concentrations are (a) there is translocation from the mature leaves towards the apex, and (b), as just mentioned, there appears to be little translocation away from the young rapidly expanding leaves (Bonner, 1942).

---

* Girdling involves destruction of a small region of stem or petiole by a jet of steam, thus blocking translocation through the phloem, although movement of water and salts through the xylem is unimpaired.

In tomatoes there is a decreasing concentration of thiamine in each successive lower leaf and a similar gradient in the stem. Maximal thiamine content, however, occurs in the eighth leaf, owing to (a) the increasing weight of the older leaves, and (b) the fact that the older leaves continue to synthesize the vitamin. The thiamine concentration tends to reach a maximum at the time of flowering (Kohler, 1944).

(ii) *Reproductive tissues*

Thiamine is well distributed in the reproductive tissues of plants; it has been detected in flower buds, calices, corolla, stamens and pistils of peas and tulips (von Rytz, 1939), and also in many pollens and seeds.

In the case of the wheat plant, Geddes and Levine (1942) found that during seed production, the thiamine of the glumes, rachides, stems and leaves decreased to an extent that equalled the increased amounts found in the developing seeds. It would appear from these observations that around seeding time thiamine synthesis in the vegetative tissues of wheat stops and the vitamin already present is transferred to the seeds. In the pea plant, however, vegetative synthesis continues during seed formation, and von Rytz (1939) could not decide unequivocally whether translocation to the developing seeds, which reached their maximal concentration just before drying out, did or did not occur.

There is considerable differential distribution of thiamine within the seeds of cereals. Von Rytz (1939) found the concentration to

TABLE 3. Quantitative Distribution of Thiamine in Rice Seeds (Hinton, 1948)

Tissue	Concentration mg/100 g
Plumule	4·65
Radicle	6·45
Epiblast	7·80
Coleorhiza	9·45
Scutellum	18·90
Pericarp and aleurone layer	3·15
Endosperm, outer	0·14
Endosperm, inner	0·30

be relatively low in the endosperm, high in the embryo and highest (150 $\mu g/g$) in the scutellum where about 50% of the total seed thiamine is located. Quantitative values for rice are given in Table 3. Further details for other plants are reported by Holman (1956). This distribution pattern is maintained throughout maturation of the seed (Pollock and Geddes, 1951).

(iii) *Synthesis during seed germination*

Light is necessary for thiamine synthesis in germinating seeds of many species. Bonner and Greene (1938), for example, demonstrated that cotyledonectomized pea embryos kept in the dark synthesized no thiamine for at least eight days following the onset of germination. Similar results have been obtained with tomatoes (Bonner and Bonner, 1948), wheat (Hoffer *et al.*, 1946) and soya and mung beans (Burkholder and McVeigh, 1945). Although there is no net synthesis of thiamine in the dark, considerable redistribution occurs in the developing seedling. After 18 days germination in the dark, the thiamine content of the wheat embryo increased from 11 to 60% of the total; there was a corresponding decrease in the amount of the endosperm (Hoffer *et al.*, 1946). Even in the light there is occasionally a lag period of some 36 hr before thiamine synthesis begins and this is clearly seen in germinating black-eyed peas and lima beans, but not in cotton seedlings (Cheldelin and Lane, 1943).

(iv) *Effect of trace elements*

Bluzmanas (1961) reported that addition of Zn, Cu, Mn and B singly to sand cultures of *Lupinus luteus* stimulated thiamine synthesis. For example Zn (0·5 mg/kg sand) increased the thiamine concentration by 43–58% whilst at the same time stimulating growth by 68%. Spraying the plants with solutions of salts of the trace elements had similar effects.

(v) *General*

Treatment of red kidney bean plants with 2,4-dichlorophenoxyacetic acid (2,4-D) reduces the thiamine levels in the leaves but increases the levels in the stems (Luecke *et al.*, 1949). Thiamine synthesis in *Tradescantia* leaves varied with the wavelength of light illuminating them; active wavelengths were between 435 and 505 mμ and above 630 mμ (Ruge, 1959). These observations suggest that the extent of thiamine synthesis was closely related to the intensity of photosynthetic activity.

B. *Micro-organisms*

(i) *Bacteria*

The constitution of the basal medium often has a profound effect on the synthetic ability of a bacterium. *Bacillus paaralvei*, for example, normally requires thiamine–thiazole when cultured on a medium devoid of cystine, phenylalanine, valine and leucine. However, in the absence of these constituents but in a reducing medium (containing thioglycocholate, $Na_2S_2O_4$ or ascorbic acid), neither the thiazole nor an external source of thiamine is required (Katznelson, 1947).

In the presence of small amounts of biotin the requirement of *Micrococcus pyogenes* var. *aureus* for thiamine (and nicotinic acid) is reduced by a factor of ten (Kögl and Wagtendonk, 1938); the reason for this is not yet forthcoming. On the other hand, the presence of vitamin B_{12} is said to inhibit thiamine synthesis in *Esch. coli* without affecting growth (Saxena *et al.*, 1954). In a study of thiamine synthesis in the various phases of development of *Azotobacter chroococcum* Pakarskite (1961) found that the maximum value for bound thiamine was achieved at the very beginning of the logarithmic phase; free thiamine only appeared during the stationary phase.

Some bacteria which normally require thiamine for growth can be induced to synthesize it (Silverman and Werkman, 1939). The synthesis of thiamine by 12 species of bacteria isolated from maize and potato rhizospheres was stimulated by the addition of Mo, Zn, or Mn, but not by B, Cu, or Co (Bershova and Kozlova, 1962).

(ii) *Fungi*

Rather more work with fungi than with bacteria has been carried out on the general factors controlling thiamine biosynthesis. The effects of the alteration of various medium constituents have been examined in detail. According to Fromageot and Tschang (1938), *Rhodotorula sanniei* requires thiamine when glucose is the carbon source but can dispense with it when glycerol is the carbon source. It has also been reported that the amino acids present in the medium affect the thiamine requirement of many fungi (Leonian and Lilly, 1940). It is perhaps desirable to view these early reports with a little scepticism; the experiments were carried out before the development of modern methods of purification of amino acids and sugars which may have been contaminated with traces of thiamine.

Low concentrations of minerals appear to stimulate thiamine synthesis, because high yields of thiamine from *Aspergillus oryzae* are obtained on media low in chloride (Wirth and Nord, 1942); furthermore *Phythium butleri*, which requires thiamine for growth when the culture medium contain 1·64% of minerals, requires only thiamine – thiazole when this concentration is reduced ten times (Robbins and Kavanagh, 1938). Thiamine synthesis is much increased in *Torula utilis* in the absence of iron (Lewis, 1944).

The pH optimum for thiamine synthesis in yeasts in 4·3 (Pavcek *et al.*, 1937, 1938). In some other fungi the thiamine requirement of the organisms is pH-dependent. For example, *Sodaria fimicola* when grown in the pH range 3·4–3·8 requires thiamine, whilst at pH 4·0 and above, thiamine is not required (Lilly and Barnett, 1947).

Early work appeared to establish the fact that thiamine synthesis is stimulated by anaerobic conditions (see, e.g. Lewis *et al.*, 1944; Maizel, 1946), although it is claimed that the coupling of the thiazole and pyrimidine fragments is enhanced by aeration (van Lanen *et al.*, 1942). In the latter case aerobiosis presumably stimulates the synthesis of the ATP required for the condensing reaction (p. 6) However, it has recently been reported that the fungus *Mucor rouxii* requires an exogenous source of thiamine if grown under anaerobic conditions (Bartnicki–Garcia and Nickerson, 1961).

It is interesting that pyridoxal phosphate (X) inhibits the synthesis

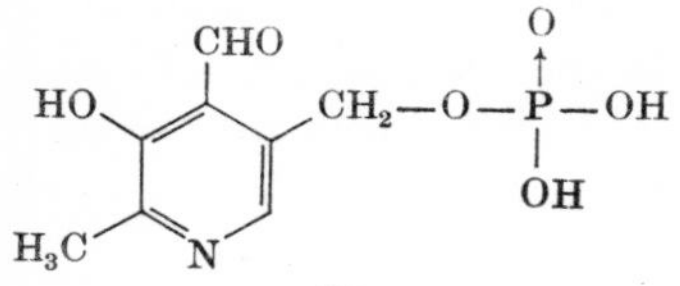

(X)

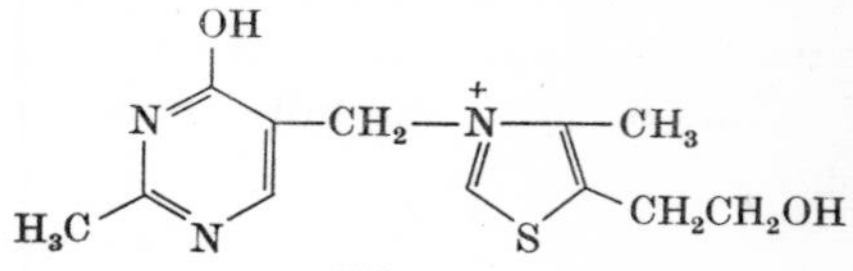

(XI)

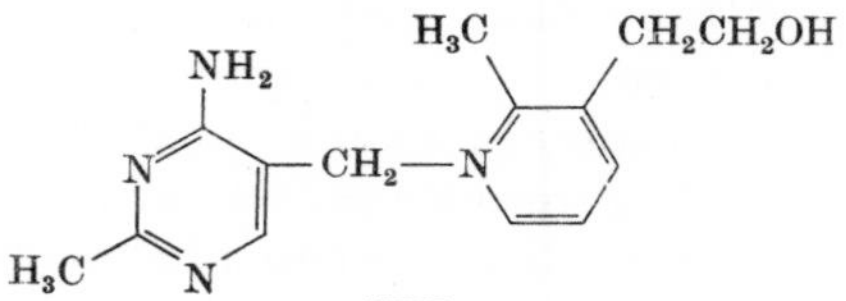

(XII)

of thiamine in *Neurospora* (Harris, 1956). This appears to be a true competitive inhibition for it is overcome competitively by the pyrimidine residue of thiamine; presumably pyridoxal interferes with the synthesis of this residue. It remains to be seen whether this relationship is important in the metabolic control of thiamine synthesis. Conversely, Harris (1953) earlier found that pyridoxine auxotrophs of *N. crassa* and *N. sitophila* grew better when thiamine was present in the medium. This was eventually found to be due to the fact that thiamine inhibited the destruction of pyridoxine in the medium.

Ascorbic acid also has a thiamine-sparing action in *Lactobacillus casei* (Fang and Butts, 1953), but the mechanism of this action is unknown.

Algae

Most algae are able to synthesize their own thiamine but a number do require an exogenous source. These follow the same pattern observed in the bacteria and fungi: for example, the colourless *Polytoma ocellatum* requires only the thiazole residue preformed (Lwoff, 1947), whilst both residues must be supplied to two other colourless algae, *Chilomonas paramoecium* and *Prototheca zopfii* (Anderson, 1945, Lwoff, 1947). *Euglena gracilis* requires only the pyrimidine residue (Lwoff, 1947) and this requirement remains irrespective of whether the organism is growing heterotrophically or photosynthetically. A mutant of *Chlamydomonas moewusii* has been obtained by ultraviolet treatment which responds to as little as 10^{-4} μg/ml of thiamine in the medium (Lewin, 1952). The quantitative requirements of the native algal species which require thiamine have not been investigated in detail, but if they are as low as with the *Chlamydomonas* mutant, then it is not difficult to believe that there is sufficient thiamine in natural waters to supply the demands of these algae.

IV. BIOSYNTHESIS OF THIAMINE PHOSPHATES
A. *Thiamine Monophosphate (TMP)*

It has already been pointed out (p. 6) that thiamine is synthesized at the monophosphate level in micro-organisms. There is no well-documented enzymatic evidence that TMP can be synthesized by the phosphorylation of free thiamine by a thiamine kinase, but FMN phosphatase purified from green gram seeds will act as a transphosphorylase and transfer the phosphate group from FMN to thiamine (reaction 12) (Kumar, 1962).

$$FMN + thiamine \rightleftharpoons TMP + riboflavin \qquad (12)$$

$[^{35}S]$-TMP is present in the liver of rats injected with $[^{35}S]$thiamine, but the kinetics of the appearance of label in this compound and into thiamine diphosphate indicate that TMP is formed from TDP (Rindi *et al.*, 1962).

B. *Thiamine Diphosphate (TDP: Co-carboxylase)*

(i) *Micro-organisms*

In the late 1930's von Euler and Vestrin (1937) and Weil-Malherbe (1939) obtained acetone-dried powders of brewers' yeast which would convert thiamine into TDP in the presence of ATP (reaction 13). This has since been confirmed by many investigators, including Lipton and Elvehjem (1940), Westenbrink *et al.* (1947), Kiessling, (1956), Shimazona *et al.* (1959) and Mano (1960), who used intact and plasmolysed cells and also partly purified systems. The enzyme responsible has been termed *thiamine pyrophosphokinase* [ATP: thiamine pyrophosphotransferase] and the mechanism of action outlined in reaction 13 has been demonstrated by Forsander (1956), Greiling (1958) and Kaziro *et al*, (1961) who used [γ-^{32}P]-ATP to show that the distribution of label in TDP was consistent only with the direct transfer of a pyrophosphate group. Weil–Malherbe

$$\text{Thiamine} + \text{ATP} \xrightarrow{\text{Mg}^{2+}} \text{TDP} + \text{AMP} \qquad (13)$$

(1939) made the important observation that TMP was a less effective substrate than free thiamine. This has now been explained at the enzyme level by Camiener and Brown (1959) and Kaziro *et al.* (1961) who found that TMP was not a substrate for purified thiamine pyrophosphokinase prepared from bakers' yeast.

Steyn-Parvé (1952) found that thiamine pyrophosphokinase could be activated by Mn^{2+}, but that at concentrations above 2×10^{-3}M Mn^{2+} was inhibitory. Similarly the reaction is stimulated by traces of orthophosphate but inhibited completely by molar concentrations. The enzyme has a broad pH optimum stretching between 6 and 9 (Steyn-Parvé, 1952). A purified preparation free from adenylate kinase, adenine triphosphatase, nucleoside diphosphokinase and thiamine pyrophosphatase, will use the nucleoside triphosphates of uracil, cytosine, hypoxanthine and guanine in place of ATP as pyrophosphate donor (Kaziro and Shimazono, 1959).

The ability of intact yeast cells to phosphorylate thiamine is considerable and, in the presence of excess substrate, can continue for up to 14 hr (Westenbrink *et al.*, 1947; Kiessling, 1953). Thiamine pyrophosphokinase is inhibited by the pyrimidine residue of thiamine (V) (Westenbrink *et al.*, 1947) and by oxythiamine (XI) (Eusebi and Cerecedo, 1950) but not by pyrithiamine (XII) (Eich and Cerecedo, 1954). The enzyme from animal sources responds differently to these inhibitors (see below).

With one possible exception, all organisms which require thiamine must possess thiamine pyrophosphokinase, because their requirements can be satisfied by the free base. The exception is *Neisseria gonorrhaeae* which requires preformed TDP, thiamine itself being completely ineffective (Lankford and Skeggs, 1946). Indeed thiamine competitively inhibited the utilization of TDP.

(ii) *Animals*

The enzymatic synthesis of TDP from thiamine was demonstrated in many animal tissues about the same time as in micro-organisms (see Tauber, 1938; Goodhart and Sinclair, 1939; Ochoa, 1939). The formed elements (e.g. red blood cells) have a particularly active enzyme (Westenbrink, 1958).

Leuthart and Nielsen (1952) demonstrated that the liver enzyme was not present in the mitochondria, and then proceeded to purify it considerably. The mechanism of the reaction was shown to be the same as that occurring in yeast (reaction 13; p. 18). ATP was required in excess, and ADP and AMP inhibited the synthesis. Similar preparations have been obtained from rat intestinal mucosae (Cerecedo *et al.*, 1954; Eich and Cerecedo, 1954). The pH optimum for the liver enzyme is 6·8–6·9 (Leuthart and Nielsen, 1952).

In experiments with rat kidney particles Bartley (1954) showed that synthesis of TDP by phosphorylation of either thiamine or TMP did not occur; however, slow incorporation of $^{32}P_i$ into added TDP did occur. Kiessling (1957), on the other hand, found that $^{32}P_i$ was incorporated into endogenous TDP in liver mitochondria, but that added thiamine phosphates became labelled only to a slight extent.

Pyrithiamine, but not oxythiamine, inhibits the liver enzyme (Eich and Cerecedo, 1954); this is opposite to the observations made with the yeast enzyme. Pyrithiamine is actually converted into its pyrophosphate by the liver enzyme (Koedam, quoted by Westenbrink, 1958).

C. *Diphosphothiamine Disulphide*

Diphosphothiamine disulphide (XIII) has been reported in bakers' yeast grown under anaerobic conditions (Suomalainen *et al.*, 1949; Olivo *et al.*, 1962) but not in brewers' yeast or in animal tissues. It is almost certainly formed by the oxidation of TDP, but no investigations on this point have been reported.

(XIII)

D. *Thiamine Triphosphate (TTP)*

Kiessling (1953, 1956) showed that bakers' yeast accumulated TTP as well as TDP when incubated with excess thiamine. Experiments with $^{32}P_i$ and with $[^{32}P]$-ATP indicate that TTP is formed by the transfer of an orthophosphate group from ATP to TDP (Greiling, 1958; Kiessling, 1959) (reaction 14). For example, with a purified yeast extract in the presence of $[\gamma\text{-}^{32}P]$-ATP, Greiling

$$TDP + ATP \rightarrow TTP + ADP \qquad (14)$$

found that the ratio of the radioactivity in the α- and β-phosphorus atoms in TDP was $1:3$, and in the α, β, and γ atoms of TTP $1:3:3$.

E. *Hydroxyethylthiamine Pyrophosphate*

α-Lactyl-2-thiamine pyrophosphate and hydroxyethylthiamine pyrophosphate, "active acetaldehyde", are formed enzymatically from TDP and pyruvate in the presence of purified yeast carboxylase (Carlson and Brown, 1960, 1961; Holzer and Beaucamp, 1959, 1961; Holzer *et al.*, 1960). If α-oxobutyrate replaces pyruvate then a different compound, probably α-hydroxypropylthiamine pyrophosphate is formed (Carlson and Brown, 1960, 1961)

F. *Thiamine sulphate esters*

When isolated rat livers are perfused with a mixture of blood and Ringer's solution containing relatively large amounts (1 – 3 mg) of thiamine, up to one half of the vitamin is converted into thiamine disulphate and the remainder into the di- and tri-phosphates (Barnabei and Wildemann, 1961). The reason for this unexpected observation is not clear.

REFERENCES

Anderson, E. H. (1945). *J. gen. Microbiol.* **28**, 287, 297.

Barker, H. A. (1961). *Fed. Proc.* **20**, 956.

Barnabei, O., and Wildemann, L. (1961). *Hoppe-Seyl. Z.* **395**, 1.

Bartnicki-Garcia, S. and Nickerson, W. J. (1961). *J. Bact.*, **82**, 142

Bartley, W. (1954). *Biochem. J.* **56**, 379.

Bershova, O. I., and Kozlova, I. A. (1962). *Mikrobiol. Zh. Akad. Nauk. Ukr. R. S.* **24**, 30

Bluzmanas, P. (1961). *In* "Proceedings of the 5th International Congress of Biochemistry, Moscow", p. 498. Pergamon Press, London.

Bonner, J. (1938). *Amer. J. Bot.* **25**, 543.

Bonner, J. (1940). *Amer. J. Bot.* **27**, 692.

Bonner, J. (1942). *Amer J. Bot.* **29**, 136.

Bonner, J., and Bonner, H. (1948). *Vitam. & Horm.* **6**, 225.

Bonner, J., and Buchman, E. R. (1938). *Proc. nat. Acad. Sci.*, *Wash.* **24**, 431.

Bonner, J., and Greene, J. (1938). *Botan. Gaz.* **100**, 226.

Breslow, R. (1957). *J. Amer. chem. Soc.* **79**, 1762.

Breslow, R. (1958). *J. Amer. chem. Soc.* **80**, 3719.

Buchman, E. R., and Richardson, E. M. (1939). *J. Amer. chem. Soc.* **61**, 891.

Burkholder, P. R., and McVeigh, I. (1940). *Amer. J. Bot.* **27**, 853.

Burkholder, P. R., and Snow, A. G. (1942). *Bull. Torrey Bot. Club* **69**, 421.

Burkholder, P. R., and McVeigh, I. (1945). *Plant Physiol.* **20**, 301.

Camiener, G. W., and Brown, G. M. (1959). *J. Amer. chem. Soc.* **81**, 3800.

Camiener, G. W., and Brown, G. M. (1960). *J. biol. Chem.* **235**, 2404, 2411.

Carlson, G. L., and Brown, G. M. (1960). *J. biol. Chem.* **235**, PC 3.

Carlson, G. L., and Brown, G. M. (1961). *J. biol. Chem.* **236**, 2099.

Cerecedo, L. R., Eich, S., and Bresnick, E. (1954). *Biochim. biophys. Acta.* **15**, 144

Cheldelin, V., and Lane, R. L. (1943). *Proc. Soc. exp. Biol. Med.* **54**, 53.

David, S., and Estramareix, B. (1960). *Biochim. biophys. Acta* **42**, 562

David, S., and Estramareix, B. (1961). *Biochim. biophys. Acta* **49**, 411.

Eberhart, B. M., and Tatum, E. L. (1959). *J. gen. Microbiol.* **20**, 43

Eich, S., and Cerecedo, L. R. (1954). *J. biol. Chem.* **207**, 295.

Emmett, A. D., and Luros, G. O. (1920). *J. biol. Chem.* **43**, 265.

Eusebi, A. J., and Cerecedo, L. R. (1950). *Fed. Proc.* **9**, 169.

Fang, S. C., and Butts, J. S. (1953). *Proc. Soc. exp. Biol.*, *N. Y.* **82**, 617.

Forsander, O. (1956). *Soc. sci. fenn., Comm. phys. math.* **19**, no. 22.

Fromageot, C., and Tschang, J. L. (1938). *Arch. Mikrobiol.* **9**, 434.

Funk, C. (1911). *J. Physiol.* **43**, 395.

Geddes, W. F., and Levine, M. N. (1942). *Cereal Chem.* **19**, 547.

Goodhart, R. S., and Sinclair, H. M. (1939). *Biochem. J.* **23**, 1099.

Goodwin, T. W. (1960). "Recent Advances in Biochemistry". Churchill, London.

Goodwin, T. W., and Howells, D. J. (1961). Unpublished observations.

Greiling, H. (1958). "Abstract of the 4th International Congress of Biochemistry Vienna", p. 46. Pergamon Press, London.

Harington, C. R., and Moggridge, R. C. G. (1939). *J. chem. Soc.* 443.

Harington, C. R., and Moggridge, R. C. G. (1940). *Biochem. J.* **34**, 685.

Harris, D. L. (1953). *Arch. Biochem. Biophys.* **41**, 294.

Harris, D. L. (1955). *Arch. Biochem. Biophys.* **57**, 240

Harris, D. L., and Yavit, J. (1957). *Fed. Proc.* **16**, 192.

Hinton, J. J. C. (1948). *Brit. J. Nutr.* **2**, 237.

Hitchcock, C. H. S., and Walker, J. (1961). *Biochem. J.* **80**, 137.

22   THE BIOSYNTHESIS OF VITAMINS AND RELATED COMPOUNDS

Hoffer, A., Alcock, A. W., and Geddes, W. F. (1946). *Cereal Chem.* **23,** 76.
Holman, W. I. M. (1956). *Nutr. Abstr. Rev.* **26,** 277.
Holzer, H., and Beaucamp, K. (1959). *Angew. Chem.* **71,** 776.
Holzer, H., and Beaucamp, K. (1961). *Biochim. biophys. Acta* **46,** 225.
Holzer, H., Goedder, H. W., Göggel, K. H. and Ulrich, B. (1960). *Biochem. Biophys. Res. Comm.* **3,** 599.
Howells, D. J. (1962). Ph. D. Thesis. University of Wales.
Jansen, B. C. P., and Donath, W. F. (1926). *Proc. Acad. Sci. Amst* **29,** 1390.
Johnson, D. B., and Goodwin, T. W. (1963). *Biochem J.* (in press)
Katznelson, H. (1947). *J. biol. Chem.* **167,** 615.
Kawasaki, T., and Fujita, T. (1961). *Seikagaku,* **33,** 742.
Kaziro, Y. (1959). *J. Biochem, Tokyo* **46,** 1523, 1587.
Kaziro, Y., Tanaka, R., Mano, Y., and Shimazono, N. (1961). *J. Biochem. Japan* **49,** 472
Kaziro, Y. and Shimazono, N. (1959). *J. Biochem., Tokyo* **46,** 963.
Kiessling, K. H. (1953). *Nature, Lond.* **172,** 1187.
Kiessling, K. H. (1956). *Ark. Kemi,* **10,** 279.
Kiessling, K. H. (1957). *Acta chem. scand.* **11,** 97.
Kiessling, K. H. (1959). *Acta chem. scand.* **13,** 1358.
Kögl, F., and Wagtendonk, W. J. (1938). *Rec. Trav. chim. Pays-Bas* **57,** 747.
Kohler, G. O. (1944). *J. biol. Chem.* **152,** 215.
Korte, F., and Weitkamp, H. (1959). *Liebigs Ann.* **622,** 121.
Korte, F., Weitkamp, H., and Vögel, J. (1959). *Liebigs Ann.* **628,** 158.
Korte, F., Paulus, W., Vögel, J., and Weitkamp, H. (1961). *Liebigs Ann.* **648,** 124.
Koser, S. A., and Wright, M. H. (1942). *J. infect. Dis.* **71,** 86.
Krampitz, L. O., Greull, G., Miller, C. S., Bicking, J. B., Skeggs, H. R., and Sprague, J. M. (1958). *J. Amer. chem. Soc.* **80,** 5893.
Krampitz, L. O., Suzuki, I., and Greull, G. (1961). *Fed. Proc.* **20,** 941.
Kumar, S. A. (1962). Ph. D. Thesis. Indian Institute of Scince.
Lankford, C. E., and Skeggs, P. K. (1946). *Arch. Biochem.* **9,** 265.
Leder, I. G. (1959a). *Fed. Proc.* **18,** 270.
Leder, I. G. (1959b). *Biochem. Biophys. Res. Comm.* **1,** 63.
Leder, I. G. (1961). *J. biol. Chem.* **236,** 3066.
Leonian, L. H., and Lilly, V. G. (1940). *Amer. J. Bot.* **27,** 18.
Leuthart, F., and Nielsen, H. (1952). *Helv. chim. Acta* **35,** 1196.
Lewin, R. A. (1952). *J. gen. Microbiol.* **6,** 233.
Lewin, L. M., and Brown, G. M. (1961). *Fed. Proc.* **20,** 447.
Lewis, J. C. (1944). *Arch. Biochem.* **4,** 217.
Lewis, J. C., Stubbs, J. J., and Noble, W. M. (1944). *Arch. Biochem.* **4,** 389.
Lilly, V. G., and Barnett, H. K. (1947). *Amer. J. Bot.* **34,** 131.
Lipton, M. A., and Elvehjem, C. A. (1940). *Nature, Lond.* **145,** 226.
Lohmann, K., and Schuster, K. (1937). *Biochem. Z.* **294,** 188.
Louis, R. (1951). *Mitt. naturf. Ges. Bern* **10,** 1.
Luecke, R. W., Hamner, C. L., and Sell, H. M. (1949). *Plant Physiol.* **21,** 546.
Lutz, A. (1948). *Bull. Soc. Chim. biol., Paris* **30,** 330.
Lwoff, A. (1947). *Annu. Rev. Microbiol.* **1,** 101.
Maizel, B. (1946). *U. S. Pat. Syst. Leafl.* **2,** 411, 445.
Mano, Y. (1960). *J. Biochem., Tokyo,* **47,** 283.
McClary, J. E. (1940). *Proc. nat. Acad. Sci., Wash.* **26,** 581.
Mizuhara, S., and Handler, P. (1954). *J. Amer. chem. Soc.* **76,** 571.
Nakayama, H. (1956). *Vitamins (Kyoto),* **10,** 356, 417.
Nakayama, H. (1957). *Vitamins (Kyoto)* **11,** 20, 169.
Nobécourt, P. (1940). *C. R. Soc. Biol., Paris* **133,** 530.

Nose, Y., Ueda, K., and Kawasaki, T. (1959). *Biochim. biophys. Acta* **34**, 277
Nose, Y., Ueda, K. Kawasaki, T., Iwashima, A. and Fujita, T. (1961). *J. Vitaminol. (Osaka)* **7**, 98
Ochoa, S. (1939). *Biochem. J.* **33**, 1262.
Olivo, F., Rossi, C. S., and Siliprandi, N. (1962). *Biochim. biophys. Acta*, **56**, 158.
Pakarskite, K. Y. (1961). *In* "Proceedings of the 5th International Congress of Biochemistry", p. 292. Pergamon Press, London.
Pavcek, P. L. Peterson, W. H., and Elvehjem, C. A. (1937). *Industr. Engng Chem.* **29**, 536.
Pavcek, P. L., Peterson, W. H., and Elvehjem, C. A. (1938). *Industr. Engng Chem.* **30**, 802.
Pine, M. J., and Guthrie, R. (1959). *J. Bact.* **78**, 545.
Plaut, G. W. E. (1961). *Annu. Rev. Biochem.* **30**, 409.
Pollock, J. M., and Geddes, W. F. (1951). *Cereal Chem.* **28**, 289.
Rindi, G. and de Giuseppe, L. (1961). *Biochem. J.* **78**, 602
Rindi, G., Perri, V., Venture, U., and Breccia, A. (1962). *Nature, Lond.* **193**, 582.
Robbins, W. J. (1940). *Plant Physiol.* **15**, 547.
Robbins, W. J., and Bartley, M. A. (1937). *Proc. nat. Acad. Sci., Wash.* **23**, 385.
Robbins, W. J., and Kavanagh, F. (1937). *Proc. nat. Acad. Sci., Wash.* **23**, 499.
Robinson, F. A. (1951). "The Vitamin B. Complex". Chapman and Hall, London.
Rossi-Fanelli, A., Siliprandi, N., and Fasella, P. (1952). *Science* **116**, 711.
Ruge, U. (1959). *Z. Naturforsch.* **14b**, 582.
Sarrett, H. P., and Cheldelin, V. H. (1944). *J. biol. Chem.* **156**, 91.
Saxena, K. C., Ghatak, S., and Agarwala, S. C. (1954). *Experientia* **10**, 488.
Schopfer, W. H. (1938). *Protoplasma*, **31**, 105.
Schopfer, W. H. (1943). "Plants and Vitamins". Chronica Botanica, Waltham, Massachusetts.
Schopfer, W. H., and Jung, A. (1937). *C. R. Acad. Sci., Paris*, **204**, 1500.
Shimazono, N., Mano, Y., Tanaka, R., and Kaziro, Y. (1959). *J. Biochem., Tokyo* **46**, 959.
Silverman, M., and Werkman, C. H. (1939). *J. Bact.* **38**, 25.
Steyn-Parvé, E. P. (1952). *Biochim. biophys. Acta* **8**, 310.
Sukhorukov, K., and Filippov, V. (1940). *C. R. Acad. Sci. U. R. S. S.* **29**, 347.
Suomalainen, H., Rihtniemi, S., and Oura, E. (1959). *Acta Chem. scand.* **13**, 2131
Suzuoki, J, and Kobata, A. (1960). *J. Biochem., Tokyo* **47**, 262.
Tatum, E. L., and Bell, T. T. (1946). *Amer. J. Bot.* **33**, 362.
Tauber, H. (1938). *J. biol. Chem.* **123**, 499.
van Lanen, J. M., and Tanner, F. W. Jr. (1942). *Vitam. & Horm.* **6**, 163.
von Euler, H., and Vestrin, R. (1937). *Naturwissenschaften* **25**, 416.
von Rytz, W. (1939). *Ber. schweiz. bot. Ges.* **49**, 339.
Weeks, O. B., and Beck, S. M. (1960). *J. gen. Microbiol.* **23**, 217.
Weil-Malherbe, H. (1939). *Biochem. J.* **33**, 1997.
Went, F. W., Bonner, J., and Warner, G. C. (1938). *Science* **87**, 170.
Westenbrink, H. G. (1958). *In* "Proceedings of the 4th International Congress of Biochemistry, Vienna", p. 73. Pergamon Press, London.
Westenbrink, H. G., Steyn-Parvé, E. P., and Veldman, H. (1947). *Biochim. biophys. Acta* **1**, 154.
Williams, R. R. (1938). "Vitamin B₁ and Its Use in Medicine". Macmillan.
Williams, R. R., Waterman, R. E., and Keresztesy, J. C. (1934). *J. Amer. chem. Soc.* **56**, 1187.
Wirth, J. C. and Nord, F. F. (1942). *Arch. Biochem.* **1**, 143.
Woolley, D. W., and Koehelik, I. H. (1961). *Fed. Proc.*, **20**, 359.
Watco-Manzo E., Roddy, F., Yount, R. G., and Metzler, D. E. (1959). *J. biol. Chem.* **234**, 733.

CHAPTER 2

RIBOFLAVIN AND RELATED COMPOUNDS

I. INTRODUCTION

The developments which led to the emergence of riboflavin (vitamin B_2) as a fully fledged vitamin are not simple, but they have been fully described by Robinson (1951). In essence, yellow compounds which exhibited a strong yellowish-green fluorescence in ultraviolet light and which had growth-promoting power for rats were first isolated from egg-white (Kuhn *et al.*, 1933) and whey (Ellinger and Koschara, 1933); later they were found in many other tissues (e.g. liver, kidney, urine, muscle and yeast cells). In the early stages these compounds were given separate names until it was eventually shown that they were identical; the name lactoflavin was then adopted. This name persisted until the researches of Kuhn and of Karrer and their colleagues proved that the structure of vitamin B_2 was 6,7-dimethyl-9-D-ribityl-isoalloxazine (I) (Karrer *et al.*, 1935; Kuhn *et al.*, 1935). The current name, riboflavin, dates from the time of the general acceptance of this structure.

(I)   (II)

Free riboflavin is a relatively rare natural compound for it occurs in significant amounts only in the culture media of a restricted number of micro-organisms and in the retina, urine and, occasionally, milk and seminal fluid of animals. Of particular interest is the high concentration of riboflavin in the semen of some bulls, caused apparently by a Mendelian dominant characteristic controlling the ability of the seminal vesicles to concentrate riboflavin (White and Lincoln, 1958), and the existence of crystals of riboflavin in the tapetum of the lemur (Pirie, 1959). Although some reports indicated that in animal tissues some 10–30% of the total riboflavin is in the free form (Bessey *et al.*, 1949), more sensitive tests have indicated its absence (Crammer, 1948); the same picture was revealed in a survey of riboflavin in micro-organisms (Peel, 1958). The combined forms of riboflavin which exist in living cells are riboflavin 5'-phosphate (FMN) (II) and flavin adenine dinucleotide (FAD) (III). FMN was first isolated from heart muscle (Banga and Szent-

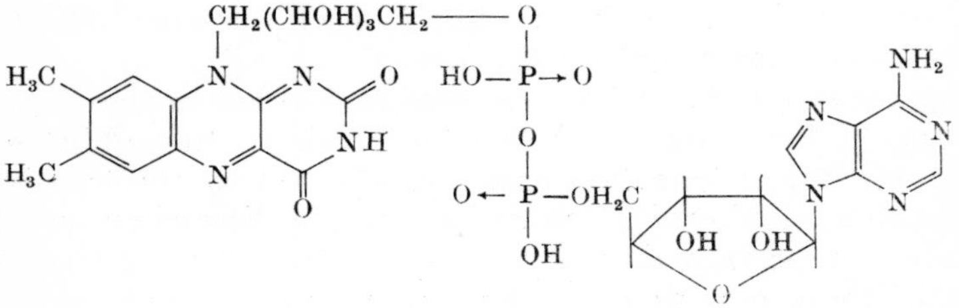

$$CH_2(CHOH)_3CH_2 \underline{\qquad} O$$

(III)

Györgyi, 1932) and from yeast, as the prosthetic group of a "yellow enzyme" (Warburg and Christian, 1932). The position of the phosphate group was established by Karrer *et al.* (1934) and by Kuhn *et al.* (1936). Warburg and Christian proposed structure III for FAD in 1938, but it was not confirmed by total synthesis until 1954 when it was achieved in Todd's laboratory (Christie *et al.*, 1954). Other syntheses have followed (Huennekens and Kilgour, 1955; Deluca and Kaplan, 1956).

II. RIBOFLAVIN FORMATION IN MICRO-ORGANISMS

A. *Fungi*

(i) *Ascomycetes*

Two closely related ascomycetes, *Ashbya gossypii* and *Eremothecium ashbyii* synthesize large amounts of riboflavin, especially in shake cultures, and excrete essentially all of it into the culture medium. On a fully defined medium riboflavin production by *A. gossypii* is negligible (Robbins and Schmidt, 1939), but it is greatly stimulated by replacement of defined growth factors by yeast extract and peptone; under such conditions titres of 1000 μg/ml culture medium can be obtained (Wickerham *et al.*, 1946). For the commercial synthesis of riboflavin by *A. gossypii* plant residues such as corn-steep liquor and distiller's solubles can replace yeast extract, animal residues such as slaughter house wastes (stick liquor) can replace peptone, and corn oil can replace a carbohydrate source; indeed good yields can be obtained with a medium containing only 2 constituents, corn oil and corn steep liquor (see Goodwin, 1959). Surface active agents also stimulate flavinogenesis (Smith *et al.*, 1957). A pilot plant for producing riboflavin by *A. gossypii* has been fully described by Pfeifer *et al.* (1950).

E. ashbyii also produces larger amounts of riboflavin on a complex medium compared with that produced on a simple, defined medium. One of the best yields reported is 2200 μg/ml on a medium consisting of whey and skim milk (1:1) fortified with sucrose (5%) (Hendrickz and de Vleeschauwer, 1955).

A. gossypii and *E. ashbyii* resemble each other in that riboflavin synthesis in both organisms is stimulated by the addition of a lipid to the culture medium and is unaffected by the iron level of the medium employed (Hendrickz and de Vleeschauwer, 1956). The latter property makes large scale manipulations of the fermentation of these moulds much less exacting than with some other flavinogenic organisms such as *Candida* spp. and *Clostridium* spp.

E. ashbyii has one considerable disadvantage compared with *A. gossypii*; it readily gives rise to stable non-flavinogenic strains, which do not revert (Schopfer and Guilloud, 1945, 1946; Arragon *et al.*, 1946). Furthermore, attempts to preserve yellow strains by storage at 3–10° or by lyophilization have not been universally successful (Moore and de Becze, 1947; Moore *et al.*, 1947), although Hoštálek (1957) has described a method of lyophilization which in his hands preserves flavinogenicity. Yellow strains of *A. gossypii* can be stored lyophilized (Wickerham *et al.*, 1946; Pridham and Raper, 1952) although their viability in this form is not great (Pridham, 1952).

(ii) *Yeasts*

Burkholder (1943) first demonstrated that *Candida guilliermondii* synthesized large amounts of riboflavin; this was soon shown to be a characteristic of many other *Candida* species including *C. tropicalis* var. *rhaggi* (Schopfer and Guilloud, 1944). *C. flareri* (Levine *et al.*, 1949), *C. arborea* (Singh *et al.*, 1948), *C. lactis (Mycotorula lactis)* (Rogosa, 1943), *C. krusei* (Hedrick and Burke, 1950), *C. ghoshii* (Mitra, 1957), *C. chalmersi, C. lypolytica, C. olea, C. pulcherrima, C. solani* and *C. melibiosi* (Shavlovsky and Fiktash, 1961).

The great attraction of *Candida* spp. is that they grow rapidly with high flavinogenesis on a simple, fully defined medium (Levine *et al.*, 1949), although aeration of the medium is required for good yields (Burkholder, 1943). The disadvantages associated with these organisms are (a) flavinogenesis is extremely sensitive to the presence of traces of iron in the medium (Tanner *et al.*, 1945), the level tolerated being only 0·005–0·07 μg/ml; this precludes the use of complex media which contain by-products such as corn-steep liquor; and (b) the riboflavin levels attained (325 μg/ml with *C. flareri*) are lower than those obtained with *E. ashbyii* and *A. gossypii* (see previous section). In spite of these difficulties Levine *et al.* (1949) produced a successful pilot plant in which plastic-coated aluminium or glass tanks are used. As the starting pH (5–6) of the medium rapidly falls to 3·0–3·5 bacterial contamination can be avoided without the necessity for sterilizing the medium.

(iii) *Other fungi*

The fungi listed in Table 1 (Goodwin, 1959, 1963) synthesize

TABLE 1. Flavinogenic Fungi (Goodwin, 1959) [Excluding *A. gossypii*, *E. ashbyii* and *Candida* spp.]

Yeasts		Higher fungi	
Genus	Riboflavin (μg/g dry cells)	Genus	Riboflavin (μg/g dry cells)
Hansenula	54	*Agropyrum*	10
Mycotorula	59	*Alternaria*	10–20
Oidium	55	*Elymus*	57
Saccharomyces	50–100	*Fusarium*	20–30
*Torulopsis**	50–90	*Hormodendrum*	10–20
		Mucor	20
		Penicillium	20–40
		Phalaris	6
		Phragmites	6
		Rhizopus	20
		Secale	17
		Trichoderma	20

* Synthesis inhibited by iron.

more than their metabolic requirement of riboflavin. The media in which these organisms were grown have not been systematically examined, but it must be assumed that the excretion of riboflavin into the medium was never spectacular. The visual appearance of media such as those on which organisms such as *Candida* spp.

grow, would certainly have attracted comment. The iron content of the media used in the experiments recorded in Table 1 was, except in the case of *Torulopsis* (Lewis, 1944), never controlled so that it is possible that some of the organisms listed have iron-sensitive pathways of flavinogenesis. Under optimum conditions *Aspergillus niger* will synthesize 39 μg/ml of riboflavin (Shukla and Prabku, 1961).

B. *Bacteria*

(i) *Clostridium spp.*

The only bacteria used commercially for riboflavin production are the various species of the anaerobic solvent-producing genus *Clostridium*. This dual function gives the fermentation added industrial attraction, and the residues from fermentations designed mainly for butanol and acetone production are good sources of riboflavin (Stiles, 1940). As the riboflavin levels in the media from acetone-butanol fermentation are low (not more than 100 μg/ml) compared with those produced by the flavinogenic fungi, the vitamin is not generally extracted from the medium but the medium, after removal of the solvents by fractional distillation, is filtered and dried, and the resulting concentrate, which can contain up to 8000 μg riboflavin per gram of dry matter (Rodgers *et al.*, 1948) is marketed. Growth of *Clostridium* spp. is good on a fully defined medium, but riboflavin production is poor; (Leviton, 1946; Obata and Tomoeda, 1953); for example *C. acidi urici* cells contain only 14·3 μg/g dry matter (Barker and Peterson, 1944). The three media used most commonly in industry are based on (a) grain products, e.g. flour mashes of 4—8% maize (Artzberger, 1943; Yamasaki, 1942); (b) milk products, usually whey (Meade *et al.*, 1945); and (c) molasses (Hickey, 1945). A medium based on potato starch has also been recommended (Dyr and Munk, 1954).

As is the case with *Candida* spp., riboflavin synthesis by the Clostridia is inhibited by the presence of iron in the medium, although these organisms can tolerate 50–100 times more iron than can *Candida* spp. Media low in iron but not free from iron, must be used if high riboflavin levels are sought (Hickey, 1945; Saunders and McClung, 1943). Iron can be removed from grain products mechanically by using magnets (Artzberger, 1943), or by addition of the appropriate amount of α,α-dipyridyl to chelate most of the iron and thus render it biologically unavaliable (Hickey, 1945). Moderate levels of iron can be dealt with by the addition of sodium hydrosulphite or catalase to the medium (Leviton, 1946). The improved yields noted on adding $CaCO_3$ to media based on grain products are probably due to the adsorption of iron on to the $CaCO_3$ (Yamasaki, 1941; Sebek, 1947). When media which contain whey are used, the whey must not be prepared in steel or iron vessels because this can increase its iron content from 1·5—4·0 $\mu g/ml$ to 10—12 $\mu g/ml$ (Meade et al., 1945). It follows that vessels made of iron or steel are excluded when riboflavin is required in addition to solvents from the fermentation of the Clostridia; glass and aluminium equipment is recommended (Artzberger, 1943).

(ii) Aerobacter spp.

Various Aerobacter spp. produce small amounts of riboflavin (110 $\mu g/g$ dry cells; 10 $\mu g/ml$ medium) on synthetic media but stimulation, up to 4 times with some species (e.g. A. aerogenes), occurs when stillage is added to the media (Tittsler and Whittier, 1941). The design of a small pilot plant (100 gal scale) for this fermentation has been reported (Novak et al., 1943; Novak, 1948).

(iii) Azotobacter

Azotobacter spp. are potentially useful as sources of riboflavin because, although they only produce low levels, no nitrogen is required in the medium; this reduces both running costs and risks of contamination. Lee and Burris (1943) have produced cultures on a pilot plant scale (200 gal) in which the cells contained 350 μg of riboflavin per gramme of dry matter; however, the medium contained only 1 $\mu g/ml$. Maximum synthesis with A. chroococcum occurs during the transition from the latent to logarithmic phase of growth (Pakarskite, 1961).

(iv) Mycobacteria

Certain Mycobacteria synthesize high levels of riboflavin (up to 36,000 $\mu g/g$ dry cells and 57 $\mu g/ml$ medium; see Goodwin, 1959, for full references). There are, however, many good reasons why these organisms have not been exploited industrially; these include (a) long incubation times, up to 42 days at 37°; (b) low gross yields of cells, and (c) the pathogenicity of some strains.

(v) Other flavinogenic bacteria

Pridham (1952) has collected information available on riboflavin synthesis by a large number of bacteria. Only those which synthesize more than 10 $\mu g/ml$ medium and/or 100 $\mu g/g$ of dry cells are listed in Table 2. Many of the data recorded by Pridham have been obtained with cells growing on defined synthetic media; use of com-

TABLE 2. Moderately Flavinogenic Bacteria
(Pridham, 1952)

Organism	$\mu g/ml$ medium	$\mu g/g$ dry cells
Corynebact. diphtheriae	25	—
Escherichia coli	505	106
Pseudomonas fluorescens	22—34*	310
Rhizobium trifolii	—	300
Serratia marcescens	—	160

* According to strain employed.

plex natural products and/or careful control of the iron levels in the media might in many cases increase the synthesis of riboflavin.

(vi) *Intestinal synthesis of riboflavin*

(a) *Non-ruminant mammals.* It is well established that isolated bacterial cultures of intestinal inhabitants such as *Proteus vulgaris, Bacillus lactoaerogenes* and *Escherichia coli* can synthesize riboflavin (Burkholder and McVeigh, 1942). It is also true that they synthesize the vitamin *in situ*, because in many animal species faecal excretion is greater than the dietary intake. This has been repeatedly demonstrated in rats (e.g. Mannering *et al.*, 1944), guinea-pigs (Yasuda, 1951), horses (Carroll, 1950), humans (e.g. Najjar *et al.*, 1944) and fowls (Lamoureux and Schumacher, 1940).

(b) *Ruminants.* The investigations of McElroy and Goss (1940) strongly suggested that the rumen organisms of cattle synthesized riboflavin; the output of riboflavin in the milk was frequently up to ten times greater than the intake in the food. However, it is possible that some of the riboflavin in the milk was not true riboflavin, because Pearson and Schweigert (1947) made the important observation that there is a marked discrepancy in the riboflavin levels in the urine and milk of goats when assayed fluorimetrically and microbiologically, the values with the former method being some five times greater than those obtained microbiologically. As the discrepancy is not observed in human or rat urine it appears that the microbiologically inactive material is a fluorescing metabolite of riboflavin produced by the rumen microflora. Recently, such a metabolite, probably 6,7-dimethyl-9-(2-hydroxyethyl)isoalloxazine, has been isolated from goat urine (Owen *et al.*, 1962). This compound had previously been obtained by Stadtman (1958) by bacterial degradation of riboflavin.

(c) *Insects*. It is appropriate to consider here some insects which harbour intracellular symbiotic micro-organisms. For example, the fact that the Coleoptera *Sitodrepa panicea* and *Ladioderma serricorne* do not require a dietary source of riboflavin is almost certainly due to the flavinogenic activity of these micro-organisms, because neither insect grew in the absence of riboflavin when reared from bacteria–free eggs (Fraenkel and Blewett, 1943, 1944). The same explanation probably accounts for the observation that *Periplaneta americana* and *Tineola bisselliella* accumulate much more riboflavin in their malpighian tubules than they consume in their food (Busnel and Drilhon, 1943; Metcalf and Patton, 1942).

C. *Algae*

It is known that algae synthesize riboflavin (see Fogg, 1953) but no detailed work has been reported.

D. *Protozoa*

Chilomonas paramoecium synthesizes riboflavin when cultured on a medium containing only acetate and inorganic salts (Holz, 1950). Seaman (1953) demonstrated that *Tetrahymena gleii* synthesizes riboflavin, although it does not secrete any into the medium.

III. GENERAL FACTORS CONTROLLING FLAVINOGENESIS IN MICRO-ORGANISMS

A. *Ashbya gossypii*

Riboflavin synthesis in *A. gossypii* is a strongly aerobic process and for high yields it is necessary to aerate the cultures either by shaking or by bubbling air through the medium (Ganguly, 1954; Tanner *et al.*, 1949). However, excessive shaking, which interferes with mycelial development, reduces riboflavin synthesis (Pfeifer *et al.*, 1950). At the optimal temperature of 26–28° and the optimal pH of 6·0–7·5 maximal riboflavin levels are achieved after 90–130 hr (Tanner *et al.*, 1949; Pfeifer *et al.*, 1950).

With glucose as carbohydrate source maximum flavinogenesis is obtained with a concentration of 3% (Wickerham *et al.*, 1946) and this is not improved by substituting crude carbohydrates such as molasses (Tanner *et al.*, 1949; Smiley *et al.*, 1951). Almost all the glucose in the medium is utilized during the first 24 hr of the fermentation during which time the pH drops from 6·3 to 4·5 and no significant amounts of riboflavin are formed; thereafter up to 90—130 hr after inoculation riboflavin is rapidly synthesized and the pH of the medium gradually rises (Fig. 1) (Pfeifer *et al.*, 1950).

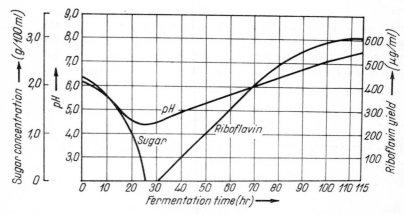

Fig. 1. Metabolic changes in the medium of *Ashbya gossypii* during growth (Pfeifer *et al.*, 1950).

Glycine stimulates flavinogenesis in *A. gossypii* (Plaut, 1961a,b); this contrasts sharply with the situation in *E. ashbyii*.

B. *Eremothecium ashbyii*

The pattern of flavinogenesis in *E. ashbyii* closely resembles that in *A. gosypii*. Aeration of the medium increases yields at least three-fold (Goodwin, 1959).

The optimum pH of the medium is 5·5–6·8 (Hickey, 1953) and maximum yields are achieved 72–120 hr after inoculation (see Goodwin, 1959, for references to patent literature). The metabolic changes in the medium of shake cultures of *E. ashbyii* (Fig. 2 ; Kaprálek, 1957) are very similar to those in *A. gossypii* (Fig. 1). Growth and glucose utilization are essentially complete within 30 hr of inoculation and the accompanying drop in pH is due to the accumulation of pyruvate. Active flavinogenesis occurs only after growth

2. RIBOFLAVIN AND RELATED COMPOUNDS

is complete and coincides with the onset of sporulation. Flavinogenesis is also accompanied by an increase in pH which is due to
the disappearance of pyruvate and the appearance of ammonium
ions (Kaprálek, 1962).

The effect of various amino acids on flavinogenesis in *E. ashbyii*
has been examined in detail (Goodwin and Pendlington, 1954).

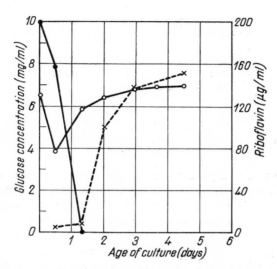

FIG. 2. Metabolic changes in the medium of *Eremothecium ashbyii* during
growth (Kaprálek, 1957).

The amino acid under test was added at a level of 0·20 mg N/ml
to a basal medium containing 0·05 mg/ml of peptone nitrogen. The
basal medium provided reasonable growth but low riboflavin production. The response to the amino acid was compared with that
produced in a medium containing 0·25 mg/ml peptone N. The amino
acids fell into three main groups, examples of which are given in
Table 3. The first group, which includes the majority of amino
acids, stimulated neither growth nor flavinogenesis; the second group,
asparagine, aspartate and glutamate (glutamine was not examined) stimulated both growth and flavinogenesis, whilst the
third group, consisting of serine and threonine, but not glycine,
greatly stimulated flavinogenesis without having any effect on
growth. The stimulatory effect of serine and threonine is explained
on p. 45. The observation of the strong positive effect of aspartate
and glutamate falls into line with those of Hickey (1953) and Chin
(1947) but not with those of Schopfer and Guilloud (1945)
and Minoura (1950). Schopfer and Guilloud (1945) found that

TABLE 3. Growth and Flavinogenesis by *E. ashbyii* in the Presence of Various Amino Acids* (Goodwin and Pendlington, 1954)

Medium	Dry wt (mg)	Riboflavin (µg)
Control A	13·7	230
L-Asparagine	27·2	506
DL-Serine	14·5	342
DL-Threonine	10·9	428
Glycine	13·7	141
Control B	22·6	473

* Dry wt and riboflavin production per 15 ml medium in 50 ml conical flasks; temperature 28°; 5-day static cultures; controls A and B contain a basal medium plus 5 mg/100 ml and 25 mg/100 ml peptone-B respectively; other media contain 5 mg peptone-N and 20 mg amino acid N per 100 ml.

in their medium aspartate and glutamate would not support growth of *E. ashbyii*, although asparagine and glutamine were effective. Minoura's results indicated that although asparagine was equal to peptone in promoting growth, it was less effective in stimulating flavinogenesis.

Maclaren (1952) first noted that purines were strongly flavinogenic in *E. ashbyii* and these observations have been confirmed and extended (Minoura, 1953a,b; Goodwin and Pendlington, 1954; McNutt, 1954; Brown *et al.*, 1958). Guanine is always the most effective purine (Table 4).

TABLE 4. Effect of Various Purines on Flavinogenesis by *E. ashbyii* (Brown *et al.*, 1958)*

Purine added	Dry wt (mg)	Riboflavin (µg)
None	12·0	583
Uric acid	12·8	715
Hypoxanthine**	12·5	742
Adenine***	12·5	920
Xanthine	11·8	930
Guanine	12·2	1010

* Purines added to a basal medium at a level of 0·37 mM; 5-day static cultures; temperature 28°; amount produced in 15 ml medium in 50 ml conical flasks.
  ** Inosine has the same effect as hypoxanthine.
*** Adenosine and adenosine 3'-phosphate have the same effect as adenine.

In marked contrast to the purines, no pyrimidine or pyrimidine precursor (e.g. orotic acid) has any flavinogenic action in *E. ashbyii* (Maclaren, 1952; Goodwin and Pendlington, 1954; Table 4). When cultured on a synthetic medium *E. ashbyii* requires inositol, thiamine and biotin as growth factors (Hickey, 1953). For maximal riboflavin synthesis, two additional unidentified factors are required. One occurs in yeast extract and can be partly replaced by oleic acid. The other is associated with certain "vitamin-free" caseins; it does not appear to be strepogenin (Hickey, 1953).

C. *Candida spp.*

In *Candida flareri* flavinogenesis is a strongly aerobic process and, as is the case with *A. gossypii* and *E. ashbyii* cultures have to be aerated if high yields of riboflavin are required (Levine *et al.*, 1949). In shake cultures maximum growth and flavinogenesis occurs within 48–72 hr of inoculation (Goodwin and McEvoy, 1959).

In the basic culture medium in which $(NH_4)_2SO_4$ is the nitrogen source, 7·5 mg of $(NH_4)_2SO_4$–N per 100 ml produces maximal growth, whilst maximal flavinogenesis is only achieved when the $(NH_4)_2SO_4$–N level is 15 mg/100 ml (Goodwin and McEvoy, 1959). Replacement of $(NH_4)_2SO_4$ by most amino acids greatly stimulates growth but reduces flavinogenesis considerably; on the other hand, glycine, serine, ornithine and arginine stimulate growth and flavinogenesis. Urea is similarly effective (Goodwin and McEvoy, 1959). Xanthine, guanine and uric acid when added to a medium containing $(NH_4)_2SO_4$ greatly stimulated flavinogenesis; adenine and hypoxanthine were ineffective. In the absence of $(NH_4)_2SO_4$, xanthine, guanine and uric acid supported growth but not flavinogenesis; adenine and hypoxanthine did not support growth. Flavinogenesis was not stimulated by any pyrimidines tested, nor by orotic acid (Goodwin and McEvoy, 1959). The significance of these observations in relation to the mechanism of flavinogenesis is discussed on p. 42.

The most critical constituent of the medium for flavinogenesis in *Candida* spp. is iron; concentrations above 1·0–2·0 μg/100 ml are strongly inhibitory (Tanner *et al.*, 1945; Levine *et al.*, 1949; Goodwin and McEvoy, 1959). The early reports that high concentrations of glucose and phosphate inhibited flavinogenesis in *Candida* spp. (Burkholder, 1943, 1944) were due to the iron present in these compounds (Goodwin and McEvoy, 1959). According to Enari (1955) and Enari and Kauppinen (1961) the permissible concentration of iron can be increased ten times if the cobalt level in the medium is maintained at 10 μg/ml. Levine *et al.* (1949) found that manganese, copper, zinc, tin, nickel and aluminium at concentrations up to 10 μg/100 ml had no inhibitory effects on flavinogenesis However, zinc at slightly higher concentrations (20–80 μg/100 ml) is inhibitory (Schopfer and Knüsel, 1956). Riboflavin synthesis in *C. tropicalis* var. *rhagii* is not sensitive to the presence of iron in the medium (Shavlovsky *et al.*, 1962).

Although most *Candida* species accumulate only free riboflavin in the medium, *C. tropicalis* var. *rhagii* accumulates some FMN and FAD as well (Shavlovsky and Fiktash, 1961).

D. *The Action of Inhibitors on Microbial Flavinogenesis*

Various sulphonamides inhibit both growth and flavinogenesis in *E. ashbyii* but inhibition of riboflavin synthesis is always first observed; the inhibition is overcome by *p*-aminobenzoic acid (Schopfer *et al.*, 1947). Dichloroflavin (methyls at C-6 and C-7 replaced by chlorine) in large amounts (Schopfer, 1944) and Gammexane (γ-hexachlorocyclohexane) in low concentration (0·01 mg/ml) (Schopfer and Guilloud, 1946; Minoura, 1953b) inhibit flavinogenesis in the same organism. In the concentration range 0·001–0·01 mg/ml Gammexane stimulates flavinogenesis. The α-, β- and δ-isomers of hexachlorocyclohexane are inactive (Minoura, 1953b).

Biotin sulphone inhibits riboflavin synthesis in *Aspergillus oryzae;* this is overcome by biotin but not by inositol (Tirunarayanan and Sarma, 1954). In *E. ashbyii* biotin sulphone did not appear to be antiflavinogenic (Goodwin, 1959).

A number of 4,5-disubstituted (mainly phenyl and ethyl) pyrimidines, 1,2-dihydro-*s*-triazines (IV), antibiotics as well as *iso*-riboflavin (methyls at C-5 and C-6 instead of C-6 and C-7) and azaserine (V) exerted no specific inhibition on flavinogenesis in *E. ashbyii*. (Brown *et al.*, 1958). Aminopterin (VI) at very low concentrations (0·02 μg/ml) inhibits growth but strongly stimulates flavinogenesis in *E. ashbyii* (Brown *et al.*, 1955). At substrate concentrations isoguanine inhibits growth but stimulates flavinogenesis (Horton, 1960). 8-Azaxanthine but not 8-azahypoxanthine inhibits flavinogenesis in *E. ashbyii* (Brown *et al.*, 1958), and the pyrimidines which can be considered as arising from adenine (4,5,6-triaminouracil) and isoguanine (4,5,6-triamino-6-hydroxypyrimidine) are also inhibitory (Brown *et al.*, 1955).

E. *A Possible Explanation of Flavinogenicity in Micro-organisms*

In *Candida* spp. a reasonable explanation of the high level of flavinogenesis in the absence of iron would be the switching of terminal oxidation from the normal cytochrome pathway to a pathway involving a flavin oxidase, with a concomitant lack of metabolic control of the stimulated synthesis of riboflavin resulting from the increased requirement for flavin-containing coenzymes. No direct evidence exists for this conclusion, but McEvoy (1959) has shown that *C. flareri* will grow in the absence of iron (8 subcultures on iron-free media) and that on his normal flavinogenic medium, which contained 1 μg Fe/100 ml the cytochrome *c* levels of the cells were only approximately one half those in cells grown on a medium containing 100 μg Fe/100 ml. Furthermore, the presence of a flavoprotein oxidase and the absence of cytochromes have also been reported in *Streptococcus faecalis* (Smith, 1954; Dolin 1953, 1955; Niederpruem and Hackett, 1958) and in certain *Lactobacillus* spp. (Strittmatter, 1958), and a flavoprotein oxidase/peroxidase system capable of transferring electrons from NADH to oxygen is present in *Bacillus subtilis* (Lightbown and Kogut, 1959).

The recent observations of Kaprálek (1962) indicate that the same switch of oxidative metabolism occurs in *E. ashbyii* even in the presence of iron. In this organism excessive riboflavin synthesis occurs only after growth is completed, and during this period there are also indications that a flavin-linked oxidase takes over from the cytochrome system.

A well-known objection to terminal flavo-oxidases is that the resultant is H_2O_2 which, conventionally, is metabolized by catalase or peroxidase. As both these enzymes are iron prophyrin-containing proteins, they cannot exist in cells of *Candida* species grown on an iron-free medium. However, it should be pointed out that a flavin-dependent enzyme which will oxidize NADH and reduce H_2O_2 and which increases in amount in iron-deficient media, has been obtained from *S. faecalis* (Dolin, 1955). In *E. ashbyii* this problem does not arise and the organism deals with the situation by increasing its catalase activity during the period when riboflavin is being rapidly synthesized (Dikanskaya, 1953; Kaprálek, 1962).

The influence of iron on flavinogenesis in the anaerobic *Clostridium* spp. obviously cannot be related to control of terminal oxidation. Leviton (1946) found that addition of catalase or sodium hydrosulphite to the medium in which *Cl. acetobutylicum* was growing increased production of riboflavin in the presence of amounts of iron which would normally inhibit flavinogenesis. As he found that riboflavin is stable in pure solutions of hydrogen peroxide but is rapidly oxidized if iron is added, and that riboflavin added to a culture of *Cl. acetobutylicum* containing high levels of iron was rapidly oxidized, he postulated that metabolic H_2O_2 would rapidly oxidize metabolic riboflavin in the presence of iron and that added catalase and hydrosulphite protect the metabolic riboflavin by destroying H_2O_2 as it is formed. Although this may be an acceptable explanation for the *Clostridia*, it does not apply to *Candida* spp. (Shavlovsky and Chistiakova, 1956; Knüsel, 1957; Enari, 1958; McEvoy, 1959).

IV. FLAVINOGENESIS IN HIGHER PLANTS

As is the case with all water-soluble vitamins of the B complex, riboflavin is synthesized by green leaves. However, in contrast to some of the other water-soluble vitamins, riboflavin is also synthesized by other regions of the plant. Bonner (1942), for example, first showed that excised roots of tomato, sunflower and *Datura* produced riboflavin grown on a normal root-culture medium. This was substantiated by the observations of Bonner and Dorland (1943) that no translocation of riboflavin from leaves to roots occurs in intact tomato plants. In fact, translocation of riboflavin did not appear to occur in any direction. It was probably these observations which led Bonner and Bonner (1948) to suggest that riboflavin is also synthesized *in situ* by developing seeds and embryos. The histology of riboflavin distribution in the kernel of rice during the ripening period has been described by Sone (1959).

A. *Germinating Seeds*

Synthesis of riboflavin has been demonstrated many times in germinating seedlings. Cheldelin and Lane (1943) showed that germination for 36–48 hr in the light resulted in considerable production of riboflavin in black-eyed peas and in lima beans, but much less in cotton seeds. Burkholder (1943) germinated the seeds of a number of species for 5–6 days and found similar quantitative variations in riboflavin synthesis; the amount in oats, wheat, barley and corn increased fourteen, four, eight, and four times respectively. Very similar observations have been made with various other seedlings (Klatzin *et al.*, 1949; Petit, 1950; Wai *et al.*, 1947; Nandi and Banerjee, 1950; Burkholder and McVeigh, 1942; Raut and Chitre 1961.)

The experiments of Burkholder and McVeigh (1945) clearly demonstrated that light is not essential for riboflavin synthesis in developing seedlings, and this has been confirmed by Povolotskaya and Zaitseva (1951); indeed in some cases light appears to inhibit synthesis (Gustafson, 1955; Naik and Narayana, 1960; Kumar, 1962).

Povolotskaya and Zaitseva (1951) also reported that crushed cotyledons of peas synthesize 2·5 times more riboflavin than do intact cotyledons. Similar increases are observed with potato slices, especially at the surface of the cuts. Furthermore, whilst the intact tissues synthesize mainly bound riboflavin, the riboflavin in the injured tissues is mostly free. This is probably due to the action of an FAD-ase liberated on disintegration of the cells. The reason for this stimulation of riboflavin synthesis following trauma is not known, but it is paralleled by an increase in respiration.

Infiltration of purines into germinating *Cicer arietinum* (Bengal gram) stimulated riboflavin synthesis. Glycine was the only effective amino acid examined (Naik and Narayana, 1960).

The riboflavin synthesized is entirely in the form of FAD and FMN in the case of *Phaseolus radiatus* (green gram) and *Vigna catjang* (cow pea) (Kumar, 1962) and is concentrated in the growing plumule and radicle. The synthesis almost certainly takes place in the growing regions, because in *Cicer arietinum* removal of the radicle after the first day of germination prevents further riboflavin formation by the remaining parts of the seed (Naik and Narayana, 1960).

B. *Synthesis by Isolated Tissues*

Only one investigation has been reported on the problem of riboflavin synthesis by isolated leaves (Povolotskaya and Zaitseva, 1951). Isolated begonia and oat leaves actually lose riboflavin. Similarly outer cabbage leaves lose riboflavin; the white inner leaves, on the other hand, synthesize it.

C. *Synthesis in the Intact Plant*

(i) *General observations*

The youngest leaves of the tomato plant always contain the greatest concentration of riboflavin, and a gradient exists in the stem (Bonner and Dorland, 1943). There is more in the blade of the leaf than in the rachis or petiole (Gustafson, 1947). The concentration in the root is always higher than in the stem (Bonner and Dorland, 1943), and is generally equal to that in the middle part of the plant taken as a whole, but always lower than that in the apical regions (Gustafson, 1947). Mature leaves always contain more riboflavin than mature fruit (Gustafson, 1947).

The riboflavin content of the root nodules in leguminous plants is, however, much higher than in any other part of the plant (Tsujimura, 1950). The part played by the symbiotic bacteria in this synthesis is not known.

There appears to be no correlation between the riboflavin and protein content of wheat, barley and oats. In the same investigation it was found that the riboflavin levels in plants grown on gray soils were always slightly lower than those in plants grown on black or brown soils (McElroy *et al.*, 1948).

When winter wheat is vernalized at 2° and cultured under an 8 hr photoperiod it grows only vegetatively; under a 14 hr photoperiod, however, the plants joint and produce grain. Under the first set of conditions, the riboflavin content varied rhythmically with a period of about 12 days, whilst under the second condition, the rhythmicity was considerably speeded up and a full "wave" was completed in about 4 days (Noggle, 1946).

The riboflavin content of the leaves of red kidney bean plants treated with 2,4-dichlorophenoxyacetic acid (2,4-D) was decreased compared with non-treated plants. On the other hand, the levels in the stems of the treated plants were higher than normal (Luecke *et al.*, 1949).

(ii) *Effect of culture conditions*

(a) *Nutrients.* Watson and Noggle (1947) found that, in water culture, deficiencies of K^+, Ca^{2+}, NO_3^-, SO_4^{2-} and PO_4^{3-} all reduced riboflavin synthesis by oat plants; nitrate deficiency had the most marked effect.

The riboflavin content of the leaves of turnips grown in nutrient solutions increased with increasing concentrations of the trace elements Mn and Zn. With Fe, Mo and Co, however, a unimodal curve was obtained when riboflavin production was plotted against micronutrient concentration (Lyon *et al.*, 1948).

(b) *Temperature.* Gustafson (1950) showed that some plants, e.g. tomato and soya bean, produced more riboflavin when cultivated at 28—30° than at 10–15°, whilst with others (broccoli, cabbage, spinach, clover, pea and wheat) the situation was reversed.

(c) *Light.* In a large number of plants (tomato, potato, bean, pea, maize etc.) light stimulated riboflavin production, even though plants cultured in the dark were provided with all necessary nutrients. An albino strain of oats was the only exception to this observation. It was suggested that in this case there was photodestruction of riboflavin by light which would normally have been absorbed by the chloroplast pigments (Gustafson, 1948).

V. MECHANISM OF BIOSYNTHESIS

A. *Origin of Rings B and C*

Riboflavin (I), can formally be considered to arise either (a) from a pyrimidine such as alloxan (VII) condensing with a compound

(VII)   (VIII)

(IX)

such as 4-amino-5-(D-1-ribitylamino)-*o*-xylene (VIII), or (b) from a purine such as xanthine (IX), which after loss of C-8 could condense with the ribityl side-chain and ring A precursors. The first indication that the second pathway was the more probable one arose from reports that certain purines, but not pyrimidines or active pyrimidine precursors such as orotic acid (X), stimulated flavinogenesis in *E. ashbyii* (Maclaren, 1952; Goodwin and Pendlington, 1954; Pendlington, 1954; McNutt, 1954), *A. gossypii* (Broberg, 1954) and *Candida flareri* (Goodwin and McEvoy, 1957, 1959). Although these observations pointed strongly to a purine precursor of riboflavin they were not conclusive, and could have been the result of an indirect effect of the added compounds on the metabolic pathways of the organisms. For example, purine-stimulated flavinogenesis was not observed in *E. ashbyii* by Yaw (1952) or by Minoura (1951), although under Minoura's conditions intact nucleic acid was somewhat effective. Furthermore 2-methyl-adenine (XI) and 2-methyl-hypoxanthine (XII) as well as aminopterin (VI) are strongly flavinogenic in *E. ashbyii* (Brown *et al.*, 1955). The last compound, which is

(X)   (XI)   (XII)

effective at very low concentrations, was assumed to act by inhibiting purine nucleotide synthesis and thus releasing available precursors for channelling into riboflavin production. It is possible that the methyl purines may act in the same way; alternatively they may be incorporated after demethylation, as suggested by Plaut (1961b). The danger of assuming too much from stimulation experiments is emphasized by the observation that whilst urea stimulates riboflavin production in *C. flareri* (Goodwin and McEvoy, 1957, 1959), [14C]urea is not incorporated into the flavin molecule (Audley *et al.*, 1959; see p. 46).

However, direct evidence that purines are precursors of riboflavin has been provided by studies with labelled materials. McNutt (1954) demonstrated that [U-14C]adenine (XIII) was rapidly incorporated into riboflavin by *E. ashbyii*; on the other hand no significant incorporation occurred when [8-14C]adenine was the substrate. This has recently been confirmed with [2-14C]adenine (Smith, 1962). The activity in the riboflavin derived from [U-14C]adenine, was confined to rings B and C (I) and was equally distributed between C-2,4,4a

and 9a; this indicated that after removal of C-8, the purine residue
is incorporated into riboflavin without further degradation (McNutt,

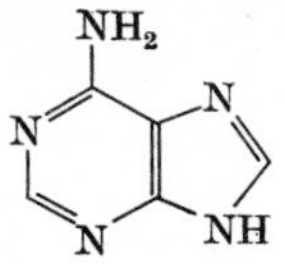

(XIII) 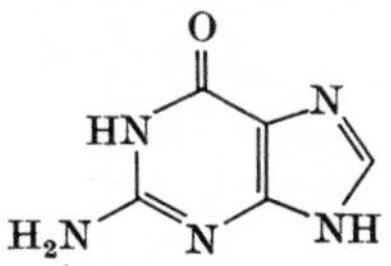   (XIV)

1956). Furthermore, with the help of [U-^{15}N]xanthine and adenine,
McNutt (1960, 1961) showed that all four nitrogen atoms of the
purines were transferred intact to riboflavin. Further support for
the view that purines are direct precursors of riboflavin is provided
by the observations that (a) the incorporation of [^{14}C]serine into
riboflavin by *E. ashbyii* is strongly diluted out by the addition of
unlabelled adenine, although the amount of serine metabolized is

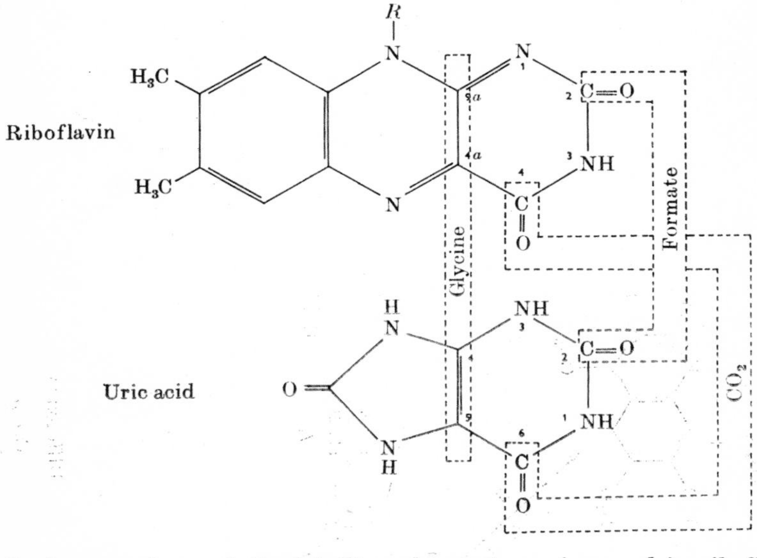

FIG. 3. A comparison of the labelling pattern in purines and in riboflavin
(Goodwin, 1960).

unchanged (Goodwin and Jones, 1956), and (b) under suitable conditions up to 80% of added [^{14}C]guanine (XIV) is incorporated into
riboflavin by *C. flareri* (Audley et al., 1959; Audley and Goodwin, 1962).
In experiments carried out simultaneously with those of McNutt,
Plaut (1954 a,b, 1956) showed that [^{14}C]formate, $^{14}CO_2$, [1-^{14}C]-

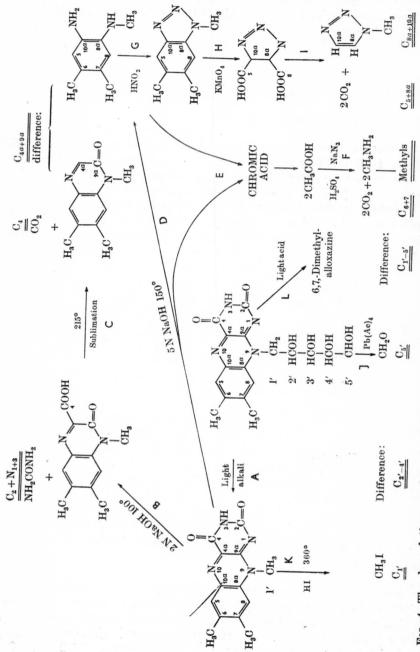

FIG. 4. The degradations used in determining isotope distribution in the riboflavin molecule (after Plaut, 1961b).

and [2-^{14}C]glycine and [^{15}N]glycine were incorporated into ribo-flavin by *A. gossypii* and yielded a labelling pattern (Fig. 3) identical to that expected if rings B and C arise from purine precursors (see Goodwin, 1960). The chemical degradations involved in locating the isotopes in the riboflavin molecule are summarized in Fig. 4. Confirmatory results were also obtained in other micro-organisms; Klungsøyr (1954) showed that [^{14}C]formate was exclusively incor-porated into C-2 of riboflavin by *E. ashbyii*, and McEvoy (1959) obtained the same results with *C. flareri*; Goodwin and Jones (1956) showed that in *E. ashbyii* [3-^{14}C]serine was incorporated almost en-tirely into C-2 whilst generally ^{14}C-labelled serine provided label in C-4a + C-9a as well as in C-2. This labelling pattern could arise from the breakdown of serine into "formate" (C-3) and glycine (C-1 and C-2) which were then incorporated as expected from a purine pattern of labelling. Similarly, Goodwin and Horton (1960) showed that the label from [U-^{14}C]threonine was incorporated only into C-4a + 9a of riboflavin. This is consistent with the breakdown of threonine by threonine aldolase into acetaldehyde (C-3 and -4) and glycine (C-1 and -2) (reaction 1), followed by incorporation of the latter into C-4a + 9a of riboflavin. In support of this view the enzyme threonine aldolase is present in *E. ashbyii* (Goodwin and Horton, 1960).

$$CH_3CHOHCHNH_2COOH \longrightarrow CH_3CHO + CH_2NH_2COOH \qquad (1)$$

The recent results with labelled serine and threonine can now explain the earlier observations that serine and threonine, but not glycine, are flavinogenic in *E. ashbyii* (Goodwin and Pendlington, 1954). Presumably the metabolite which under normal cultural conditions is present in limiting amounts for riboflavin synthesis is "active glycine", which is formed rapidly during the metabolism of serine and threonine, whilst glycine itself is either not activated at all or only slowly compared with the rate of formation of endogenous "active glycine". This view is borne out by the recent report by Kaprálek (1962) that glycine is not metabolized by *E. ashbyii*. [^{14}C]Glycine is, however, incorporated into riboflavin in the closely related *A. gossypii* (Plaut, 1954b) and flavinogenesis is also stimul-ated by glycine in this micro-organism (Plaut, 1961b). This must be one of the few metabolic differences between *E. ashbyii* and *A. gossypii*.

All the evidence just discussed points away from the view that pyrimidines biosynthesized by the accepted pathway (see Goodwin, 1960) are precursors of riboflavin; this conclusion is borne out by the fact that orotic acid (X), an intermediate in pyrimidine bio-synthesis (see, Goodwin, 1960) does not stimulate flavinogenesis in a number of organisms (Maclaren, 1952; Minoura 1953a; Pendlington, 1954; Osman and Soliman, 1960) and that [6-^{14}C]orotic acid is not incorporated into riboflavin in any organism so far investigated (Broberg, 1954; Plaut, 1956; Korte *et al.*, 1958).

In *Candida flareri* urea, arginine, ornithine, but not citrulline were flavinogenic (Goodwin and McEvoy, 1959). This immediately suggested that some modified Krebs-Henseleit urea cycle was operating. However, all efforts to detect arginase in extracts of *C. flareri* failed; this supported the results of Roche and Lacombe (1952) who had been unable to confirm the observation of Eldbacher and Baur (1938) that arginase occurs in bakers' yeast.

Experiments in which *C. flareri* was cultured in the presence of [^{14}C]urea quickly ruled out any direct effect of the carbon atoms of urea on flavinogenesis; no activity was found either in the riboflavin or in the PNA purine bases. An investigation with [^{15}N]urea should prove most illuminating.

B. *The Nature of the Purine Derivative Incorporated into Riboflavin*

The loss of C-8 from purines before incorporation into riboflavin indicates that a 4,5-diaminopyrimidine, or a derivative, is the intermediate involved. The compound most closely related to riboflavin would be 4,5-diaminouracil (XV) which could be derived from xanthine (IX) by removal of C-8. This compound has been

(XV)   (XVI)

detected in cultures of *E. ashbyii* (Goodwin and Treble, 1957) but the methods used in its isolation would not preclude its existence *in vivo* as a ribose or ribitol derivative.

There is some evidence that purine nucleosides are not directly involved in flavinogenesis; for example, in stimulation experiments purine ribosides were no more effective than free purines (Goodwin and Pendlington, 1954; McNutt, 1954). Furthermore, [U-^{14}C]guanosine is incorporated much more effectively into the ring system than into the ribitol side chain of riboflavin (Forrest and McNutt, 1958);

this latter observation strongly suggests that the ribityl residue of riboflavin does not arise from the ribose residue of guanosine. However, as recently pointed out (Goodwin and Horton, 1961), guanosine could, in the presence of a nucleoside phosphorylase, be in equilibrium with guanine and ribose 1-phosphate (reaction 2) and if the pool size of ribose 1-phosphate were much larger than that of guanine (this is highly probable because it is "active glycine"

$$\text{Guanosine} + P_i \rightleftharpoons \text{guanine} + \text{ribose 1-phosphate} \qquad (2)$$

and thus purine,which is the limiting factor in flavinogenesis in *E. ashbyii*, then this could lead to the observed results. Thus it is reasonable to conclude that either (a) a free purine is the immediate precursor and this is ribitylated possibly by transfer from a nucleotide ribitol derivative (e.g. CDP-ribitol) (Shaw, 1962) (p. 56) as indicated in reaction (3); or (b) a free purine is the

$$\text{Purine} + \text{CDP-ribitol} \rightleftharpoons \text{9-ribitylpurine} + \text{CDP} \qquad (3)$$

immediate precursor and this is converted into a phosphoribityl derivative according to reaction (4).

$$\text{Purine} + \text{ribitol 5'-phosphate} \rightleftharpoons \text{9-(5-phosphoribityl)purine} \qquad (4)$$

An unknown phosphorylated derivative of guanine (P) accumulates in *Candida guilliermondii* and *C. flareri* grown in the presence of iron; this is converted into riboflavin by cells of these organisms grown in the absence of iron and in the corresponding cell-free systems (Korte and Ludwig, 1961). It is a possibility that P is a compound similar to that envisaged in reaction (4). A logical consequence of the acceptance of the views that free purines are the precursors of riboflavin, and that there is only one *de novo* mechanism of purine biosynthesis (Fig. 5), which occurs at the nucleoside monophosphate level (see Goodwin, 1960), is that an active nucleotidase splitting nucleotides into free bases is present in flavinogenic organisms. It is possible that the control point of flavinogenesis is at this stage; any excess production of purine nucleotides caused by an "unbalanced" medium could be channelled into riboflavin production. The effective incorporation of added purines into flavinogenesis rather than into growth (PNA synthesis) is presumably due to the relatively high speeds of reactions like (3) or (4) compared with reactions concerned with converting purines into nucleotides, which involve the appropriate phosphoribosylpyrophosphate (PRPP) nucleotide pyrophosphorylase (reaction 5).

$$\text{Purine} + \text{PRPP} \rightleftharpoons \text{purine nucleoside 5'-phosphate} + \text{P-P} \qquad (5)$$

Although the conclusion that a free purine is the immediate precursor of rings B and C has not been unequivocally established,

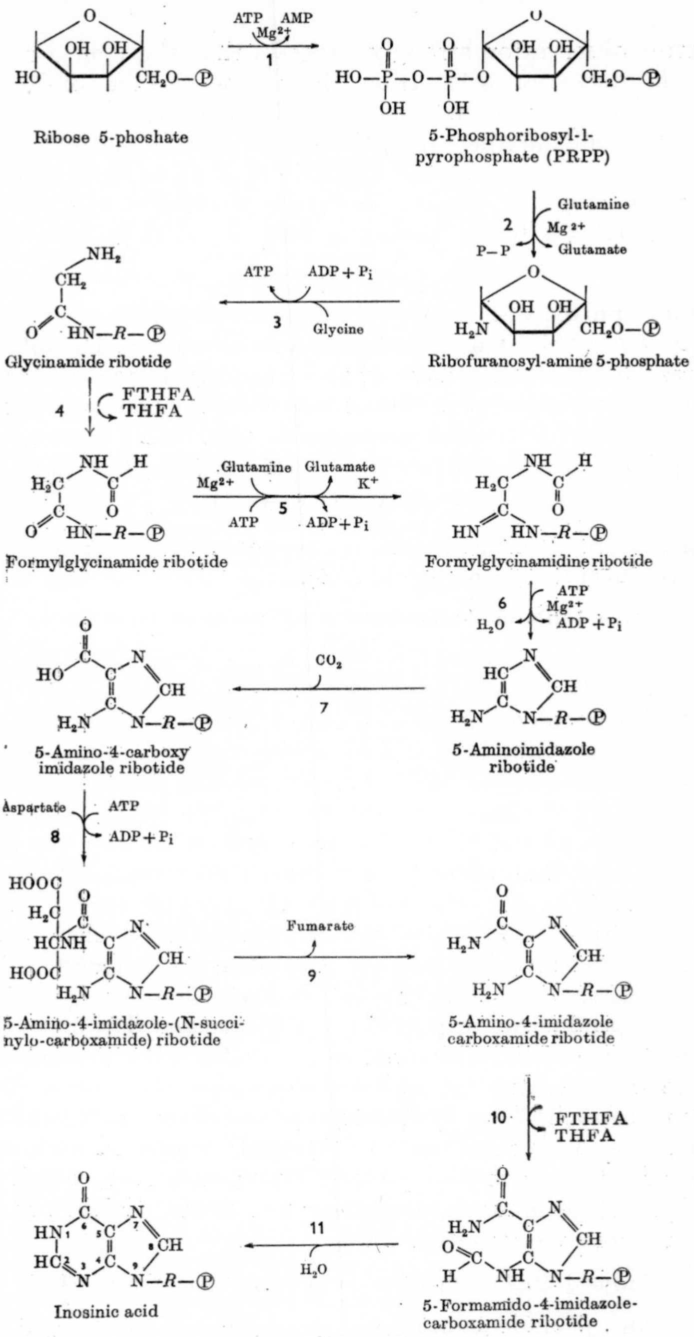

FIG. 5. The pathway of purine biosynthesis.

it is interesting to recall that a very similar situation exists in thi-amine biosynthesis. The condensation of the pyrimidine residue of thiamine with the thiazole base occurs with the phosphorylated base and not with the nucleoside monophosphate, at which level pyri-midines are synthesized (see Chapter 1).

The question next arises as to which purine is the immediate precursor; xanthine is the purine most closely related in chemical structure to riboflavin and it is an effective stimulant in both *E. ashbyii* and *C. flareri*; guanine is, however, quantitatively more effective. The reason for this is not apparent, but the greater effectiv-eness of guanine compared with adenine may be due in part to the fact that in both organisms adenine is incorporated into both PNA-adenine and guanine, whilst guanine is incorporated only into PNA-guanine (Audley, 1961). However, it should be noted that in *E. ashbyii* most adenine added is deaminated to hypoxanthine, which has only slight flavinogenic activity (Brown *et al.*, 1958); on the other hand *C. flareri* cannot deaminate adenine and does not utilize hypoxan-thine for flavinogenesis (McEvoy, 1959). The problem will only be solved by studies with isolated enzymes.

As it is now well established that 6,7-dimethyl-8-ribityllumazine (XVI) is a precursor of riboflavin (see p. 52) it is reasonable to assume from the foregoing discussion that 4-ribitylamino-5-aminouracil(XVII) or 4-(5′-phosphoribitylamino)-5-aminouracil (XVIII) might be the active intermediate in the conversion of purines into riboflavin. 4-Ribitylamino-5-aminouracil, which is very unstable, has been

(XVII)   (XVIII)

synthesized in a number of laboratories and tested for precursor activity under varying conditions. Katagiri *et al.* (1958, 1959) and Kishi *et al.* (1959) claim that in extracts of *E. ashbyii* and *Aerobacter aerogenes* it is converted into (XVI) in the presence of acetoin (XIX). Furthermore, extracts of leuco strains of *E. ashbyii* do not carry out this condensation (Asai *et al.*, 1961). However, Plaut's results with this compound were most inconclusive (see Goodwin and Horton, 1961) and Goodwin and Horton (1961) could not demonstrate its conversion into either (XVI) or riboflavin by extracts of *C. flareri* under many experimental conditions. Plaut (1961b) suggests that an explanation of the results of Katagiri *et al.*, (1958, 1959) is that their enzyme preparation converts acetoin into diacetyl (butanedione) (XX) which then condenses nonenzymatically with (XVI). The

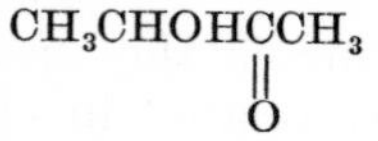

$$CH_3CHOHCCH_3$$
$$O$$
(XIX)

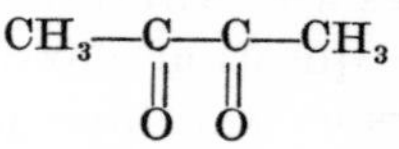

$$CH_3-C-C-CH_3$$
$$O \quad O$$
(XX)

observations that *E. ashbyii* (Masuda, 1957) and *Candida flareri* (McEvoy, 1959) produce acetoin support this view. Furthermore, although [2-^{14}C]acetate is incorporated into ring A of riboflavin, the label is much more randomized than is the label from [1-^{14}C] glucose or [6-^{14}C]glucose (Plaut, 1954b) (Table 5). This means that the C-2 unit arising from glucose does not pass through an acetate pool. The formation of acetoin, formally indicated in reactions (6) and (7), from [3-^{14}C]pyruvate would explain

$$*CH_3COCOOH \xrightarrow{CO_2} *CH_3CHO \qquad (6)$$

$$*CH_3COCOOH + *CH_3CHO \xrightarrow{CO_2} *CH_3COCHOH*CH_3 \qquad (7)$$

the non-randomization of the label from [1-^{14}C]- or [6-^{14}C]glucose (Goodwin, 1959). The non-enzymatic nature of the condensation

TABLE 5. Distribution of ^{14}C in Ring A of Riboflavin Biosynthesized by *Ashbya gossypii* in the Presence of Various Labelled Substrates (Plaut, 1954). Values are Percentages of the Specific Activity in the Riboflavin Molecule.

	Labelled Substrate			
	[1-^{14}C] Acetate	[2-^{14}C] Acetate	[1-^{14}C] Glucose	[6-^{14}C] Glucose
O-Xylene residue	55	44	60	61
C-Methyls	2	15	1	21
C_{6+7}	24	7	3	1
C_{5+8}	2	13	35	38
C_{8a+10a}	23	7	1	1

of diacetyl with (XVI) probably accounts for the lack of specificity of the reaction because a number of related 4,5-diaminopyrimidines can substitute for (XVII). However, unequivocal demonstration of (XVII) as an intermediate remains to be achieved. It is possible that the phosphate derivative is the true intermediate and, as indicated previously, that the purine is ribitylated before loss of C-8.

C. *The Immediate Precursor of Ring A*

During his investigations into the chemical constituents of the mycelium of *E. ashbyii*, Masuda (Masuda, 1956, 1957; Masuda *et al.*, 1957) isolated two compounds, one fluorescing violet (compound V) and one fluorescing green (compound G). Structure (XVI : 6,7-dimethyl-8-ribityllumazine) was assigned to compound G by Masuda (1957). Maley and Plaut (1958, 1959a) synthesized this compound and showed that it was identical with the green fluorescent material which they had also obtained from *A. gossypii;* Masuda (1957) also synthesized (XVI) and demonstrated its identity with compound G (Masuda *et al.*, 1959); it has also been isolated from *Cl. acetobutylicum* (Katagiri *et al.*, 1958) and wheat leaves (Mitsuda *et al.*, 1961a). Other aspects of the chemical synthesis of compound G have been considered by Cresswell and Wood (1959) and Pfleiderer and Nubel (1960).

The structure of 6,7-dimethyl-8-ribityllumazine made it a strong candidate for the position of intermediate in riboflavin biosynthesis.* This view was supported by a number of observations: (a) condensation of the compound with diacetyl to form riboflavin is easily achieved chemically (Masuda, 1957); (b) in *A. gossypii* [14C]formate is incorporated specifically into C-2 of compound G, as it is into riboflavin (Maley and Plaut, 1959a); (c) the extent of incorporation of various labelled substrates into the lumazine and riboflavin by *A. gossypii* was always greater in the lumazine during the early stages of the fermentation (Maley and Plaut, 1959a). More direct evidence for this conversion was obtained when it was found that the synthesis of riboflavin was enhanced by the addition of 6,7-dimethyl-8-ribityllumazine to cell-free preparations of *E. asbhyii* (Kuwada *et al.*, 1958; Katagiri *et al.*, 1959; Korte and Aldag, 1959; Asai *et al.*, 1961), *A. gossypii* (Korte and Aldag, 1959; Maley and Plaut, 1959b). *C. flareri* (Goodwin and Horton, 1961), *Esch. coli* (Katagiri *et al.*, 1959), *Neurospora crassa* (Katagiri *et al.*, 1959), *Lactobacillus plantarum* (Katagiri *et al.*, 1959), *Mycobact.* spp. (Korte and Aldag, 1959) and wheat leaves (Mitsuda *et al.*, 1961b). None of the organisms listed requires

---

* It is possible that riboflavin is synthesized *in vivo* at the FAD level and that the true intermediate is 4,5-diaminouracil adenine dinucleotide.

riboflavin as a growth factor; on the other hand *Lactobacillus casei*, which does require riboflavin as a growth factor, cannot convert 6,7-dimethyl-8-ribityllumazine into riboflavin (Maley and Plaut, 1958; Korte and Aldag, 1959; Katagiri *et al.*, 1958).

6,7-Dimethyl-8-ribityllumazine is not converted into riboflavin by intact cells of *E. ashbyii* (Korte and Aldag, 1959; Korte *et al.*, 1958; Goodwin and Horton, 1961) or *A. gossypii* (Maley and Plaut, 1959b), presumably because of a permeability barrier.

Unequivocal confirmation of the precursor activity of 6,7-dimethyl-8-ribityllumazine was obtained when Maley and Plau-(1959b) showed that the specific activity of the riboflavin formed from [2-^{14}C]-6,7-dimethyl-8-ribityllumazine was similar to that of the substrate. A purely chemical conversion of 6,7-dimethyl-8-ribityllumazine into riboflavin has been reported recently by Rowan and Wood (1963) who obtained riboflavin in 55% yield by refluxing the lumazine dissolved in phosphate buffer (pH 7·3) under nitrogen for 15 hr.

D. *Mechanism of the Conversions of 6,7-Dimethyl-8-ribityllumazine into Riboflavin*

Four additional carbon atoms are required to convert 6,7-dimethyl-8-ribityllumazine into riboflavin. Masuda (1957) suggested that acetoin might be the source of these carbon atoms because, according to him, acetoin will react chemically with 6,7-dimethyl-8-ribityllumazine to form riboflavin. However, Birch and Moye (1957, 1958) who synthesized lumichrome by condensing 4,5-diaminouracil with a dimer of diacetyl (reaction 8) and Cresswell and

(8)

Wood (1959) who used the same reaction to synthesize riboflavin, obtained no flavins when lumazine derivatives were treated with acetoin. Furthermore, Katagiri *et al.* (1958) found that acetoin did not stimulate the synthesis of riboflavin from 6,7-dimethyl-8-ribityllumazine in preparations from *Cl. acetobutylicum* and *Esch. coli neapolitanus*. However, they did claim a stimulation when either acetaldehyde, acetate or pyruvate was used instead of acetoin, and they eventually concluded that acetate, ATP, CoASH and NADH were essential components for the condensation. However, their blank values were high and their conclusions were not entirely convincing. Soon it became clear that 6,7-dimethyl-8-ribityllumazine was converted into riboflavin as effectively in crude extracts of *C. flareri* from which all possible endogenous substrates had been removed by dialysis (Goodwin and Horton, 1961) and in a 100-fold purified enzyme system from *A. gossypii* (Plaut, 1960), as it was in untreated crude extracts. The activity of the extracts was unaffected by the addition of possible 4-carbon precursors: − acetoin, diacetyl, DL-β-hydroxybutyrate, pyruvate, acetate, acetyl phosphate, acetyl CoA, ribose 5-phosphate, glucose-6-phosphate − or by possible co-factors, ATP, ADP, CoASH, lipoic acid, thiamine, NAD$^+$, NADH. NADP$^+$, NADPH, Ca^{2+}, Mg^{2+} (Plaut, 1960; Goodwin and Horton, 1961). Furthermore, Plaut (1960) demonstrated that radioactivity from [^{14}C]acetate or [^{14}C]glucose was not incorporated into the riboflavin synthesized from the lumazine in the presence of the purified enzyme.

Both groups of workers concluded that the 4-C unit (or two 2-C units) was probably being provided by 6,7-dimethyllumazine itself. Plaut (1960) showed that 2·3 molecules of the lumazine disappeared for every molecule of riboflavin synthesized and this was confirmed by Asai *et al.* (1961) in extracts of *E. ashbyii*. Plaut further demonstrated that [6,7-^{14}C]dimethyl-8-ribityllumazine yielded labelled riboflavin, which on degradation by the Kuhn-Roth procedure gave [^{14}C]acetic acid from C-6 and C-7 and their attached methyl groups. Goodwin and Horton (1961) used 6,7-dimethyl-8-ribityllumazine labelled in both methyl groups and in C-6 and C-7 and obtained the same results. If the mechanism indicated in reaction (9) is functional, then the specific molar activities of the dimethyl-8-ribityllumazine, riboflavin and acetic acid should be in the ratio 1 : 2 : 0·5. These were essentially the values observed in both series of experiments. The nature of the active 2-C or 4-C unit involved in this reaction remains to be investigated. The earlier observation of Goodwin and Treble (1958) that [1-^{14}C]-3-hydroxy-2-butanone (acetoin) was exclusively incorporated into ring A with one half of the activity in the methyl groups and the remainder in C-5 and C-8, supports Plaut's (1961) view that 6,7-dimethyl-8-ribityllumazine is formed by condensation of 4-amino-5-ribitylaminouracil, or a phosphate derivative, with diacetyl, formed from acetoin (see p. 50). Reaction (9) would then produce the observed labelling pattern. Although the conversion of 6,7-dimethyl-8-ribityllumazine into riboflavin is now well establish in *in vitro* experiments, the possibility that the synthesis may occur at the FAD level *in vivo* should be borne in mind. The recent kinetic studies of Korte and Ludwig (1961) on FAD and riboflavin synthesis

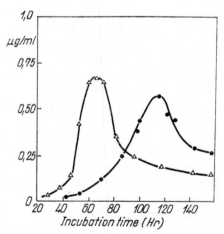

(9)

by growing *C. guilliermondii* are consistent with the view that FAD is first formed and then hydrolysed to riboflavin which is excreted into the culture medium (Fig. 6.).

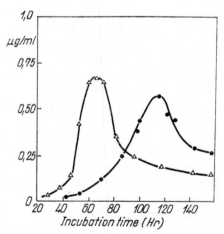

FIG. 6. Synthesis of riboflavin in (●—●—●) and FAD (△—△—△) in growing cells of *Candida guilliermondii* (Korte and Ludwig, 1961).

E.   *6-Methyl-7-hydroxy-8-ribityllumazine*

The blue fluorescing compound, first observed by Masuda in *E. ashbyii* has been isolated from *E. ashbyii* (Masuda *et al.*, 1957; Forrest and McNutt, 1958), *A. gossypii* (Maley and Plaut, 1959 a,b) and *Cl. acetobutylicum* (Katagiri *et al.*, 1958). Its structure (XXI) has been well established (Maley and Plaut, 1959b; Masuda *et al.*, 1958a,b, 1959; Forrest and McNutt, 1958). Its biosynthesis is

(XXI)

clearly related to that of riboflavin because label from [^{14}C]adenine, [^{14}C]guanine and [^{14}C]formate is incorporated into the molecule (McNutt and Forrest, 1958; Maley and Plaut, 1959b; McNutt, 1960). Masuda *et al.* (1958a,b) suggest that (XXI) arises by the condensation of 4-amino-5-ribitylaminouracil with pyruvate, as in the chemical synthesis, but Plaut (1961b) reports that [1-^{14}C]pyruvate is not incorporated into (XXI) by *A. gossypii*, although [3-^{14}C]pyruvate is. Another claim is that (XXI) is formed enzymatically from 6,7-dimethyl-8-ribityllumazine (Kuwada *et al.*, 1958; Plaut, 1960); however, it has been pointed out that this conversion can occur non-enzymatically (Maley and Plaut, 1959a,b), probably by an oxidative or peroxidative process, because the conversion is accelerated by aeration or by the addition of H_2O_2 (Korte *et al.*, 1958; Korte and Aldag, 1959).

F. *The Source of the Ribitol Side Chain*

It is not known when or in what form the ribitol side chain is attached to N-10 during the biosynthesis of riboflavin. All that can be said is that it is already present by the time the known intermediate 6,7-dimethyl-8-ribityllumazine is formed (see p. 51). Plaut (1956) and Plaut and Broberg (1956) examined the incorporation of [1-^{14}C]-, [2-^{14}C]- and [6-^{14}C]glucose into the ribitol side chain of riboflavin by *A. gossypii;* the results (Table 6) indicated that at least two pathways of carbohydrate metabolism, the hexose monophosphate shunt and the transaldolase-transketolase system, contribute to the formation of ribitol. If a different distribution is observed in other organisms, this would not necessarily mean the existence of different precursors but merely different glycolytic pathways in the various organisms.

TABLE 6. The Incorporation of Labelled Glucose into the Ribityl Side Chain of Riboflavin by *Ashbya gossypii* (Plaut, 1956; Plaut and Broberg, 1956). The values are the percentage of the activity of intact riboflavin.

Source of ^{14}C	Carbon atoms of ribitol		
	1	2 + 3 + 4	5
D-[1-^{14}C]glucose	19	1	15
D-[2-^{14}C]glucose	18	34	1
D-[6-^{14}C]glucose	1	1	29

It has already been suggested (p. 47) that a possible ribityl or phosphoribityl intermediate exists at the purine level. Plaut (1961b) has indicated how CDP-ribitol could arise. The first step would be the reduction of ribulose to ribitol either at the phosphate level (reaction 10) by an enzyme similar to mannitol 1-phosphate dehydrogenase which has been found in a number of bacteria (see e.g. Wolff and Kaplan, 1956) or at the free sugar level in a reaction catalysed by ribitol dehydrogenase, an enzyme which has been extracted and purified from cells of *Aerobacter aerogenes* (Fromm, 1958) (reaction 11). In this case the ribitol could be phosphory-

$$\text{Ribulose 5-phosphate} + \text{NADH} + \text{H}^+ \rightleftharpoons \text{ribitol 5-phosphate} + \text{NAD}^+ \quad (10)$$

$$\text{Ribulose} + \text{NADH} + \text{H}^+ \rightleftharpoons \text{ribitol} + \text{NAD}^+ \quad (11)$$

lated conventionally by an appropriate kinase. Reaction (12) is proposed by analogy with the reaction leading to CDP-choline (see Goodwin, 1960); the final possible reaction (3) has already been mentioned (p. 47). In support of this view the discovery of CDP-ribitol in

$$\text{Ribitol 5-phosphate} + \text{CTP} \rightleftharpoons \text{CDP-ribitol} + \text{P-P} \quad (12)$$

Lactobacillus arabinosus by Baddiley *et al.* (1956) and the purification of the enzyme concerned by Shaw (1962) may be quoted. But it should be pointed out that this compound appears to be concerned specifically with the biosynthesis of the teichoic acids, which are important constituents of the bacterial cell wall. Baddiley (personal communication) could not find CDP-ribitol in *E. ashbyii* and, furthermore, the cell walls of fungi are chitinous and, as far as is known, do not contain teichoic acids.

G. *Other Possible Pathways of Riboflavin Synthesis*

It has been claimed that alloxan (VII) and 4-amino-5-ribityl-amino-*o*-xylene (VIII) combine to form riboflavin in *Mycobacterium tuberculosis* (Smith and Emmart, 1949), and the fact that (VII) and 4,5-diamino-*o*-xylene have slight riboflavin activity (1/10,000 and 1/100,000 of that of riboflavin itself, respectively) in *L. casei* and other bacteria also led to the suggestion that they are ribo-flavin precursors (Woolley, 1950, 1951); this claim appears to be very tenuously based. The first conclusion may be the result of a mis-interpretation of the results; Brown *et al.* (1955) found that (VII) and (VIII) reacted spontaneously when incubated in uninoculated sterile media for 5 days at 28°. However, only minute amounts of riboflavin, if any, were formed, the major product being a com-pound, probably (XXII), which, like riboflavin, exhibited an in-tense green, alkali-labile, fluorescence in ultraviolet light, and which could be reduced by dithionite and reoxidized by shaking in

(XXII)

air; it could easily be distinguished from riboflavin by spectro-scopic and chromatographic study. The same results were obtained when (VII) and (VIII) were incubated with growing cells of *E. ash-byii*. Furthermore, no *o*-xylene derivatives have ever been found to stimulate flavinogenesis. (Plaut, 1956; Goodwin and Pendling-ton, 1954; Yaw, 1952; Schopfer, 1955).

In contrast to these observations it should be emphasized that 4,5-diamino-*o*-xylene derivatives are rapidly incorporated into the dimethylbenzimidazole residue of vitamin B_{12} (see Chapter 8).

H. *Partial Synthesis in Animals*

Experiments by Katagiri *et al.* (1958) and Kuwada *et al.* (1960) indicate that the last step in the biosynthesis of riboflavin, the con-version of 6,7-dimethyl-8-ribityllumazine into riboflavin (p. 52), oc-curs in extracts of bovine liver. The conversion does not, however, take place in rat liver or rabbit liver homogenates (Kuwada *et al.*, 1960). Furthermore the feeding of 6,7-dimethyl-8-ribityllum-azine to riboflavin-deficient rats did not cure the deficiency (Suzu-oki *et al.* 1960) and did not result in the excretion of urinary riboflavin (Kuwada *et al.*, 1960).

VI. Riboflavin Derivatives

A. *Riboflavin-5'-Phosphate (FMN)*

(i) *Synthesis in animal tissues*

Rudy (1935) first claimed to have demonstrated the phosphorylation of riboflavin in animal tissues by incubating riboflavin with intestinal phosphatase. The claim of Laszt and Verzár (quoted by Robinson, 1951) that phosphorylation of riboflavin was controlled by the adrenocortical hormones was not substantiated by Ferrebee (1940) who found that phosphorylation of riboflavin occurred as efficiently in adrenalectomized as in normal rats. A further claim of Hubner and Verzár (quoted by Robinson, 1951) that riboflavin could be phosphorylated by incubation with inorganic phosphate and intestinal mucosae could also not be confirmed (Kearney and Englard, 1951); and it is now apparent that the reaction involves a typical kinase, *flavokinase* [ATP: riboflavin 5'-phosphotransferase], with ATP as the mandatory phosphate donor. Phosphorylation of riboflavin takes place in the intestinal mucosae only in the presence of ATP and Mg^{2+} and at a pH of 7·4 (Yagi,

$$\text{Riboflavin} + \text{ATP} \xrightarrow{\ \ Mg^{2+}\ \ } \text{Riboflavin 5'-phosphate} + \text{ADP} \qquad (13)$$

1951; reaction 13). The mucosal enzyme has not been purified. The enzyme has, however, been purified from rat liver (McCormick, 1961). It is present in the supernatant fraction of the cell, has a pH optimum of 4·0 when assayed using 10^{-4}M Zn^{2+}, 10^{-3}M ATP, 10^{-4}M riboflavin and 0·075 M phosphate and an optimum temperature of 50°. The K_m values for riboflavin and ATP are 5×10^{-5}M and 2×10^{-4}M, respectively. Its substrate specificity which has been examined in considerable detail is similar to that of yeast flavokinase (see below) (McCormick, 1962; McCormick and Butler, 1962a). McCormick and Butler consider that the minimum attachment of riboflavin to liver flavokinase is that given in Fig. 7. Flavokinase activity cannot be detected in crude liver homogenates under normal conditions because of the activity of a particulate phosphatase. However, at high pH values and in the presence of Zn^{2+} and phosphate, which inhibit phosphatase activity, FMN synthesis can be demonstrated.

Yagi and Okuda (1958) claim that formation of FMN from ribo-flavin by phosphate esters (e.g. β-glycerophosphate, AMP) will take place in the presence of intestinal phosphate (reaction 14). However, McCormick and Butler (1962b) report that although acid phosphata-

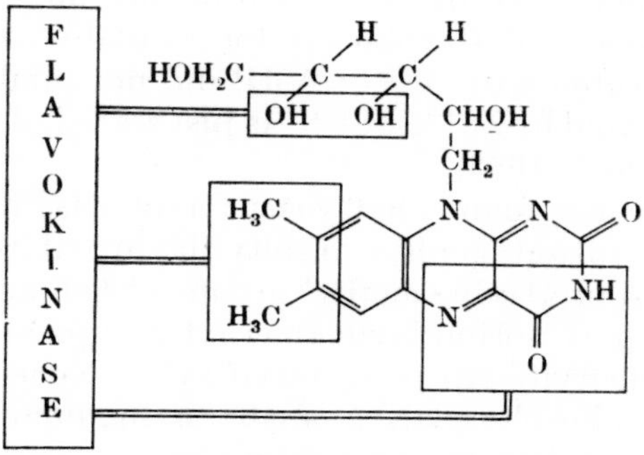

FIG 7. The minimum attachment of riboflavin to liver flavokinase.

ses which hydrolyse FMN are widespread in animal tissues none will catalyse transphosphorylation between riboflavin and the usual phosphate esters.

FMN is synthesized from free riboflavin during the incubation of eggs, most of it being found in the embryo (Kubota, 1951; Matsuura, 1951).

$$\beta\text{-Glycerophosphate} + \text{riboflavin} \rightarrow \text{FMN} + \text{glycerol} \qquad (14)$$

(ii) Synthesis by higher plants

Flavokinase, which is widely distributed in plants has been ex-tracted from mung beans and purified 75-fold; it has an optimum pH of 7·2. The activity of the enzyme increases concomitantly with riboflavin levels in germinating seedlings (Giri et al., 1958).

(iii) Synthesis by micro-organisms

Phosphorylation of riboflavin to form FMN has been obtained with a purified flavokinase isolated from yeast (Kearney and Eng-lard, 1951). It was originally thought that ADP (adenosine diphos-phate) was also a phosphate donor in the reaction, but it is now known that even the purest preparations of flavokinase used contained traces of myokinase, which converts ADP into ATP. This was demon-strated by replacing Mg^{2+} as the co-factor by Zn^{2+}, which activates flavokinase but not myokinase; in the presence of Zn^{2+}, ADP was ineffective as a phosphate donor (Englard, 1953). Mn^{2+} and Co^{2+} can also replace Mg^{2+} as stimulators of flavokinase but are less ef-fective. The optimal temperature for the reaction is 38° and the optimal pH 8·0. The K_S values for ATP and ADP are $1·7 \times 10^{-5}$ M and $1·6 \times 10^{-5}$M, respectively (Kearney, 1955).

Adenylic acid (AMP) competitively inhibited the reaction and inosine triphosphate was completely inactive as either stimulator or inhibitor. The inhibition by AMP is probably due to competition between myokinase and flavokinase for available ATP when the enzymes are activated with Mg^{2+}; AMP did not inhibit flavokinase when it was activated by Zn^{2+}, which, as just stated, does not activate myokinase (Englard, 1953).

Kearney (1952) has found that yeast flavokinase also phosphorylates the riboflavin antagonists arabitylflavin (ribitol replaced by arabitol) and dichloroflavin (methyl groups at C-6 and C-7 replaced by chlorine) but not isoriboflavin (methyl groups at C-5 and C-6), galactoflavin, dulcitylflavin or sorbitylflavin. None of these, however, inhibits the phosphorylation of riboflavin; lumiflavin in excess does inhibit this reaction to some extent.

An enzyme, distinct from flavokinase, with an optimum pH of 5·4, which catalyses the transfer of phosphate from glucose 1-phosphate to riboflavin has been reported in unnamed flavinogenic micro-organisms (Katagiri and Imai, 1961).

B. *Flavin Adenine Dinucleotide (FAD)*

(i) *Synthesis in animals*

The first claim to have synthesized FAD *in vitro* was made by Klein and Kohn (1940) who incubated riboflavin with human red cells at 30–34°; *in vivo* synthesis by human red cells could also be demonstrated after the subject consumed a dose of riboflavin. About the same time, Trufanov (1941, 1942) obtained FAD synthesis in mouse liver slices.

More recent studies on the synthesis of FAD by various animal tissues indicate some apparent discrepancies which should eventually be resolved. Itoh and Ohta (1950) and Makino *et al.* (1950) claimed that FAD can be synthesized from riboflavin, ATP and Na_2HPO_4 by an acetone-dried powder of pig kidney. Yagi (1951), on the other hand, found that FMN, but not free riboflavin, was converted into FAD by acetone-dried powders of liver and kidney in the presence of ATP and Mg^{2+} at pH 7·4. It is interesting that, although Yagi showed that the intestinal mucosa could convert riboflavin into FMN, he found that it could not synthesize FAD. It is thus possible that FAD is synthesized in two steps, the first (to FMN) occurring in the intestinal wall and the second (FMN→FAD) in the liver or kidney.

The mechanism of synthesis of FAD from FMN in animal tissues has not been fully elucidated, but a pyrophosphorylase reaction is probably involved (equation 15); this has been clearly demonstrated with the enzyme isolated from yeast (see next section). Watarai *et al.* (1955) observed that [^{32}P]-FAD synthesized by rat liver homogenates from [^{32}P]-FMN had the same specific activity as the starting material. This would support the mechanism indicated in equation 15, but a net synthesis of FAD was not obtained in these

$$FMN + ATP \rightleftarrows FAD + P\text{-}P \qquad (15)$$

experiments. The difficulty in achieving a net synthesis of FAD is due to the high FAD-ase activity of most extracts. Deluca and Kaplan (1958) removed this activity by differential centrifugation of homogenates, and to demonstrate FAD synthesis in many mouse and rat tissues, e.g. liver, brain, heart, spleen and skeletal muscle. The purified preparation from rat liver required Mg^{2+} or Mn^{2+} for activation, and riboflavin would not substitute for FMN. The final requirement for proof of reaction (15), pyrophosphorolysis of FAD, could not be demonstrated.

As in the case of FMN, FAD is produced from free riboflavin in the developing chick embryo (Kubota, 1951; Matsuura, 1951). It is not known whether or not FMN is an obligatory intermediate.

(ii) *Synthesis in micro-organisms*

Preparations which carry out reaction 15 (see previous section) have been obtained by Schrecker and Kornberg (1950) from bakers' yeast. The reaction was shown to be reversible and to require Mg^{2+} for activation. ATP cannot be replaced by ADP or AMP. The very slight activity with riboflavin as substrate was ascribed to the presence in the preparation of traces of flavokinase. The analogy between this reaction and that concerned with the synthesis of NAD (Chapter 3) should be emphasized. A similar enzyme has been prepared from *Lactobacillus arabinosus* 17-5 (Snoswell, 1957) and a flavinogenic yeast (Giri and Krishnaswamy, 1956). As indicated on p. 54 the recent kinetic studies of Korte and Ludwig (1961) on the production of FAD and riboflavin in growing cells of *C. guilliermondii* suggest that riboflavin may be synthesized at the FAD level.

(iii) *Synthesis in higher plants*

An enzyme which synthesizes FAD from FMN, but not riboflavin, and ATP has been demonstrated in a number of plants, and purified some 83-fold from *Phaseolus radiatus* (Giri *et al.*, 1960). The enzyme has an optimum pH of 7·4, and K_m values for FMN and ATP are 0·043 mM and 0·75 mM, respectively. The enzyme is activated by Mg^{2+} and Zn^{2+} at all concentrations and by Mn^{2+} at low concentrations (0·1 mM); Ni^{2+}, Cu^{2+}, Hg^{2+} and CN^- inhibited at a concentration of 0·1 mM, whereas Co^{2+}, Fe^{2+} were without effect even at a concentration of 10mM. It would appear that this FAD-synthesizing enzyme is a phosphorylase, but this has not yet been clearly esablished.

The activity of the enzyme and the FAD levels increased in parallel during germination of *P. radiatus* seeds (Giri *et al.*, 1960).

C. *Riboflavinyl Glycosides*

Whitby (1950, 1952, 1954) found that rat liver preparations can convert riboflavin into riboflavinyl-α-D-glucoside. The enzyme responsible catalyses transglycosidation of D-glucose from maltose, maltulose, turanose and, in crude liver extracts, glycogen (reaction 16). The enzyme also exhibits hydrolytic activity (reactions 17

$$\text{Maltose} + \text{riboflavin} \rightleftarrows \text{riboflavin-}\alpha\text{-D-glucoside} + \text{D-glucose} \qquad (16)$$

and 18). The corresponding anomers (cellobiose and riboflavin-β-D-glucoside) are not substrates for this enzyme.

$$\text{Maltose} + H_2O \rightleftarrows 2 \text{ D-Glucose} \qquad (17)$$
$$\text{Riboflavin } \alpha\text{-D-glucoside} \rightleftarrows \text{D-glucose} + \text{riboflavin} \qquad (18)$$

The specificity of the donor molecule is considerable, the disaccharide must contain an α-glucopyranose residue, and the aglycone must contain a reducing group; furthermore the position of linkage of the aglycone to the α-glucopyranose residue is critical, for example, as indicated above, maltulose (α-glucopyranoside -4-0--D-fructofuranose) and turanose (α-glucopyranoside-3-0-D-fructofuranose) are active, whilst isomaltose (α-glucopyranoside-6-0-D-glucopyranose) is not. The specificity of the acceptor molecule is not great; a large number of flavins with different stereoisomers replacing ribitol are active to about the same extent. However, lengthening of the side chain to C-6 (D-galactoflavin) and shortening to C-3 (9-dihydroxypropylisoalloxazine) reduces activity considerably, whilst shortening the side chain still further to C-2 (9-oxyethylisoalloxazine) leads to complete inactivity.

Riboflavin glycosides are synthesized by growing cells of *Cl. acetobutylicum* and *A. oryzae* (Tachibana and Katagiri, 1955; Tachibana, 1955). The nature of the glycoside residue depends on the carbohydrate present in the medium, and compounds formed include the maltoside, galactoside melibioside, dextrantrioside and dextrantetraoside (Katagiri and Imai, 1961).

The significance of riboflavin glycoside formation in animal tissues remains to be assessed, because their natural occurrence has not yet been demonstrated.

A. oryzae can utilize riboflavin glycoside for formation of glycogen (Tachibana, 1955) but, again, the significance of the reaction under normal cultural conditions is uncertain.

REFERENCES

Arragon, G., Mainil, J., Refait, R., and Velu, H. (1946). *Ann. Inst. Pasteur* **72**, 300.
Artzberger, F. C. (1943). *U. S. Pat. Syst. Leafl.* **2**, 326, 425.
Asai, M., Masuda, T. and Kuwada, S. (1961). *Chem. & Pharm. Bull.* 9, 85, 496, 503.
Audley, B. G. (1961). Ph. D. Thesis. University of Liverpool.
Audley, B. G., and Goodwin, T. W. (1962). *Biochem. J.* **84**, 587.
Audley, B. G., Goodwin, T. W., and McEvoy, D. (1959). *Biochem. J.* **72**, 8P.
Baddiley, J., Buchanan, J. G., Carss, B., and Mathias, A. P. (1956). *Biochim. biophys. Acta* **21**, 191.
Banga, I., and Szent-Györgyi, A. (1932). *Biochem. Z.* **246**, 203.
Barker, H. A., and Peterson, W. H. (1944). *J. Bact.* **47**, 307.
Bessey, O. A., Lowry, O. H., and Love, R. H., (1949). *J. biol. Chem.* **180**, 755.
Birch, A. J., and Moye, C. J. (1957). *J. chem. Soc.* 412.
Birch, A. J., and Moye, C. J. (1958). *J. chem. Soc.* 2622.
Bonner, J. (1942). *Bot. Gaz.* **103**, 581.
Bonner, J., and Dorland, R. (1943). *Amer. J. Bot.* **30**, 414.
Bonner, J., and Bonner, H. (1948). *Vitam. & Horm.* **6**, 225.
Broberg, P. L. (1954). M. S. Thesis. University of Wisconsin.
Brown, E. G., Goodwin, T. W., and Pendlington, S. (1955). *Biochem. J.* **61**, 37.
Brown, E. G., Goodwin, T. W., and Jones, O. T. G. (1958). *Biochem. J.* **68**, 40
Burkholder, P. R. (1943). *Science*, **97**, 562; *Arch. Biochem.* **3**, 121; *Proc. nat. Acad. Sci., Wash.* **29**, 166.
Burkholder, P. (1944). *Arch. Biochem.*, **4**, 217.
Burkholder, P. R., and McVeigh, I. (1942). *Proc. nat. Acad. Sci., Wash.* **28**, 285, 1440.
Burkholder, P. R., and McVeigh, I. (1945). *Plant Physiol.* **20**, 276, 301.
Busnel, R. G., and Drilhon, A. (1943). *C. R. Acad. Sci., Paris,* **216**, 213.
Carroll, F. D. (1950). *J. Anim. Sci.* **9**, 139.
Cheldelin, V. H., and Lane, R. L. (1943). *Proc. Soc. exp. Biol. Med.* **54**, 43.
Chin, C. (1947). *J. Ferment. Technol.* **25**, 140.
Christie, S. M. H., Kenner, G. W., and Todd, A. R. (1954). *J. chem. Soc.* 46.
Crammer, J. K. (1948). *Nature, Lond.* **161**, 349.
Cresswell, R. M., and Wood, H. C. S. (1959). *Proc. chem. Soc.* 387.
Deluca, C., and Kaplan, N. O. (1956). *J. biol. Chem.* **223**, 569.
Deluca, C., and Kaplan, N. O. (1958). *Biochim. biophys. Acta*, **30**, 6.
Dikanskaya, E. (1953). *Microbiology, Moscow*, **22**, 256.
Dolin, M. I. (1953). *Arch. Biochem.* **46**, 483.
Dolin, M. I. (1955). *Arch. Biochem.* **55**, 415.

Dyr, J., and Munk, V. (1954). *Čsl. Biol.* **3**, 17.
Eldbacher, S., and Baur, H. (1938). *Hoppe-Seyl. Z.* **254**, 275.
Ellinger, P., and Koschara, W. (1933). *Ber. dtsch. chem. Ges.* **66**, 315.
Enari, T. M. (1955). *Acta chem. scand.* **9**, 1726.
Enari, T. M. (1958). *Ann. Acad. Sci. fenn.* **90**, 7.
Enari, T. M. and Kauppinen, V. (1961). *Acta chem. scand.* **15**, 1513.
England, S. (1953). *J. Amer. chem. Soc.* **75**, 6048.
Ferrebee, J. W. (1940). *J. biol. Chem.* **136**, 719.
Fogg, G. E. (1953). "The Metabolism of Algae". Methuen, London.
Forrest, H. S., and McNutt, W. S. (1958). *J. Amer. chem. Soc.* **80**, 739.
Fraenkel, G., and Blewett, M. (1943). *Biochem. J.* **37**, 686.
Fraenkel, G., and Blewett, M. (1944). *Proc. roy. Soc.* B. **132**, 212.
Fromm, H. J. (1958). *J. biol. Chem.* **233**, 1049.
Ganguly, S. (1954). *Nature, Lond.* **174**, 559.
Giri, K. V., and Krishnaswamy, P. R. (1956). *J. Indian Inst. Sci.* **38**, 232.
Giri, K. V., Krishnaswamy, P. R., and Appaji Rao, N. (1958). *Biochem. J.* **70**, 66.
Giri, K. V., Appaji Rao, N., Cama, H. R., and Mumar, S. A. (1960). *Biochem. J.* **75**, 381.
Goodwin, T. W. (1959). *In* "Progress in Industrial Microbiology", **1**, 137 (D. J. D. Hockenhull Ed.). Heywood, London.
Goodwin, T. W. (1960). "Recent Advances in Biochemistry". Churchill, London.
Goodwin, T. W. (1963). *In* "Biochemistry of Industrial Micro–organisms", (A. L. Rose and C. Rainbow, eds.). Academic Press, London and New York.
Goodwin, T. W., and Pendlington, S. (1954). *Biochem. J.* **57**, 631.
Goodwin, T. W., and Jones, O. T. G. (1956). *Biochem. J.* **64**, 9.
Goodwin, T. W., and McEvoy, D. (1957). *Biochem. J.* **67**, 17P.
Goodwin, T. W., and Treble, D. H. (1957). *Biochem. J.* **67**, 10P.
Goodwin, T. W., and Treble, D. H. (1958). *Biochem. J.* **70**, 14P.
Goodwin, T. W., and McEvoy, D. (1959). *Biochem. J.* **71**, 742.
Goodwin, T. W., and Horton, A. A. (1960). *Biochem. J.* **75**, 52.
Goodwin, T. W., and Horton, A. A. (1961). *Nature, Lond.* **191**, 772.
Gustafson, F. G. (1947). *Plant Physiol.* **22**, 620.
Gustafson, F. G. (1948). *Plant Physiol.* **23**, 373.
Gustafson, F. G. (1950). *Plant Physiol.* **25**, 150.
Gustafson, F. G. (1955). *Plant Physiol.* **25**, 150.
Hedrick, L. R., and Burke, G. C. (1950). *J. Bact.* **59**, 481.
Hendrickz, H., and de Vleeschauwer, A. (1955). *Meded. Landb Hoogesch, Gent,* **20**, 229.
Hendrickz, H., and de Vleeschauwer, A. (1956). *Meded. Landb Hoogesch, Gent,* **21**, 663.
Hickey, R. J. (1945). *Arch. Biochem.* **8**, 439.
Hickey, R. J. (1953). *J. Bact.* **66**, 22, 27.
Holz, G. G. (1950). *Physiol. Zoöl.* **23**, 213.
Horton, A. A. (1960). Ph. D. Thesis. University of Liverpool.
Hoštáleck, Z. (1957). *J. gen. Microbiol.* **17**, 267.
Huennekens, F. M., and Kilgour, G. L. (1955). *J. Amer. chem. Soc.* **44**, 6716.
Itoh, F., and Ohta, K. (1950). *Vitamins (Kyoto)* **3**, 27.
Kaprálek, F. (1957). *Preslia,* **29**, 113.
Kaprálek, F. (1962). *J. gen. Microbiol.* **29**, 403.
Karrer, P., Salomon, H., Schöpp, K., Schlitler, E., and Fritzsche, H. (1934). *Helv. chim. acta* **17**, 1010.

Karrer, P., Schöpp, K., and Benz, F. (1935). *Helv. chim. acta* **18,** 426.
Katagiri, H., and Imai, K. (1961). *In* "Proceedings of the 5th International Congress of Biochemistry, Moscow", p. 283. Pergamon Press, London.
Katagiri, H., Takeda, I., and Imai, K. (1958). *J. Vitaminol.*, *Japan* **4,** 207, 211, 278, 285.
Katagiri, H., Takeda, I., and Imai K. (1959). *J. Vitaminol.*, *Japan* **5,** 81, 287.
Kearney, E. B. (1952). *J. biol. Chem.* **194,** 747.
Kearney, E. B. (1955). *In* "Methods in Enzymology", Vol. 2, p. 640. (S. P. Colowick and N. O. Kaplan, eds.). Academic Press, New York and London.
Kearney, E. B., and Englard, S. (1951). *Arch. Biochem. Biophys.* **32,** 222.
Kishi, J., Asai, M., Masuda, T., and Kuwada, S. (1959). *Chem. pharmacol. Bull.* **7,** 515.
Klein, J. R., and Kohn, H. I. (1940). *J. biol. Chem.* **136,** 177.
Klatzin, C., Norris, F. W., and Wokes, F. (1949). *Comm. lst. International Congress of Biochemistry*, Cambridge, England p. 26.
Klungsøyr, L. (1954). *Acta chem. scand.* **8,** 723.
Knüsel, F. (1957). *Arch. Mikrobiol.* **27,** 252.
Korte, F., and Aldag, H. V. (1959). *Liebigs Ann.* **628, 144.**
Korte, F., and Ludwig, G. (1961). *Liebigs Ann.* **648,** 131.
Korte, F., Aldag, H. V., Ludwig, G., Paulus, W., and Storiko, K. (1958). *Liebigs Ann.* **619,** 70.
Kubota, H. (1951). *Igaku to Seibutsugaku*, **18,** 202.
Kuhn, R., Rudy, H., and Weygand, F. (1936). *Ber. dtsch. chem. Ges.* **69,** 1543.
Kuhn, R., György, P., and Wagner-Jauregg, T. (1933). *Ber. dtsch. chem. Ges.* **66,** 315.
Kuhn, R., Reinemund, K., Kalkschmidt, H., Strobele, R., and Trischmann, H. (1935). *Naturwiss.* **23,** 260.
Kumar, S. A. (1962). Ph. D. Thesis. Indian Institute of Science. Bangalore.
Kuwada, S., Masuda, T., Kishi, T., and Asai, M. (1958). *Chem. pharmacol. Bull.* **6,** 618.
Kuwada, S., Masuda, T., and Asai, M. (1960). *Chem. pharmacol. Bull.* **8,** 792.
Lamoureux, W. F., and Schumacher, R. S. (1940). *Poultry Sci.* **19,** 418.
Lee, S. B., and Burris, R. H. (1943). *Industr. Engng Chem.* **35,** 354.
Levine, R., Oyaas, J. E., Wasserman, L., Hoogeheide, J. C., and Stern, R. M. (1949). *Industr. Engng Chem.* **41,** 1665-1668.
Leviton, A. (1946). *J. Amer. chem. Soc.* **68,** 835.
Lewis, J. C. (1944). *Arch. Biochem.* **4,** 217.
Lightbown, J. W., and Kogut, M. (1959). *Biochem. J.* **73,** 14 P.
Luecke, R. W., Hamner, C. L., and Snell, H. M. (1949). *Plant Physiol.* **24,** 546.
Lyon, C. B., and Beeson, K. C. (1948). *Bot. Gaz.* **109,** 506.
Maclaren, J. A. (1952). *J. Bact.* **63,** 233.
Makino, K., Itoh, F., and Ohta, K. (1950). *J. Biochem.*, *Tokyo* **37,** 459.
Maley, G. F., and Plaut, G. W. E. (1958). *Fed. Proc.* **17,** 268.
Maley, G. F., and Plaut, G. W. E. (1959a). *J. biol. Chem.* **234,** 641.
Maley, G. F., and Plaut, G. W. E. (1959b). *J. Amer. chem. Soc.* **81,** 2025.
Mannering, G. J., Orgini, D., and Elvehjem, C. A. (1944). *J. Nutr.* **28,** 141.
Masuda, T. (1956). *Pharmacol. Bull. (Tokyo)* **4,** 71, 375, 382.
Masuda, T. (1957). *Pharmacol. Bull. (Tokyo)* **5,** 28, 136.
Masuda, T., Kishi, T., and Asai, M. (1957). *Pharmacol. Bull. (Tokyo)* **5,** 598.
Masuda, T., Kishi, T., Asai, M., and Kuwada, S. (1959). *Chem. Pharmacol. Bull.* **7,** 361.
Matsuura, K. (1951). *Igaku to Seibutsugaku*, **18,** 202.
McCormick, D. B. (1961). *Fed Proc.* **20,** 447; *Proc. Soc. exp. Biol.*, *N.Y.* **104,** 54.
McCormick, D. B. (1962). *Fed. Proc.* **21,** 239; *J. biol. Chem.* **234,** 959.

McCormick, D. B. and Butler, R. C. (1962a). *Biochim. biophys. Acta* **65**, 326.
McCormick, D. B. and Butler, R. C. (1962b). *Comp. Biochem. Physiol.* **5**, 113.
McElroy, L. W., and Goss, H. (1940). *J. Nutr.* **20**, 527.
McElroy, L. W., Kastelic, J., and McCalla, A. G. (1948) *Canad. J. Res.* **26 F**, 191.
McEvoy, D. (1959). Ph. D. Thesis. The University of Liverpool.
McNutt, W. (1954). *J. biol. Chem.* **210**, 511.
McNutt, W. (1956). *J. biol. Chem.* **219**, 363.
McNutt, W. (1960). *Fed. Proc.* **19**, 157; *J. Amer. chem. Soc.* **82**, 217.
McNutt, W. (1961). *J.,Amer. chem. Soc.* **83**, 2303.
McNutt, W. and Forrest, H. S. (1958). *J. Amer. chem. Soc.* **80**, 951.
Meade, R. E., Pollard, H. L., and Rodgers, N. E. (1945). *U. S. Pat. Syst. Leafl.* **2**, 369, 680.
Metcalf, R. L., and Patton, R. L. (1942). *J. cell. comp. Physiol.* **19**, 373.
Minoura, K. (1950). *J. Ferment. Technol.* **28**, 60, 186.
Minoura, K. (1951). *J. Ferment. Technol.* **29**, 124.
Minoura, K. (1953a). *Vitamins (Kyoto)* **7**, 407.
Minoura, K. (1953b). *Vitamins (Kyoto)* **6**, 62.
Mitra, K. K. (1957). *Experientia* **13**, 356.
Mitsuda, H., Kawai, F. and Moritaka, S. (1961a). *J. Vitaminol. (Japan)* **7**, 128.
Mitsuda, H., Kawai, F., Suzuki, Y., and Nakayama, Y. (1961b). *J. Vitaminol. (Japan)*, **7**, 243, 247.
Moore, H. N., and de Becze, G. (1947). *J. Bact.* **54**, 41.
Moore, H. N., de Becze, G., and Schraffenberger, E. (1947). *J. Bact.* **53**, 502.
Naik, M. S. and Narayana, N. (1960). *Ann. Biochem. exp. Med. (India)*, **20**, 237.
Najjar, V. A., Johns, G. A., Medairy, G. C., Fleischmann, G., and Holt, L. E. (1944). *J. Amer. med. Ass.* **126**, 357.
Nandi, N., and Banerjee, S. (1950). *Indian Pharm.* **5**, 202.
Niederpruem, D. J., and Hackett, D. P. (1958). *Plant Physiol.* **33**, 113.
Noggle, G. R. (1946). *Plant Physiol.* **21**, 492.
Novak, A. F. (1948). *U. S. Pat. Syst. Leafl* **2**, 447, 814.
Novak, A. F., Stark, W. H., and Kolachov, P. (1943). *J. Bact.* **45**, 34.
Obata, Y., and Tomoeda, M. (1953). *J. agric. chem. Soc. Japan*, **27**, 867, 869.
Osman, H. G., and Soliman, M. H. M. (1960). *Biochem. Z.* **333**, 351.
Owen, E. C., Montgomery, J. P., and Proudfoot, R. (1962). *Biochem J.* **82**, 8P.
Pakarskite, K. Y. (1961). *In* "Proceedings of the 5th International Congress of Biochemistry, Moscow", p. 292. Pergamon Press, London.
Pearson, P. B., and Schweigert, B. S. (1947). *J. Nutr.* **34**, 443.
Peel, J. L. (1958). *Biochem. J.* **69**, 403.
Pendlington, S. (1954). Ph. D. Thesis. University of Liverpool.
Petit, M. (1950). *Industr. agric.* **67**, 43.
Pfeifer, U. F., Tanner, F.W., Vojnovich, C., and Traufler, D. J. (1950). *Industr. Engng. Chem.* **42**, 1776.
Pfleiderer, W., and Nubel, G. (1960). *Ber. dtsch. chem. Ges.* **93**, 1406.
Pirie, A. (1959). *Biochem. J.* **71**, 29P; *Nature, Lond.* **183**, 985.
Plaut, G. W. E. (1954a). *J. biol. Chem.* **208**, 513.
Plaut, G. W. E. (1954b). *J. biol. Chem.* **211**, 111.
Plaut, G. W. E. (1956). *Nutrition Symp. Ser. No.* **13**, 20.
Plaut, G. W. E. (1960). *J. biol. Chem.* **235**, PC41.
Plaut, G. W. E. (1961a). *In* "Metabolic Pathways", Vol. II. (D. Greenberg, ed.). Academic Press, New York.
Plaut, G. W. E. (1961b). *Ann. Rev. Biochem.* **30**, 409.
Plaut, G. W. E., and Broberg, P. L. (1956). *J. Biol. Chem.* **219**, 131.

2. RIBOFLAVIN AND RELATED COMPOUNDS

Povolotskaya, K. L., and Zaitseva, N. I. (1951). *C. R. Acad. Sci. U. R. S. S.* **77**, 317.
Pridham, T. G. (1952). *Econ. Bot.* **6**, 185.
Pridham, T. G., and Raper, K. B. (1952). *Mycologia*, **44**, 452.
Raut, V. S. and Chitre, R. G. (1961). *J. Postgrad. Med.*, **7**, 35.
Robbins, W. J., and Schmidt, M. B. (1939). *Bull. Torrey Bot. Cl.* **66**, 139.
Robinson, F. A. (1951). "The Vitamin B Complex." Chapman and Hall, London.
Roche, J., and Lacombe, G. (1952). *Biochim. biophys. Acta* **9**, 687.
Rodgers, N. E., Pollard, H. L., and Meade, R. E. (1948). *U. S. Pat. Syst. Leafl.* **2**, 449. 143.
Rogosa, M. (1943). *J. Bact.* **45**, 459.
Rowan, T., and Wood, H. C. S. (1963). *Proc. chem. Soc.* 21.
Rudy, H. (1935). *Naturwissenschaften* **23**, 286.
Saunders, A., and McClung, L. S. (1943). *J. Bact.* **46**, 575.
Schopfer, W. H. (1944). *Helv. chim. acta*, **27**, 1017.
Schopfer, W. H. (1955). *Bull. Ass. Dipl. Microb., Nancy*, **61**, 3.
Schopfer, W. H., and Guilloud, M. (1944). *Arch. Sci. phys. nat.* **61**. 232.
Schopfer, W. H., and Guilloud, M. (1945). *Schweiz. Z. Path.* **8**, 521.
Schopfer, W. H., and Guilloud, M. (1946). *Ber. schweiz. bot. Ges.* **56**, 700.
Schopfer, W. H., and Knüsel, F. (1956). *Schweiz. Z. Path.* **19**, 659.
Schopfer, W. H., Posternak, T. and Boss, M. L. (1947). *Schweiz. Z. Path.* **10**, 443.
Schrecker, A W., and Kornberg, A. (1950). *J. biol. Chem.* **182**, 795.
Seaman, G. R. (1953). *Physiol. Zoöl.* **26**, 22.
Sebek, O. (1947). *Chem. Listy* **41**, 238.
Shavlovsky, G. M., and Chistiakova, U. S. (1956). *C. R. Acad. Sci. U. R. S. S.* **111**, 887.
Shavlovsky, G. M., and Fiktash, I. S. (1961). *In* "Proceedings of the International Congress of Biochemistry, Moscow", p. 305. Pergamon Press, London.
Shavlovsky, G. M., Tsarenko, E. M., and Fiktash, I. S. (1962). *C. R. Acad. Sci., U. R. S. S.* **142**, 940.
Shaw, D. R. D. (1962). *Biochem. J.* **82**, 297.
Shukla, J. P. and Prabku, K. A. (1961). *J. sci. industr. Res.* **20**, 40.
Singh, K., Agarwal, G. N., and Peterson, W. H. (1948). *Arch. Biochem.* **18**, 181.
Smiley, K. L., Sobolov, M., Austin, F. L., Rasmussen, R. A., Smith, M. B., van Lanen, J. M., Stone, L., and Boruff, C. S. (1951). *Industr. Engng Chem.* **43**, 1380.
Smith, C. G. (1962). *Biochim. biophys. Acta* **61**, 380.
Smith, L. (1954). *Bact. Rev.* **18**, 106.
Smith, M. I. and Emmart, E. W. (1949). *J. Immunol.* **61**, 259.
Smith, C. G., Smith, G. A., and Papadopoulou, Z. (1957). *Fed. Proc.* **16**, 251.
Sone, K. (1959). *Nippon Nogei Kaish Kagaku*, **33**, 949.
Stadtman, E. R. (1958). *In* "Proceedings of the 4th International Congress of Biochemistry, Vienna", **11**, 19. Pergamon Press, London.
Stiles, H. R. (1940). *Amer. Miller*, 54.
Strittmatter, P. (1958). *Fed. Proc.* **17**, 318.
Suzuoki, J. *et al.* (1960). *J. Vitaminol.* **6**, 145.
Tachibana, S. (1955). *Vitamins (Kyoto)* **8**, 356, 363; **9**, 119.
Tachibana, S., and Katagiri, H. (1955). *Vitamins (Kyoto)* **8**, 304.
Tanner, F. W., Vojnovich, C., and van Lanen, J. M. (1945). *Science*, **101**, 180.
Tanner, F. W., Vojnovich, C., and van Lanen, J. M. (1949). *J. Bact.* **58**, 737.
Tirunarayanan, M. O., and Sarma, P. S. (1954). *J. sci. industr. Res.* **13B**, 488.
Tittsler, R. P., and Whittier, F. O. (1941). *J. Bact.* **42**, 151.
Trufanov, A. V. (1941). *Biochemistry, Leningr.* **6**. 391.

Trufanov, A. V. (1942). *Biochemistry, Leningr.* **7**, 188.
Tsujimura, K. (1950). *J. agric. chem. Soc. Japan* **24**, 97.
Wai, K. N. T., Bishop, J. C., Mack, P. B., and Cotton, R. H. (1947). *Plant Physiol.* **22**, 546.
Warburg, O., and Christian, W. (1932). *Biochem. Z.* **254**, 438
Warburg, O., and Christian, W. (1938). *Biochem. Z.* **298**, 150.
Watarai, K., Uchida, J., Ishikawa, E., Itaya, J., and Katsunuma, N. (1955). *Vitamins (Kyoto)* **8**, 331.
Watson, S. A., and Noggle, G. R. (1947). *Plant Physiol.* **22**, 228.
Whitby, L. G. (1950). *Nature, Lond.* **166**, 479.
Whitby, L. G. (1952). *Biochem. J.* **50**, 433.
Whitby, L. G. (1954). *Biochem. J.* **57**, 390.
White, I. G., and Lincoln, G. J. (1958). *Nature, Lond.* **182**, 667.
Wickerham, L. J., Flickinger, M. H., Johnston, R. M. (1946). *Arch. Biochem.* **9**, 95.
Wolff, J. B., and Kaplan, N. O. (1956). *J. biol. Chem.* **218**, 849.
Woolley, D. W. (1950). *Proc. Soc. exp. Biol., N. Y.* **77**, 745.
Woolley, D. W. (1951). *J. exp. Med.* **93**, 13.
Yagi, K. (1951). *Igaku to Seibutsugaku*, **18**, 96.
Yagi, K., and Okuda, J. (1958). *Nature, Lond.* **181**, 1663.
Yamasaki, I. (1941). *Biochem, Z.* **307**, 431.
Yamasaki, I. (1942). *Rep. Jap. Ass. Adv. Sci.* **16**, 556.
Yasuda, T. (1951). *Vitamins (Kyoto)* **4**, 436, 440.
Yaw, K. E. (1952). *Mycologia* **44**, 307.

CHAPTER 3

THE BIOSYNTHESIS OF NICOTINIC ACID AND ITS DERIVATIVES

I. INTRODUCTION

The history of the emergence of nicotinamide (I) or nicotinic acid (II) (they are equally effective) as the pellagra-preventive factor is, as with the history of most vitamins, tortuous and complex. It has, however, been discussed in detail by Robinson (1951) and it is sufficient here to note that it was Elvehjem *et al.* (1937) who first isolated nicotinamide as the active factor from liver and who further showed that nicotinic acid is also a highly effective pellagra-preventive factor.

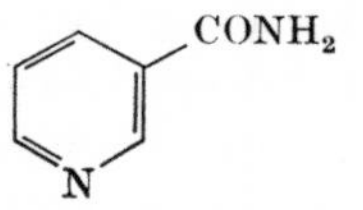

(I) 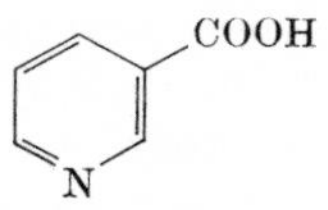   (II)

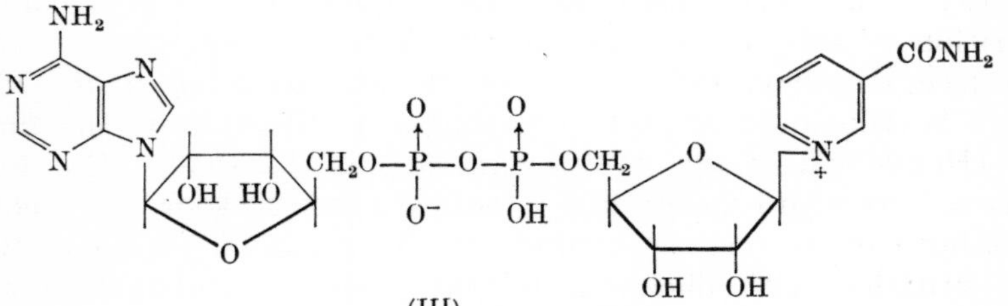

(III)

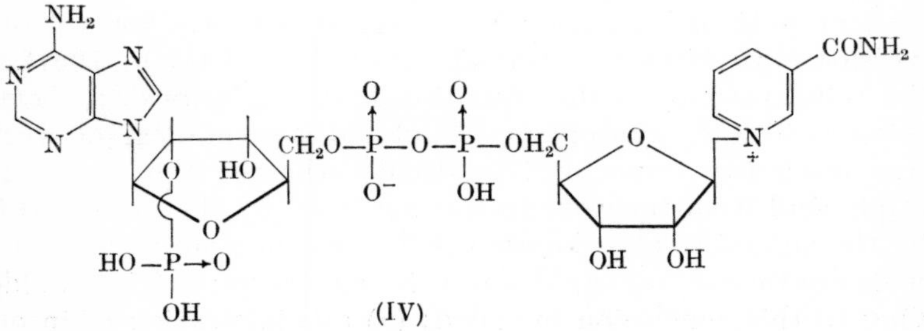

(IV)

The nature and biological significance of the derivatives of nicotin-amide, coenzyme I and coenzyme II, now more usually known as diphosphopyridine nucleotide or nicotinamide adenine dinucleotide (DPN, NAD; III) and triphosphopyridine nucleotide, nicotinamide adenine dinucleotide phosphate (TPN, NADP; IV), were known before the significance of the parent compound in human nutrition. Warburg and Christian in 1935 demonstrated that nicotinamide was a constituent of NAD and Albus *et al.* (1935) about the same time showed that it was also a constituent of NADP. The chemical structures of NAD and NADP were elucidated by von Euler *et al.* (1936, 1937) and Schlenk (1937, 1943).

II. GENERAL OBSERVATIONS

Investigations into the problem of the pellagragenic effect of maize (corn) led directly to the recognition of the major precursor of nicotinamide in animals. Although maize, rice and wheat contain approximately the same amounts of nicotinamide, pellagra was far more frequently encountered amongst communities whose staple diet was maize than amongst rice- or wheat-eating communities. This was found to be due to the much lower level of tryptophan in maize than in the other two cereals, for the pellagragenic effect of maize can be countered by feeding supplements of either nicotinic acid (1 mg/100 g diet) or tryptophan (50 mg/100 g diet) (Krehl *et al.*, 1945a,b). Tryptophan can also replace nicotinic acid in the nutrition of rats, dogs, pigs, rabbits, chicks, monkeys and cotton rats (see Hundley, 1954), but not of cats (da Silva *et al.*, 1952). There is still doubt whether tryptophan is effective in the guinea pig (Henderson *et al.*, 1949; Banerjee *et al.*, 1950). Ruminants (calves, horses and sheep) do not require a dietary source of nicotinic acid, but can convert tryptophan into nicotinamide (Kaplan, 1961). The situation with ducklings is that a small number of a given population on a niacin-deficient diet will respond to tryptophan in an "all or nothing" manner. This suggests genetic control of the conversion (van Reen and Kaplan, quoted by Kaplan, 1961).

The observations on the nutritional interrelationship between nicotinic acid and tryptophan stimulated a great deal of work as it was obviously important to decide whether the synthesis of nicotinic acid from tryptophan was achieved by the intestinal flora or by the animal tissues themselves. There is now no doubt that the animals are themselves capable of this conversion; the first evidence leading to this conclusion included: (a) administration of insoluble sulphonamides, which sterilize the gut, did not inhibit the cure of

human pellagra (caused by nicotinic acid deficiency) by the administration of tryptophan (Singal *et al.*, 1947); and (b) intravenous
injection of tryptophan increased the excretion of N-methylnicotinamide, a urinary metabolite of nicotinic acid (Snyderman *et al.*,
1949). Germ-free insects, e.g. *Drosophila*, *Tribolium confusum* and
Tenebrio molitor can also convert tryptophan into nicotinic acid
(Schultz and Rudkin 1948; Fraenkel and Stern, 1951). Direct evidence of conversion was first obtained in 1949 by Hurt *et al.* who
worked with isolated rat liver slices.

Indications that tryptophan was also a nicotinic acid precursor
in fungi came in 1947 when Beadle *et al.* isolated a *Neurospora*
mutant which required either tryptophan or nicotinic acid for
growth. Later experiments, in which the specific activity of [^{14}C]
tryptophan added to *Neurospora* was compared with that of the
isolated nicotinic acid, indicated that all the nicotinic acid synthesized
by the mould arose from tryptophan. In bacteria, on the other hand,
evidence that tryptophan is a precursor of nicotinic acid only exists
for one organism, *Xanthomonas pruni*; there is no evidence in many
other organisms that nicotinamide arises from tryptophan, and
this conclusion is probably also true for higher plants (p .79). This is
also true for the protozoan *Tetrahymena* (Kidder *et al.*, 1949).

Although the discovery that nicotinic acid can be synthesized from
tryptophan in animals strictly rules it out as a vitamin, it should be
remembered that it in almost certainly required preformed in most
mixed natural diets because tryptophan is only about 1–2% as
active as nicotinamide (Goldsmith *et al.*, 1956; Horwitt *et al.*, 1956).
Furthermore, other dietary constituents may affect the efficiency
of conversion, for addition of 12% gelatin to a normal diet containing
0·1% L-tryptophan, inhibited the increase in liver pyridine nucleotides
observed in the absence of the gelatin. This effect could be reproduced
by glycine and L-hydroxyproline (Savage *et al.*, 1962).

III. Biosynthesis in Animals and Fungi

The first step in the conversion of tryptophan into nicotinic
acid (1, Fig. 1) is the formation of N-formylkynurenine mediated
by the enzyme *tryptophan pyrrolase* (Tanaka and Knox, 1959); this
enzyme is an *oxygen transferase* (Mason, 1957) because both the
oxygen atoms incorporated into N-formylkynurenine are derived
from oxygen and not from water (Hayaishi *et al.*, 1957). The enzyme
has been purified from liver and from a *Pseudomonas** sp., and that

---

* Although tryptophan is not converted into nicotinic acid in most bacteria (p. 77),
the first steps in its bacterial oxidation are the same as those leading to nicotinic
acid formation in animals and fungi.

F<small>IG</small>. 1. The conversion of tryptophan into nicotinic acid in animals and fungi from the latter has been examined in detail. It is an iron-porphyrin enzyme and the obligatory requirement of the reaction for H_2O_2, which has been known for some time, is ascribed to the necessity of converting the inactive ferric enzyme into the active ferrous enzyme in the presence of the substrate (Tanaka and Knox, 1959). The probable mechanism is outlined in Fig. 2.

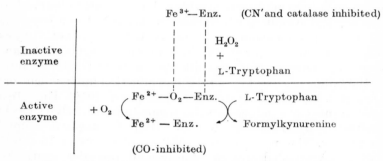

FIG. 2. Mechanism of action of tryptophan pyrrolase.

An important property of tryptophan pyrrolase is that in animals it appears to be an induced enzyme; a tenfold increase in the liver levels is observed after feeding tryptophan (Knox and Mehler, 1951). Induction is also demonstrable in rat – liver homogenates and appears to depend on the permeability of the mitochondrial membrane, for disruption of mitochondria causes a fall in the degree of induction; on the other hand, isotonic solutions of substances which are known to alter mitochondrial permeability increase the degree of induction in the presence of the substrate (Clouet and Gordon, 1959; Gordon and Rydziel, 1959).

Dubnoff and Dimick (1959) do not accept the idea of enzyme induction; they assume that the enzyme is extremely unstable except in the presence of its substrate; they argue that as there is normally a 'turn over' of enzyme, the presence of tryptophan stabilizes the newly formed enzyme and thus there is no need to assume that the presence of substrate induces new enzyme formation. However, Tanaka and Knox (1959) maintain that the phenomenon is a true induction; furthermore, inhibitors of protein synthesis such as ethionine and 8-azaguanine prevent the formation of the enzyme (Price and Dietrich, 1957; Kram and Parks, 1960).

More detailed investigations of the induction of tryptophan pyrrolase by Greengard (1961) and Feigelson (1961) indicate that up to two-thirds of the enzyme in liver cell sap is inactivated by an endogenous inhibitor which appears to be a protein. The observation that the enzyme is activated by the addition of haem (Green-gard and Feigelson, 1960; Feigelson and Greengard, 1961; Pitot and Cho, 1961) has been followed by purification of the apoenzyme 300–1000 times and the demonstration that haem is a co-factor (Feigelson and Greengard, 1962). Tissues, e.g. brain and kidney, which have no tryptophan pyrrolase activity have a very high concentration of an inhibitor.

An increase in tryptophan pyrrolase levels is also observed after adrenal cortical stimulation (cortisone treatment). A complete explanation of this phenomenon is still not available; it is not, however, due either to an increased stability of the enzyme or to an increase in the concentration of available substrate (Dubnoff and Dimick, 1959), but is caused by a primary induction independent of the inducing effect of the substrate (Civen and Knox, 1959). The difference between substrate-induced and cortisone-induced activity has been demonstrated by Feigelson (1961). After tryptophan administration to rats, the need for the addition of activator to the liver cell-sap preparation decreases rapidly and precedes synthesis of apoenzyme. Administration of cortisone on the other hand, does not increase the level of endogenous activator but leads to a slight increase in synthesis of active enzyme with a simultaneous large increase in inactive enzyme.

There is a deficiency of tryptophan pyrrolase activity in humans during the first days of life (Auricchio et al., 1960).

Reaction 2 (Fig. 1) is catalysed by *formamidase* [aryl-formylamine amidohydrolase] which has been found in mammalian liver (Mehler and Knox, 1950), a *Pseudomonas* sp. (Hayaishi and Stanier, 1951) and *Neurospora* (Jakoby, 1954). The resulting kynurenine* is hydroxylated at position 3 by a mitochondrial NADP-dependent enzyme, *kynurenine 3-hydroxylase* (reaction 3, Fig. 1) (De Castro et al., 1956) which is a typical *mixed function oxidase* (Mason, 1957); the one oxygen atom incorporated into kynurenine is derived from O_2, one mole of which is consumed for each mole of kynurenine hydroxylated, and not from water (Saito et al., 1957); furthermore the presence of NADPH is obligatory (Hayaishi. 1958). In step 4 (Fig. 1) 3-hydroxyanthranilic acid is formed from 3-hydroxykynurenine in the presence of a pyridoxal phosphate-requiring enzyme *kynureninase* (Jakoby and Bonner, 1956; Saran, 1958). The enzyme has been detected in the liver and kidney of a number of mammalian species (Itagaki and Nakayama, 1941; Kotake and Nakayama, 1941; Dalgliesh et al., 1951; Wiss and Weber, 1956) in a *Pseudomonas* sp. (Hayaishi and Stanier, 1952; Miller and

---

* Tryptophan can also be converted into kynurenine by ultraviolet irradiation of an aqueous solution (Hakim and Thiele, 1960).

Adelberg, 1953) and in *Neurospora* (Jakoby and Bonner, 1953). 3-Hydroxyanthranilic acid is the precursor of both quinolinic acid and nicotinic acid; Hankes and Henderson (1957) found that rats injected with [^{14}C]-3-hydroxyanthranilic acid excreted labelled quinolinic acid and N-methylnicotinamide (a metabolite of nicotinic acid) with little or no change in specific activity, and Moline *et al.* (1959) demonstrated the conversion of [3-^{14}C]-3-hydroxyanthranilic acid into quinolinic acid with all its activity located in its α-carboxyl carbon.

The first step in the conversion of the benzene ring (3-hydroxyanthranilic acid) into the pyridine ring is the formation of 1-amino-4-formylbutadiene-1,2-dicarboxylic acid (reaction 5, Fig 1); the production of this intermediate was demonstrated by Wiss and Bettendorf (1957) who incubated 3-hydroxyanthranilic acid with liver slices at 0°; at normal temperatures only quinolinic acid is formed. The question now arises whether nicotinic acid is formed from the intermediate via quinolinic acid (reactions 6 and 8, Fig. 1) or via 1-amino-4-formylbutadiene-2-carboxylic acid (reactions 7 and 9, Fig. 1), or whether both pathways exist side by side. Nutritional studies with quinolinic acid indicate that it is a source of nicotinic acid but that it is inferior in this respect to 3-hydroxyanthranilic acid; confirmation of this view was obtained when it was found that only 8–24% of a dose of [T]quinolinic acid accumulated in the urinary N-methylnicotinamide (Hankes and Segel, 1957). There is thus no doubt that quinolinic acid can be converted into nicotinic acid in intact animals, but the problem of whether it is the main *in vivo* pathway remains unsolved. Obviously the conditions in liver slices, when only quinolinic acid is produced from 3-hydroxyanthranilic acid, are abnormal and the failure to detect quinolinic during the transformation of 3-hydroxyanthranilic acid to nicotinic acid in chick embryos (Quaglieriello and Pietra, 1956) does not rule it out as an active intermediate; indeed it has recently been shown by Wilson and Henderson (1960) that [T]quinolinic acid is effectively converted into nicotonic acid in the developing chick embryo. The low precursor-efficiency of quinolinic acid administered to intact animals could be due to rapid excretion or to the possibility that "metabolic" quinolinic acid is bound to an enzyme and never appears free in the tissues. It is important to note that quinolinic acid can arise in animals from other sources, e.g. β-alanine (Hankes and Schmaeler, 1960).

An indirect argument in support of the routes not involving quinolinic acid (reactions 7 and 9, Fig. 1) is that a liver enzyme which converts 3-hydroxyanthranilic acid into picolinic acid (pyridine 2-carboxylic acid) will not decarboxylate quinolinic acid, thus indicating that decarboxylation takes place at the level of the acyclic intermediate (Mehler, 1956; Mehler and May, 1956).

The report that picolinic acid, and not quinolinic acid, is exclusively produced from 3-hydroxyanthanilic acid by cat liver preparations suggests that species differences may exist (Suhadolnik *et al.*, 1957).

The inefficient conversion of tryptophan into nicotinic acid in rats is probably due to the rapid catabolism of 3-hydroxyanthranilic acid to CO_2 and unidentified compounds which are certainly not pyridine carboxylic acids. For example, 60% of the total activity of [carboxyl-^{14}C]-3-anthranilic acid fed to intact rats appeared in the respiratory CO_2 within 3 hours and 90% appeared in the respiratory CO_2 and urine within 12 hours of dosing (Hankes and Henderson, 1956). The evidence leading to the view that 3-hydroxyanthranilic acid is an intermediate in the complete oxidative catabolism of tryptophan included: (a) [α-^{14}C]tryptophan administered to rats yields serine, alanine, aspartic acid and glutamic acid with labelling patterns consistent with the liberation of the side chain as pyruvate (Gholson *et al.*, 1959a); (b) kynurenic acid is similarly metabolized to L-glutamate, D- and L-alanine and acetate in a *Pseudomonas* sp. (Hayaishi *et al.*, 1961), and (c) that, as C-7a of tryptophan is converted into C-1 of acetate (Gholson and Henderson, 1958), C-2 of anthranilic acid should be similarly converted if it is an intermediate in the oxidation of tryptophan; this has been shown to be the case (Gholson *et al.*, 1959b). Chemically feasible routes for the oxidation of 3-hydroxyanthranilic acid which may also involve glutamate (Gholson *et al.*, 1958) have been proposed (see e.g. Dalgliesh, 1959), but the only experimental support so far available is that glutamic acid is a metabolite of 3-hydroxyanthranilic acid in the rat (Gholson *et al.*, 1959c). The enzyme, 3-hydroxyanthranilic acid oxidase, has now been extensively purified from calf liver, but the primary oxidation product still awaits identification (Vescia and di Prisco, 1962).

The transformation of tryptophan into nicotinic acid in mammals is dependent on the presence of adequate amounts of other water-soluble vitamins. Deficiency of thiamine and riboflavin interferes with the activity of tryptophan pyrrolase and kynurenine 3-hydroxylase, respectively; the function of the co-factors in these reactions is unknown. Pyridoxal phosphate is a coenzyme for kynureninase, and in its absence tryptophan metabolism is shunted into the "dead ends" kynurenic acid (V) and xanthurenic acid (VI), which are excreted in the urine (Dalgliesh, 1955). In the case of kynurenine hydroxylase, there is a three-fold diminution in activity in the livers of riboflavin-deficient rats compared with controls.

Presentation of the enzyme riboflavin phosphate or FAD did not increase the activity and no co-factor could be extracted from normal preparations. The function of riboflavin thus remains obscure (Henderson, 1958).

(V)   (VI)

The formation of nicotinic acid in moulds, especially *Neurospora*, has been shown to occur in the same way as in animals, although some of the enzymes exhibit slightly different properties.

IV. FORMATION IN BACTERIA

There is no positive evidence for the existence in bacteria of the pathway outlined in Fig. 1 for the synthesis of nicotinic acid from tryptophan; indeed there is yet no conclusive evidence that tryptophan can be converted into nicotinic acid by bacteria other than *Xanthomonas pruni* (see p. 71). Volcani and Snell (1948) found that neither kynurenine nor 3-hydroxyanthranilic acid could replace nicotinic acid in the nutrition of *Leuconostoc mesenteroides*, *Streptococcus faecalis*, and *Proteus vulgaris*. Similarly, nicotinamide auxotrophs of *Escherichia coli* and *Bacillus subtilis* for example, did not respond to tryptophan or to any of the intermediates indicated in Fig. 1, and Yanofsky (1955) concluded that if tryptophan is converted into nicotinic acid in these bacteria it can only be to a very minor extent (not more than 5%) and the conversion cannot involve the pathway followed in animals and fungi.

The probable reason for the failure of a tryptophan-adapted *Pseudomonas* to convert tryptophan into nicotinic acid is its inability to hydroxylate kynurenine to 3-hydroxyknurenine. Suda and Takeda (1950) and Hayaishi and Stanier (1951) found that this organism can oxidize tryptophan to *cis-cis*-muconic acid via N-formylkynurenine, kynurenine, anthranilic acid and catechol (Fig. 3), but cannot convert it into 3-hydroxykynurenine and 3-hydroxyanthranilic acid. Furthermore, a *kynureninase* isolated from a related strain of *Pseudomonas* will convert 3-hydroxykynurenine into 3-hydroxyanthranilic acid, but it attacks kynurenine very much faster; this is the reverse of the situation observed with the enzymes isolated from *Neurospora* (Jakoby and Bonner, 1953) and from animal tissues (Wiss and Fuchs, 1951).

An early report that tryptophan and nicotinic acid were interchangeable as a growth factor for *Xanthomonas pruni* suggested that tryptophan can be converted into nicotinic acid via the conventional pathway in this organism (Davis *et al.*, 1951). Isotope experiments with [5-^{14}C]tryptophan, [T]-5-hydroxyanthranilic acid

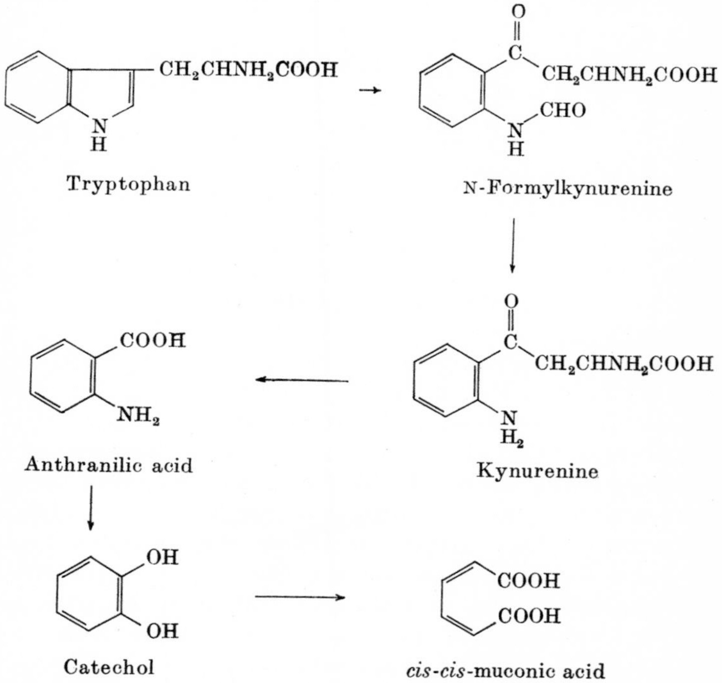

FIG. 3. The oxidation of tryptophan to *cis—cis* muconic acid by *Pseudomonas* spp.

and [T]quinolinic acid have recently confirmed this view (Wilson and Henderson, 1961).

Guavacine (tetrahydronicotinic acid, N-desmethylarecaidine) (VII), and nipolinic acid (hexahydronicotinic acid) (VIII) will substitute for nicotinic acid in the nutrition of *Staphylococcus aureus* (Woolley *et al.*, 1938; Ellinger and Kader, 1948); whether these are intermediates in the formation of nicotinic acid in this organism remains to be investigated. Guavacine, but not nipolinic acid, is also active in *Proteus vulgaris*.

Ortega and Brown (1959, 1960) have recently shown that [^{14}C] succinate and glycerol but not pyruvate are incorporated into nicotinic acid by *Escherichia coli*. In the case of [1,3-^{14}C]glycerol the label appeared exclusively in the pyridine ring, with [1,4-^{14}C]succinate the label was only in the carboxyl group, whilst with [2,3-^{14}C] succinate the label was predominantly in the pyridine ring. It is interesting that pyruvate and propionate stimulate nicotinic acid synthesis without themselves being incorporated into the molecule. Furthermore, Mothes *et al.* (1961) demonstrated that the label from DL-[4-^{14}C] aspartic acid appeared only in the carboxyl group of nicotinic acid in *Mycobact. tuberculosis*. These investigations clearly demonstrate the existence of a non-tryptophan pathway, in which a 3-C compound (glycerol or a related metabolite) combines with a 4-C carboxylic acid in such a way that one carboxyl-C is lost and the other becomes the carboxyl-C of nicotinic acid.

V. INTESTINAL FLORA

There seems little doubt that the intestinal flora of many animals can synthesize nicotinic acid. This has been demonstrated in a number of ways, for example (a) directly, by showing that bacteria isolated from human faeces at caecectomy synthesize nicotinic acid (Benesch, 1945) and (b) indirectly, by showing that rats on a protein (tryptophan)-free diet containing 7 mg of nicotinic acid per day, excrete 40–90 mg nicotinic acid per day in the faeces (Huff and Perlzweig, 1941), and that, in humans, urinary excretion of N-methylnicotinamide is reduced after partly sterilizing the gut with sulphonamides such as sulphaguanidine or succinyl sulphathiazole (Ellinger *et al.*, 1945).

VI. HIGHER PLANTS

A. *General*

Nicotinic acid is synthesized during the germination of oats, wheat, barley and maize (Burkholder, 1943) but this may be at the expense of trigonelline (N-methylnicotinic acid; IX) which is present in seeds and which disappears as the nicotinamide nucleotides appear (Handler, 1959). The conversion of trigonelline into nicotinic acid has not been demonstrated in higher plants, but it occurs in the yeast *Torula cremoris*, probably via trigonelline adenylate as an intermediate (Joshi and Handler, 1961). In whole pea plants nicotinic acid increases in amount up to the seventh week and then decreases; the amounts in the leaves, roots and stems all fall at flowering (Zeijlemaker, 1953). If excised shoots are supplied with exogenous nicotinic acid, the endogenous levels remain constant and the excess material is converted into trigonelline (Terroine, 1948).

High levels occur in cucurbit and tomato fruit during the early growing period when cell multiplication is active; there is, however, a decrease in concentration during subsequent growth which involves cell expansion rather than cell multiplication (Wilson, 1947; Withner, 1949).

Nicotinic acid is required as a growth factor for isolated pea roots; it can be replaced by nicotinamide or nicotinuric acid (X) (Bonner, 1940). In association with pyridoxine, nicotinic acid is required for germination of orchids (Noggle and Wynd, 1942).

(IX)   (X)

B. *Mechanism of Formation*

In spite of one or two early reports to the contrary, the general opinion is that tryptophan is not a precursor of nicotinic acid in plants; for example, Henderson *et al.* (1959) found that under conditions which ensured almost complete absorption of the substrates, neither [^{14}C]tryptophan nor [T]anthranilic acid was converted into nicotinic acid by germinating maize seedlings.

The fact that Teas and Anderson (1951) found a maize mutant which accumulates anthranilic acid when tryptophan is metabolized, indicates that tryptophan is probably oxidized by a route similar to that followed in *Pseudomonas* (see p. 78), but that neither the plant nor the bacterium is able to hydroxylate the resulting kynurenine.

C. *Genetic Studies*

Some genetic investigations on the nicotinic acid content of maize kernels have been reported. For example, endosperms homozygous for the following recessive genes, sugary[1], waxy brittle[1], brittle[1], shrunken[1] and shrunken[2] have higher nicotinic acid levels than normal strains (Teas *et al.*, 1952, 1955; Teas and Newton, 1951). In sugary[1] (su_1) and starchy (st_1) kernels, the nicotinic acid levels of the embryos were the same, but the level in the su_1 endosperm was much higher than in the st_1 endosperm. This indicates that the nicotinic acid content of endosperm is correlated with endosperm genotype, but is independent of embryo genotype (Teas *et al.*, 1955).

The nicotinic acid levels in leaves of trisomic maize are higher than in the leaves of disomic maize (Giles *et al.*, 1946).

VII. BIOSYNTHESIS OF TRYPTOPHAN

The source of tryptophan for nicotinic acid synthesis in animals is, of course, their food, because tryptophan is an essential amino acid. In higher plants and most micro-organisms, however, it is synthesized *de novo* and recent investigations, particularly with micro-organisms, have indicated the main outlines of the pathway involved.

The first suggestion of the pathway involved came from the classical work of Fildes (1940) who showed that tryptophan-requiring strains of *Bacterium typhosum* and *Staphylococcus* spp. would grow if the tryptophan in the medium were replaced by indole. Snell (1943) confirmed these results in *Lactobacillus* spp. and further observed that anthranilic acid was as effective as indole. Numerous studies with isotopically labelled materials demonstrated the incorporation of these two compounds into tryptophan (see Scott, 1962). In particular it was shown that the carboxyl carbon of anthranilic acid is lost during its conversion into indole by *Neurospora* and *Esch. coli* (Nyc *et al.*, 1949; Yanofsky, 1955), that the carbons of the pyrrole ring of indole are derived, in *Esch. coli*, from C_1 and C_2 of a ribose derivative (Yanofsky, 1955) and that the amino nitrogen of anthranilic acid is retained during the conversion in *Neurospora* (Partridge *et al.*, 1952).

The overall conversion of anthranilic acid to indole has now been obtained with isolated systems from *Esch. coli* (Yanofsky, 1956) and the reaction probably involves the steps indicated in Fig. 4.

One enzyme from *Esch. coli* catalyses the formation of indolylglycerol phosphate; the steps proposed for this reaction (**A, B, C, D,**

Fig. 4) are hypothetical, but analogous reactions are known in other biochemical systems. The second enzyme splits indolylglycerol phosphate to indole and glycerol phosphate (step **E**). Tryptophan

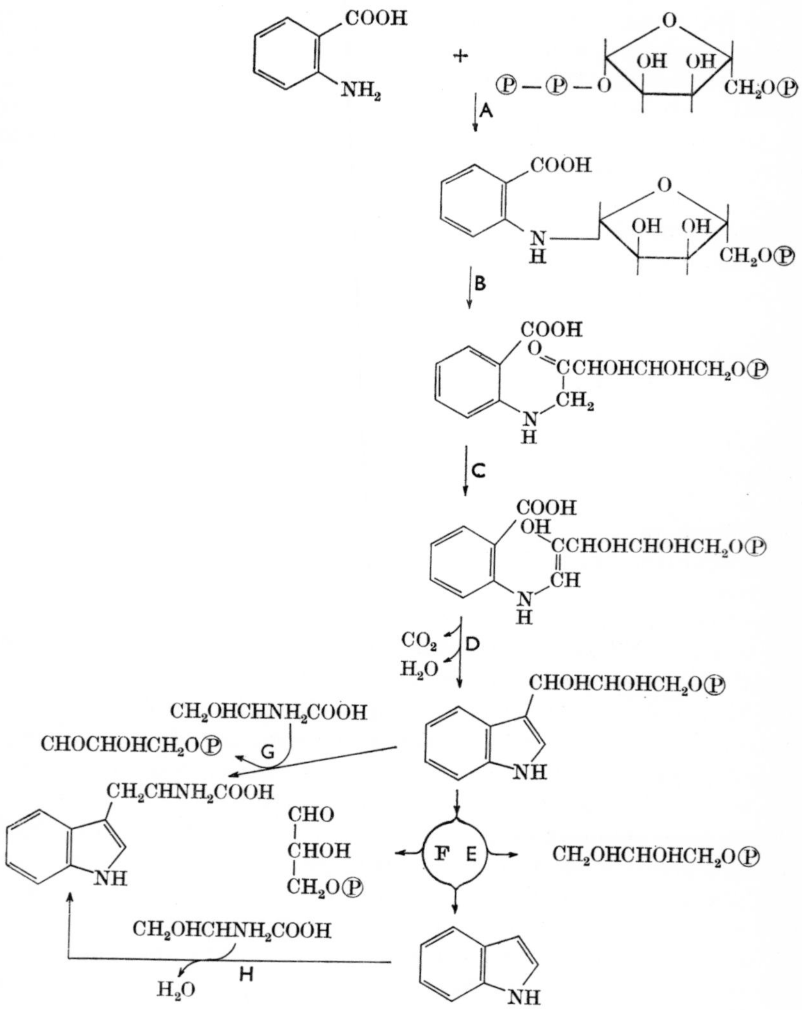

FIG. 4. The biosynthesis of tryptophan.

synthetase is also present in plants (Bengal gram) (Nair and Vaidyanathan, 1961).

Two possibilities of ring closure exist, at C-1 or C-3; this problem was settled in favour of C-1 by the enzymatic conversion of 4-methylindole into 6-methylindole (Yanofsky, 1955); ring closure at C-3 would have yielded 4-methylindole (Fig. 5). This experiment also indicates that decarboxylation occurs after ring closure; if it occured before then both 4-methylindole and 6-methylindole would be formed enzymatically. The enzyme, *tryptophan synthase* [L-serine hydro-lyase (adding indole)] which condenses indole and serine to form tryptophan (reaction H, Fig. 4) has been purified from *Neurospora*; it is a pyridoxal phosphate requiring enzyme and has a pH optimum at 7·8. It was later found that indolyl glycerophosphate was a much better substrate for this

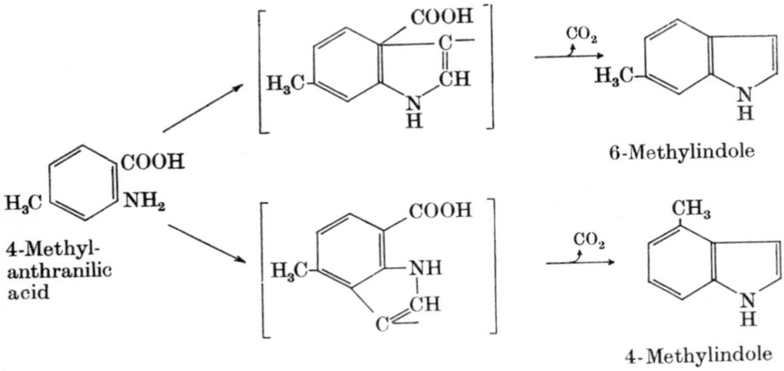

FIG. 5. Alternative pathways for the conversion of 4-methylanthranilic acid: into a methylindole by extracts of *Esch. coli*.

enzyme than indole (reaction G, Fig. 4), which does not require pyridoxal phosphate as cofactor and will also catalyse reaction F (Fig. 4) (Tatum and Bonner, 1944; Yanofsky, 1952; Yanofsky and Rachmeler, 1958).

A fascinating development in this field is the discovery that some auxotrophs of *Esch. coli* and *Neurospora*, which, although lacking tryptophan synthase activity, still contain a protein (CRM) which is immunologically similar to the parent enzyme (Suskind *et al.*, 1955; Suskind, 1957; Lerner and Yanofsky, 1957). The full genetical and biochemical implications of these observations are now being actively studied.

Although it is generally assumed that anthranilic acid arises via the shikimic acid pathway (see Goodwin, 1960) the results of a recent investigation suggest that in bean leaves shikimic acid may not be the only source of anthranilic acid (Weinstein *et al.*, 1962).

VIII. Nicotinamide

All the discussion so far has been centred on nicotinic acid, but it will be remembered that the functional form, in NAD and NADP, is nicotinamide. Amidation of nicotinic acid takes place at the dinucleotide level as described in the following section. Experiments indicating that a direct conversion of free nicotinic acid into nicotinamide takes place in various animal tissues (Porcellati, 1954) can probably by accounted for by the formation of NAD and its subsequent hydrolysis to nicotinamide by the widely distributed NAD-ase (Handler, 1959).

IX. Nicotinamide Adenine Dinucleotide (Diphosphopyridine Nucleotide) and Nicotinamide Adenine Dinucleotide Phosphate (Triphosphopyridine Nucleotide)

A. *Nicotinamide Adenine Dinucleotide*

Handler (1959) has recently described in a fascinating manner how the tenacious following up of an observation made some fifteen years ago that nicotinamide could not be synthesized from free nicotinic acid, has now borne fruit. He has now been able to show that human erythrocytes, rat liver and yeast catalyse the conversion of nicotinic acid into NAD by the following reactions:

$$\text{Nicotinic acid} + \text{phosphoribosylpyrophosphate} \longrightarrow \text{Desamido—NMN} + \text{P—P} \quad (1)$$

$$\text{Desamido—NMN*} + \text{ATP} \longrightarrow \text{Desamido—NAD} + \text{P—P} \quad (2)$$

$$\text{Desamido—NAD} + \quad \overset{\text{ATP}}{\underset{\text{glutamine}}{\nearrow}} \quad \overset{\text{AMP}}{\underset{\text{glutamate}}{\searrow}} \quad \text{NAD} + \text{P—P} \quad (3)$$

5-Phosphoribosyl 1-pyrophosphate (PRPP), first discovered as

$$\text{D-ribose 5-phosphate} \xrightarrow[\text{ATP} \quad \text{AMP}]{\text{Mg}^{2+}} \text{PRPP} \quad (4)$$

an obligatory intermediate in pyrimidine biosynthesis, is formed from D-ribose 5–phosphate in the presence of the appropriate kinase, ATP, and Mg^{2+} (equation 4). (Kornberg *et al.*, 1954; Goldthwait *et al.*, 1956).

---

* Nicotinic acid mononucleotide.

The enzyme catalysing reaction (1), *nicotinate phosphoribosyl transferase* [nicotinate nucleotide: pyrophosphate phosphoribosyl transferase] has been partly purified from human erythrocytes and yeast autolysates. The K_m value for nicotinic acid is extremely low and is thus compatible with physiological requirements. Reaction 2 is brought about by *NAD pyrophosphorylase* [ATP: NMN adenylyl transferase] which is present in red cells, the cytoplasmic fractions of yeast and the nuclei of rat liver (Kornberg, 1950; Hogeboom and Schneider 1952; Branster and Morton, 1956; Preiss and Handler, 1957, 1958). Desamido-NMN competitively inhibits the coupling of NMN with ATP (Atkinson *et al.*, 1960; Atkinson and Morton, 1960) and this may be a mechanism for controlling synthesis *in vivo*. The kinetics of the NAD-pyrophosphorylase have recently been discussed in detail (Atkinson *et al.* 1961 a, b). The enzyme from artichoke and maize will only use desamido-NMN as substrate (Atkinson and Morton, 1961). The substrate specificity of this enzyme obtained from other sources has been reported in detail (Atkinson *et al.*, 1961a).

An important observation is that [7-^{14}C]nicotinamide is a better precursor of NAD in Ehrlich ascites tumour cells than is [7–^{14}C] nicotinic acid (Holzer *et al.*, 1961). This difference is not due to differences in permeability of the cells to the substrates (Holzer and Boltze, 1961), so the possibility exists that the biosynthetic pathway of NAD is different in tumour cells from that in normal cells.

NAD synthetase [Deamido-NAD: L-glutamine amidoligase (AMP)] which completes the reaction sequence (reaction 3) has, up to the present time, been purified only from bakers' yeast (Preiss and Handler, 1957; Preiss, 1958). The reaction involves the transfer of the amide-N of glutamine to the nicotinic acid residue of desamido-NAD, and requires ATP; this situation is also observed in the formation of α-N-formylglycinamidine ribotide from α-N-formylglycinamide (Melnick and Buchanan, 1957) and guanylic acid from xanthylic acid in animal tissues (Abrams and Bentley, 1959). Although NH_4^+ is also a substrate for NAD synthetase, its intracellular concentration is so low that the *in vivo* "NH_2" donor is almost certainly glutamine. The enzyme from yeast catalysing reaction (3) is, together with other glutamine-dependent enzyme systems, inhibited by azaserine (Handler, 1959). However, azaserine (10^{-2}M) does not inhibit NAD synthesis by whole cells of *Lactobacillus arabinosus* 17-5 (Zatman, 1961). Furthermore, the reduction of the NAD levels in mouse liver by azaserine is considered to be the result of a stimulated turnover of NAD rather than an inhibition of a step in the biosynthetic pathway (Narrod *et al.*, 1961).

A characteristic of all three reactions concerned with DPN synthesis is that inorganic pyrophosphate is produced at each stage. The synthesis of DPN would thus obviously be favoured by hydrolysis of pyrophosphate and this can be easily achieved in the presence of the ubiquitous enzyme *inorganic pyrophosphatase* [pyrophosphate phosphohydrolase].

Further evidence for the sequence just discussed comes from (a) the isolation and identification of desamido-NMN and desamido-NAD following the incubation of human erythrocytes with nicotinic acid (Ballio and Serlupi-Crescenzi, 1957; Handler, 1959), and the identification of desamido-NMN in a *Fusarium* sp. (Ballio and Russi, 1959) and yeast (Wheat, 1959), and desamido-NAD in two fungi, *Penicillium chrysogenum* and *Fusarium* sp. (Serlupi-Crescenzi and Ballio, 1957), and in one bacterium *Hemophilus parainfluenzae* (R. W. Wheat, quoted by Handler, 1959).

All these observations indicate that nicotinamide is synthesized at the dinucleotide level and the following observations emphasize that free nicotinamide is not the natural precursor of NAD: (a) administration of [14C]nicotinamide to intact mice and rats results in the appearance in the liver of [14C]desamido-NAD before [14C] NAD, together with only minute traces of [14C]nicotinamide (Langan and Shuster, 1958; Handler, 1959); (b) although an enzyme exists in red cells which catalyses reaction (5) and is highly specific for nicotinamide, its K_m (nicotinamide) is high, 0·1 M; (c) NAD pyro-

$$\text{Nicotinamide} + \text{PRPP} \rightleftharpoons \text{NMN} + \text{P}{-}\text{P} \qquad (5)$$

phosphorylase from red cells will use NMN as substrate for reaction (2) either not at all (Malkin and Denstedt, 1956) or only very slightly (Handler, 1959); (d) reaction (6) can occur in animals (Rowen and Kornberg, 1951), but at physiological pH values the equilibrium is well over to the left and nicotinamide riboside formation could only be obtained with a high level of free nicotinamide and a low P

$$\text{Nicotinamide} + \text{ribose 1-P} \rightleftharpoons \text{Nicotinamide riboside} + \text{P}_i \qquad (6)$$

concentration, a situation unlikely to be realized *in vivo*. Furthermore in order to funnel nicotinamide riboside into NAD synthesis, a kinase converting it into NMN would be required; only a weakly active enzyme is known (see p. 87).

As both nutrition and tracer experiments show that nicotinamide can be incorporated into NAD, and as Handler's investigations clearly implicate nicotinic acid as the true precursor, the existence of an enzyme converting nicotinamide into nicotinic acid is necessary to reconcile these observations; such an enzyme has been reported in mammals, insects, birds and micro-organisms but it has not yet been fully characterized (Hughes and Williamson, 1953; Quaglie-riello, 1952; Oka, 1954; Porcellati, 1955; Rajagopalan *et al.*, 1958; Sundaram *et al.*, 1958, 1960; Sarma *et al.*, 1961). Bakers' yeast, which has high nicotinamide deamidase activity, will utilize nico-tinamide as effectively as nicotinic acid for NAD synthesis (Hof-mann and Peschke, 1961); on the other hand, *Leuconostoc mesen-teroides* 9135, which is devoid of deamidase activity, will utilize only nicotinic acid. The enzyme from a number of sources is inactivated by metal chelating agents; that from *Aspergillus niger* is reactiva-ted by Mg^{2+}, that from *Neurospora crassa* by Mn^{2+}, and those from pigeon liver, chicken kidney and the rice moth , *Corcyra cepha-lonica*, by Fe^{2+} (Rajagopalan *et al.*, 1960). Recently reports have been published indicating that the pathway of biosynthesis of NAD in bacteria is the same as in animals and yeasts (Sundaram *et al.*, 1960; Imsande, 1961).

Although the pathways indicated in reactions 1–3 are well established in yeast and in animal tissues, an intriguing observation on intact rats remains to be explained at the enzyme level; physio-logical levels of tryptophan are more effective than nicotinamide in stimulating the synthesis of rat liver pyridine nucleotides in previously depleted 'animals' (Williams *et al.*, 1951; Chaloupka *et al.*, 1957).

Similarly, nicotinamide is more effective than nicotinic acid in stimulating liver NAD synthesis in rats and mice, whilst only the injection of nicotinic acid increases the blood NAD levels in humans (Redetzki *et al.*, 1961); on the other hand both compounds are equally effective in chicken erythrocytes (Dietrich and Friedland, 1960). There is one bacterial genus, *Hemophilus*, which requires as a growth factor nicotinamide riboside or nicotinamide ribotide; these cannot be replaced by free nicotinic acid or nicotinamide (Gingrich and Schlenk, 1944; Bachur and Kaplan, 1955). The growth factor was originally defined as NAD or NADP, with NAD more effective (Lwoff and Lwoff, 1937), and although nicotinamide ribo-side is effective, it is less effective than is NAD. Deamido-NAD does not support growth of *Hemophilus* spp. (Lamborg *et al.*, 1958) although it is said to be present in the cells of this organism   (R. W. Wheat, quoted by Handler, 1959). One intriguing aspect of this situation is that as nicotinamide riboside is active, a phosphorylating enzyme must therefore be functioning (reaction 7); such an enzyme is present in pig liver but it has only weak activity (Kornberg, 1951).

$$\text{ATP} + \text{nicotinamide riboside} \rightleftharpoons \text{nicotinamide ribotide} + \text{ADP} \qquad (7)$$

It is interesting to find that although reaction (7) does not occur in mature rabbit erythrocytes, it does take place in reticulocytes in rabbits made anaemic with acetylphenylhydrazine, but to a much smaller extent than NAD synthesis (Jaffe and Gordon, 1961). Similary, NADPH synthesis from injected nicotinic acid is much less than NADH synthesis in rat liver (Purvis, 1961; Stollar and Kaplan, 1961).

B. *Nicotinamide Adenine Dinucleotide Phosphate (NADP)*

NADP (IV) is formed by irreversible phosphate transfer from ATP. The enzyme *NAD kinase* [ATP: NAD 2-phosphotransferase], has been purified from yeast (Kornberg, 1950) and from pigeon liver (Wang and Kaplan, 1954). NAD^+ is the specific substrate for the liver enzyme whilst the yeast enzyme will phosphorylate both NAD^+ and NADH

Although NAD kinase catalyses the irreversible phosphorylation of NAD, phosphatases have been reported which convert NADP into NAD (Kaplan *et al.*, 1952; Heppel and Whitfield, 1955).

X. N-METHYLNICOTINAMIDE AND N-METHYLNICOTINIC ACID

N-Methylnicotinamide (XI) is a characteristic urinary excretion product of nicotinic acid in animals. It is formed only in liver (Ellinger, 1948) under the influence of *nicotinamide methyltransferase* [S-adenosylmethionine: nicotinamide methyltransferase] with S-adenosylmethionine as methyl donor (reaction 8; Cantoni, 1953).

Nicotinamide + S-adenosylmethionine → N-methylnicotinamide + S-adenosyl-homocysteine

(8)

Nicotinic acid is not methylated by this enzyme, which accounts for the absence of the betaine, trigonelline (N-methylnicotinic acid; IX) from animal tissues. Trigonelline is, however, present in plants (see p. 79) but its mode of synthesis is unknown. In many animal N-methylnicotinamide is oxidized to N-methyl-6-pyridone (XII) which, in man, is the main urinary excretion product (see e.g. Hundley, 1954; Ginoulhiac *et al.*, 1962). The yeast *Torula cremoris* converts trigonelline into nicotinic acid which is used for synthesis of NAD and NADP. Trigonelline is also used slowly for the same purpose by young pea plants (Joshi and Handler, 1962).

In rats nicotinamide added at a level of 1% to the diet inhibited growth; nicotinic acid had no such effect. However, they both produced "fatty livers", a characteristic symptom of a deficiency of available labile methyl groups. Presumably the nicotinamide methyl transferase activity is so great that when high levels of nicotinamide reach the liver they trap all the available methyl groups and thus produce a methyl deficiency syndrome. Nicotinic acid is less effective than nicotinamide probably because it has first to be metabolized to nicotinamide, via NAD (Handler and Dann, 1942; Handler, 1944).

(XI)   (XII)

XI. CONJUGATES OF NICOTINIC ACID AND NICOTINAMIDE

Three characteristic "detoxication" products of nicotinic acid have been observed: nicotinuric acid (X), dinicotino-ornithine (XIII) and β-nicotinyl-D-glucuronide (XIV).

(XIII)   (XIV)

The formation of nicotinuric acid from nicotinic acid has been reported in the dog, rat, hamster and mouse (Leifer *et al.*, 1951) as well as in the rabbit, tortoise and frog (Okuda, 1960). In the first group of animals nicotinamide was not converted into nicotinuric acid according to Leifer *et al.* (1951), but later work showed that the intraperitoneal injection of [^{14}C]nicotinamide into mice resulted in the excretion of [^{14}C]nicotinuric acid (Bonavita *et al.*, 1961).

A study of the synthesis of nicotinuric acid in rat kidney slices and homogenates demonstrated that it was a two-stage process (reactions 9 and 10) involving nicotinyl-CoA (Jones and Elliott, 1959; Jones, 1959). These reactions are analogous to those leading to the synthesis of hippuric acid from glycine and benzoic acid (Schachter and Taggart, 1953, 1954).

Dinicotino-ornithine is the major excretory metabolite of nico-

$$\text{Nicotinic acid} + \text{ATP} + \text{CoASH} \rightarrow \text{nicotinyl-CoA} + P_i + \text{ADP} \qquad (9)$$
$$\text{Nicotinyl-CoA} + \text{glycine} \longrightarrow \text{nicotinuric acid} + \text{CoASH} \qquad (10)$$

tinic acid in chickens (Dann and Huff, 1947); it is probably formed in a similar fashion to nicotinuric acid but no coenzyme requirement has yet been reported (see Williams, 1959). β-Nicotinyl-D-glucuronide is excreted by the rat (van Eys et al., 1955) and chicken (Chang and Johnson 1957). This is probably synthesized, as are other glucuronides, by the transfer of glucuronic acid from UDP-glucuronic acid (see Dedonder, 1961; reaction 11).

$$\text{UDP-glucuronic acid} + \text{nicotinic acid} \rightarrow \text{UDP} + \beta\text{-nicotinyl-D-glucuronic acid} \quad (11)$$

XII. Plant Alkaloids

A. *Nicotine and Anabasine*

The reasonable assumption that the pyridine rings of nicotine (XV) and anabasine (XVI) arise from nicotinic acid has been confirmed in both compounds following the administration of [14C]nicotinic acid to *Nicotina tabacum* and *N. glauca*, respectively (Dawson et al.,

(XV)   (XVI)

1956; Dawson, quoted by Leete, 1958a). As might be expected from the conclusion drawn on p. 80 that nicotinic acid is not formed from tryptophan in plants, neither [14C]tryptophan nor [14C]anthranilic acid is incorporated into nicotine (Grimshaw and Marion, 1958; Henderson et al., 1959), but [2-14C]glycerol is incorporated and appears almost exclusively in the pyridine residue (Griffith and Byerrum, 1962). Support for this view comes from the finding that [2-14C] acetate is incorporated into the nicotinic acid residue of both nicotine (Leete, 1958a; Griffith and Byerrum, 1959) and anabasine (Leete, 1958a); if tryptophan were the source of the pyridine ring then acetate would not be incorporated (see Goodwin, 1960). β-Alanine is incorporated into both rings of nicotine (Dawson, quoted by Hankes and Schmaeler, 1960). The piperidine ring of anabasine is not formed from acetate. In some cases, however, both rings may arise from a common precursor; [1,5-^{14}C]cadaverine (discussed in detail below) is incorporated into both rings of anabasine in pea seedlings; *N. glauca,* on the other hand, incorporates cadaverine only into the pipe-ridine ring (Hasse and Berg, 1957; Mothes *et al.,* 1959). The piperi-dine ring of anabasine might be expected to arise in the same way as pipecolic acid via lysine (reaction scheme 12). Evidence in support of the pathway of biosynthesis via lysine includes: (a) administration of [ε-^{15}N]lysine to rats yields [^{15}N]pipecolic acid, whereas under the

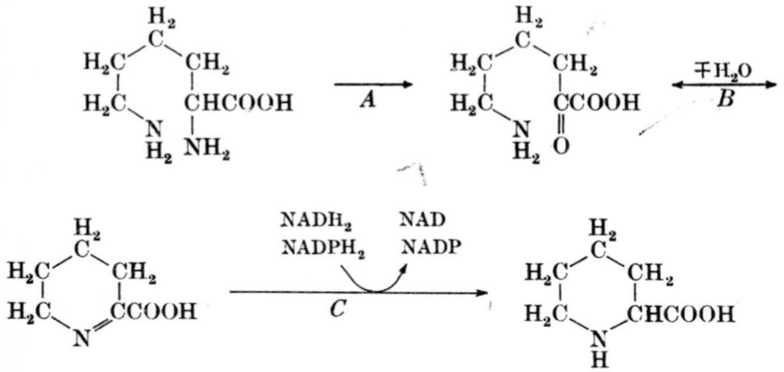

$$
\begin{array}{ccc}
\underset{\substack{H_2C \quad CH_2 \\ | \quad \quad | \\ H_2C \quad CHCOOH \\ N \quad | \\ H_2 \quad NH_2}}{\overset{H_2}{\underset{}{C}}}
& \xrightarrow{\quad A \quad}
& \underset{\substack{H_2C \quad CH_2 \\ | \quad \quad | \\ H_2C \quad CCOOH \\ N \quad \| \\ H_2 \quad O}}{\overset{H_2}{\underset{}{C}}}
\end{array}
$$

$$\xrightarrow[\text{B}]{\mp H_2O}$$

(12)

$$
\underset{\substack{H_2C \quad CH_2 \\ | \quad \quad | \\ H_2C \quad CCOOH \\ N}}{\overset{H_2}{\underset{}{C}}}
\xrightarrow[\substack{\text{NADH}_2 \quad \text{NAD} \\ \text{NADPH}_2 \quad \text{NADP}}]{\quad C \quad}
\underset{\substack{H_2C \quad CH_2 \\ | \quad \quad | \\ H_2C \quad CHCOOH \\ N \\ H}}{\overset{H_2}{\underset{}{C}}}
$$

same conditions [α-^{15}N]lysine yields unlabelled pipecolic acid; (b) α-oxo-ε-aminocaproic acid, the result of the oxidative deamina-tion of lysine (step A — scheme 12), has been isolated from *N. crassa* and exists in solution in equilibrium with Δ^1-dehydropipecolic acid (step B — scheme 12); (c) rats and *N. crassa* can convert Δ^1-dehydro-pipecolic acid into pipecolic acid (step C — scheme 12; Schweet *et al.,* 1954); (d) extracts from *N. crassa,* peas *(Pisum sativum),* beans *(Phaseolus radiatus)* and rat liver contain an enzyme which will carry out step C whilst a mutant of *N. crassa* blocked at the Δ^1-dehydropipecolic acid stage lacks this enzyme (Meister *et al.* 1957). The enzyme from rat liver has been purified and shown to require either NADPH or NADH as hydrogen donor (Meister and Buckley, 1957); it is not specific for Δ^1-dehydropipecolic acid and will catalyse a similar reaction converting Δ^1-pyrroline 5-carboxylic acid into proline (reaction 13). Lysine is incorporated into anabasine by isolated leaves of *N. glauca,* but only very slightly (0·0026%;

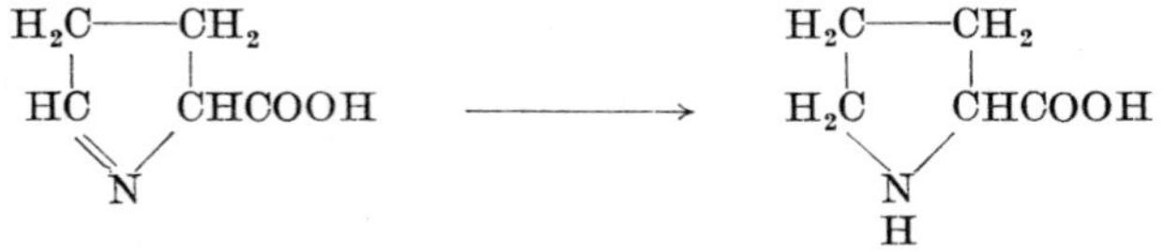

$$
\underset{\substack{HC \quad CHCOOH \\ \diagdown \quad \diagup \\ N}}{\overset{H_2C—CH_2}{\underset{}{}}}
\xrightarrow{\hspace{2cm}}
\underset{\substack{H_2C \quad CHCOOH \\ \diagdown \quad \diagup \\ N \\ H}}{\overset{H_2C—CH_2}{\underset{}{}}}
$$

(13)

Δ^1-Pyrroline 5-carboxylic acid   Proline

Leete, 1958a); this low incorporation may be due to a per-meability barrier. The non-incorporation of [^{14}C]acetate into the piperidine ring of anabasine also suggests that lysine may be the precursor because Bilinski and McConnell (1957) showed that acetate is not readily incorporated into lysine by wheat seedlings.

When [2-^{14}C]lysine is incorporated into anabasine the labelling in the piperidyl residue is confined to C-2. However, [1,5-^{14}C]cadaverine (the decarboxylation product of lysine) is much more effectively incorporated than lysine, and the label is found in C-2 and C-6 of the piperidine residue (Leete, 1958b); this labelling pattern rules out cadaverine as an intermediate in the incorporation of lysine into piperidine. The better incorporation may be discounted on permeability differences. Lysine is also the precursor of the piperidine ring in coniine (2-n-propyl piperidine) from *Conium maculatum* (Schiedt and Höss, 1962).

The most recent work on the biosynthesis of the pyrrolidine ring of nicotine confirms earlier views that metabolites such as acetate, propionate and glycerol are converted via the tricarboxylic acid cycle into glutamate, which is subsequently converted into the pyrrolidine ring (Wu *et al.*, 1962). Δ^1-Pyrroline 5-carboxylic acid (reaction 13) may be an intermediate.

The N-methyl group of nicotine presumably arises from methionine (Dewey *et al.*, 1954) probably conventionally via S-adenosylmethionine, because this compound is the source of methyl groups in hordenine (XVII) and gramine (XVIII) in barley (Mudd, 1960). However, it should be pointed out that formaldehyde and the β-carbon atom of serine were found to be better precursors of the N-methyl group of nicotine than was the methyl group of methionine (Byerrum *et al.*, 1955); it is possible that permeability effects may have been introduced into these experiments by the use of intact plants.

HO—⟨ring⟩—CH$_2$CH$_2$N(CH$_3$)$_2$

(XVII)

⟨indole ring⟩—CH$_2$N(CH$_3$)$_2$
N
H

(XVIII)

B. *Ricinine*

[7-^{14}C]Nicotinic acid gives rise to ricinine (N-methyl-3-cyano-4-methoxy-2-pyridone (XIX) labelled in the cyano group (Leete and Leitz, 1957), and ring-labelled nicotinic acid or nicotinamide gives rise to ring-labelled ricinine (Waller and Henderson, 1961 a, b) in the castor oil plant *Ricinus communis* L. Studies with nicotinamide labelled with ^{15}N in the amide nitrogen indicated that the

cyano nitrogen of ricinine arose from the amide nitrogen of nicotinamide, and experiments with nicotinamide labelled with tritium

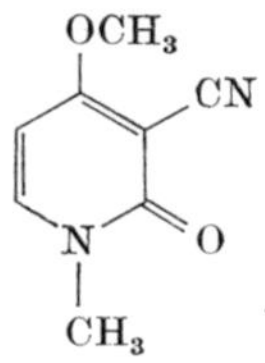

(XIX)

and with either ^{14}C in position 7 or ^{15}N in the amide nitrogen indicated
that nicotinamide is incorporated into ricinine as a unit (Waller and
Henderson, 1961b).

Experiments with possible precursors have not yet yielded a
complete answer to the problem of the origin of the nicotinic acid
ring in ricinine. The incorporation of [1,4-^{14}C]succinate into the cyano
group (Waller and Henderson, 1961a) and [2,3-^{14}C]succinate and
[3-^{14}C]aspartate into the ring (Juby and Marion, 1961; Schiedt and
Boeckh-Behrens, 1962) suggest a pathway similar to that in *E. coli* (see
p. 77). An interesting development is that Waller and Henderson
find [1,4-^{14}C] and [2-^{14}C]succinate to be incorporated into the ring to a
considerable extent in flowering plants but not in non-flowering
plants. The observed incorporation of [1-^{14}C]acetate and [2-^{14}C]
glutamate into C-7 (Anwar *et al.*, 1961, Juby and Marion, 1961;
Schiedt and Boeckh-Behrens, 1962) can be explained by their conversion into succinate via the tricarboxylic acid cycle and the gly-
oxylate cycle, which are known to be functional in *R. communis*
(Kornberg and Beevers, 1957).

An interesting variation of the picture with *E. coli* is that the
activity of both [1-^{14}C] and [2-^{14}C]glycerol is incorporated not into
the ring of ricinine but into the N- and O-methyl groups (Juby and
Marion, 1961). These groups have already been shown to arise conventionally from [CH$_3$-^{14}C]-methionine (Dubeck and Kirkwood,
1952) and recently it has been shown that formate is also a source
of these methyl groups (Schiedt and Boeckh-Behrens, 1962). The
activity arising in C-7 from labelled glycerol is as expected if glycerol were converted into acetate via the glycolytic pathway (Juby
and Marion, 1961). A possible intermediate 1-methylnicotinamide
is oxidized by extracts of *R. communis* to a pyridone, but this has
not yet been indentified (Robinson, 1962).

Labelled propionate is incorporated into ricinine (Anwar *et al.*
1961), and the general pattern is compatible with the prior conversion
of propionate into succinate via methylmalonyl-CoA (reaction 14).

There are quantitative differences in the incorporation of propio-

$$CH_3CH_2COOH \rightarrow CH_3CH_2CoSCoA \rightarrow \underset{\underset{COOH}{CH_3}}{CHCOSCoA} \rightarrow \underset{CH_3COOH}{CH_2COSCoA} \rightarrow \underset{CH_2COOH}{CH_2COOH}$$

$$(14)$$

nate in flowering and non-flowering plants (Waller and Henderson, 1961a,b). β-Alanine is incorporated into ricinine as if it were metabolized via propionate (Waller and Henderson, 1961b).

Waller and Nakazawa (1962) have recently reported that sterile cultures of excised embryos, cotyledons and roots of *R. communis* do not synthesize ricinine from nicotinic acid.

REFERENCES

Abrams, R., and Bentley, M. (1959). *Arch. Biochem. Biophys.* **79,** 91.

Albus, H., Schlenk, F., and von Euler, H. (1935). *Hoppe-Seyl. Z.* **237,** 1.

Anwar, R. A., Griffith, T., and Byerrum, R. U. (1961). *Fed. Proc.* **20,** 374.

Atkinson, M. R., and Morton, R. K. (1960). *Nature, Lond.* **188,** 58.

Atkinson, M. R., and Morton, R. K. (1961). *In* "Proceedings of the 5th International Congress of Biochemistry, Moscow", p. 99, Pergamon Press, London.

Atkinson, M. R., Jackson, J. F., and Morton, R. K. (1960). *Aust. J. Sci.* **22,** 414.

Atkinson, M. R., Jackson, J. F., and Morton, R. K. (1961a). *Biochem. J.* **80,** 318.

Atkinson, M. R., Jackson, J. F., and Morton, R. K. (1961b). *Nature, Lond.* **192,** 946.

Auricchio, S., Quaglieriello, E., and Rubino, A. (1960). *Nature, Lond.* **186,** 639.

Bachur, N. R., and Kaplan, N. O. (1955). *Bact. Proc.* **55,** 116.

Ballio, A., and Serlupi-Crescenzi, G. (1957). *R. C. Accad. Lincei* **23,** 275.

Ballio, A., and Russi, S. (1959). *Arch. Biochem. Biophys.* **85,** 567.

Banerjee, S., Banerjee, R., and Deb, C. C. (1950). *Indian J. med. Res.* **38,** 161.

Beadle, G. W., Mitchell, H. K., and Nyc, J. F. (1947). *Proc. nat. Acad. Sci., Wash.* **33,** 155.

Benesch, R. (1945). *Lancet*, 718.

Bilinski, E., and McConnell, W.B. (1957). *Canad. J. Biochem. Physiol.* **35,** 357.

Bonavita, V., Narrod, S. A., and Kaplan, N. O. (1961). *J. biol. Chem.* **236,** 936.

Bonner, J. (1940). *Plant Physiol.* **15,** 553.

Branster, M. V., and Morton, R. K. (1956). *Biochem. J.* **63,** 640.

Burkholder, P. R. (1943). *Science*, **97, 562.**

Byerrum, R. U., Ringler, R. L., Hamill, R. L., and Ball, C. D. (1955). *J. biol. Chem.* **216,** 37.

Cantoni, G. L. (1953). *J. biol. Chem.* **204,** 403.

Chaloupka, M.M., Williams, J. N. Jr., Reynolds, M. S., and Elvehjem, C. A. (1957). *J. Nutr.* **63,** 361.

Chang, M. L. W., and Johnson, B. C. (1957). *J. biol. Chem.* **226,** 799.

Civen, M., and Knox, W. E. (1959) *J. biol. Chem.* **234,** 1787.

Clouet, D. H., and Gordon, M. W. (1959). *Arch. Biochem. Biophys.* **84,** 22.

Dalgliesh, C. E. (1955). *In* "Advances in Protein Chemistry", (M. L. Anson, Kenneth Bailey, and John T. Edsall, eds.) Vol. 10, p. 31. Academic Press, New York and London.

Dalgliesh, C. E. (1959). *In* "Proceedings of the 4th International Congress of Biochemistry, Vienna", XI, p. 32. Pergamon Press, London.

Dalgliesh, C. E., Knox, W. E., and Neuberger, A. (1951). *Nature, Lond.* **168**, 20.

Dann, W. J., and Huff, J. W. (1947). *J. biol. Chem.* **168**, 121.

Da Silva, A. C., Fried, R., and de Angelis, R. C. (1952). *J. Nutr.* **46**, 399.

Davis, B. D., Henderson, L. M., and Powell, D. (1951). *J. biol. Chem.* **189**, 543.

Dawson, R. F., Christman, D. R., Anderson, R. C., Salt, M. E., D'Adamo, A. F., and Weiss, U. (1956). *J. Amer. chem. Soc.* **78**, 2645.

De Castro, F. T., Price, J. M., and Brown, R. R. (1956). *J. Amer. chem. Soc.* **78**, 2904.

Dedonder, R. A. (1961). *Annu. Rev. Biochem.* **30**, 347.

Dewey, L. J., Byerrum, R. U., and Ball, C. D. (1954). *J. Amer. chem. Soc.* **76**, 3997.

Dietrich, L. S., and Friedland, I. M. (1960). *Arch. Biochem. Biophys.* **88**, 313.

Dubeck, M., and Kirkwood, S. (1952). *J. biol. Chem.* **199**, 307.

Dubnoff, J. W., and Dimick, M. (1959). *Biochim. biophys. Acta*, **31**, 541.

Ellinger, P. (1948). *Biochem. J.* **42**, 175.

Ellinger, P., and Kader, M. M. (1948). *Biochem. J.*, **42**, ix.

Ellinger, P., Coulson, R. A., and Benesch, R. (1945). *Nature, Lond.* **154**, 270.

Elvehjem, C. A., Madden, R. J., Strong, F. M., and Woolley, D. W. (1937). *J. Amer. chem. Soc.* **59**, 1767.

Feigelson, P. (1961). *Fed. Proc.* **20**, 223.

Feigelson, P., and Greengard, O. (1961). *J. biol. Chem.* **236**, 153, 158.

Feigelson, P., and Greengard, O. (1962). *Fed. Proc.* **21**, 235.

Fraenkel, G., and Stern, H. R. (1951). *Arch. Biochem.* **30**, 438.

Fildes, P. (1940). *Brit. J. exp. Path.* **21**, 315.

Gholson, R. K., and Henderson, L. M., (1958). *Biochim. biophys. Acta*, **30**, 424.

Gholson, R. K., Rao, D. R., Henderson, L. M., Hill, R. J., and Koeppe, R. E. (1958). *J. biol. Chem.* **230**, 179.

Gholson, R. K., Henderson, L. M., and Hankes, L. V. (1959a). *Fed. Proc.* **18**, 234.

Gholson, R. K., Henderson, L. M., Mourkides, G. A., Hill. R. J., and Koeppe, R. E. (1959b). *J. biol. Chem.* **234**, 96.

Gholson, R. K., Sanders, D. G., and Henderson, L. M. (1959c). *Biochem. biophys. Res. Comm.* **1**, 98.

Giles, N. H., Burkholder, P. R., McVeigh, I., and Wilson, K. S. (1946). *Genetics*, **31**, 216.

Gingrich, W., and Schlenk, F. (1944). *J. Bact.* **47**, 535.

Ginoulhiac, E., Tenconi, L. T., and Chiancone, F. M. (1962). *Nature, Lond.* **193**, 948.

Goldsmith, G. A., Miller, O. N., and Unglaub, W. G. (1956). *Fed. Proc.* **15**, 553.

Goldthwait, D. A., Peabody, R. A., and Greenberg, G. R. (1956). *J. biol. Chem.* **221**, 569.

Goodwin, T. W. (1960). "Recent Advances in Biochemistry". Churchill, London.

Gordon, M. W., and Rydziel, I. J. (1959). *Arch. Biochem. Biophys.* **84**, 32.

Greengard, O. (1961). *Fed. Proc.* **20**, 223.

Greengard, O., and Feigelson, P. (1960). *Biochim. biophys. Acta*, **39**, 191.

Griffith, T., and Byerrum, R. U. (1959). *Science* **129**, 1485.

Griffith, T., and Byerrum, R. U. (1962). *Fed. Proc.* **21**, 398.

Grimshaw, J., and Marion, L. (1958). *Nature, Lond.* **181**, 112.

Hakim, A. A., and Thiele, K. A. (1960). *Biochem. biophys. Res. Comm.* **2**, 242.
Handler, P. (1944). *J. biol. Chem.* **154**, 203.
Handler, P. (1959). *In* "Proceedings of the 4th International Congress of Biochemistry Vienna", II. p. 39. Pergamon Press, London.
Handler, O., and Dann, W. J. (1942). *J. biol. Chem.* **146**, 357.
Hankes, L. V., and Henderson, L. M. (1956). *Fed. Proc.* **15**, 267.
Hankes, L. V., and Henderson, L. M. (1957). *J. biol. Chem.* **225**, 349.
Hankes, L. V., and Segel, I. H. (1957). *Proc. Soc. exp. Biol.* **94**, 447.
Hankes, L. V., and Schmaeler, M. A. (1960). *Biochem. biophys. Res. Comm.* **2**, 468.
Hasse, K., and Berg, P. (1957). *Naturwissenschaften*, **44**, 584.
Hayaishi, O. (1958). *In* "Proceedings of the International Symposium on Enzyme Chemistry, Tokyo", p. 207. Pergamon Press, London.
Hayaishi, O., and Stanier, R. Y. (1951). *J. Bact.* **62**, 691.
Hayaishi, O., and Stanier, R. Y. (1952). *J. biol. Chem.* **195**, 735.
Hayaishi, O., Rothberg, S., Mehler, A. H., and Saito, Y. (1957). *J. biol. Chem.*, **229**, 889.
Hayaishi, O., Taniuchi, H., Tashiro, M., and Kuno, S. (1961) *J. biol. Chem.* **236**, 2492.
Henderson, L. M. (1958). *In* "Proceedings, of the 4th International Congress of Biochemistry, Vienna", XI, p. 207. Pergamon Press, London.
Henderson, L. M., Someroski, J. F., Rao, D. R., Wee, P. H. L., Griffith, T., and Byerrum, R. U. (1959). *J. biol. Chem.* **234**, 93.
Henderson, L. M., Ramasarma, G. B., and Johnson, B. C. (1949) *J. biol. Chem.* **187**, 731.
Heppel, L. A., and Whitfield, P. R. (1955). *Biochem J.* **60**, 1.
Hoffmann, E., and Pescke, R. (1961). *Acta Biol. Med. Fer.* **6**, 453.
Hogeboom, G. H., and Schneider, W. C., (1952). *J. biol. Chem.* **197**, 611.
Holzer, H. and Boltze, H. J. (1961). *Z. Krebsforsch.* **64**, 113.
Holzer, H., Friedrich, G., and Grisebach, H. (1961). *Biochim. biophys. Acta*, **51**, 600.
Horwitt, M. K., Harvey, C. C., Rothwell, W. S., Cilter, J. L., and Haffron, D. (1956). *J. Nutr.* **60**, Suppl. 1.
Huff, J. W., and Perlzweig, W. A. (1941). *J. biol. Chem.* **142**, 401.
Hughes, D. E., and Williamson, D. H. (1953). *Biochem. J.* **55**, 851.
Hurt, W. W., Scheer, B. T., and Deuel, H. J. (1949). *Arch. Biochem.* **21**, 37.
Hundley, J. M. (1954). *In* "The Vitamins", Vol 2. (W. H. Sebrell and R. S. Harris, eds.) Academic Press, New York and London.
Imsande, J. (1961). *Fed. Proc.* **60**, 227.
Itagaki, C., and Nakayama, Y. (1941). *Hoppe-Seyl. Z.* **270**, 83.
Jaffe, E. R., and Gordon, E. E. (1961). *Fed. Proc.* **20**, 64.
Jakoby, W. B. (1954). *J. biol. Chem.* **207**, 657.
Jakoby, W. B., and Bonner, D. M. (1953). *J. biol. Chem.* **205**, 699.
Jakoby, W. B., and Bonner, D. M. (1956). *J. biol. Chem.* **221**, 689.
Jones, K. M. (1959). *J. biol. Chem.* **73**, 714.
Jones, K. M., and Elliott, W. H. (1959). *Biochem. J.* **73**, 706.
Joshi, J. G., and Handler, P. (1961). *Fed. Proc.* **20**, 228.
Joshi, J. G., and Handler, P. (1962). *J. biol. Chem.* **237**, 3185.
Juby, P. F., and Marion, L. (1961). *Biochem. biophys. Res. Comm.* **5**, 461.
Kaplan, N. O. (1961). *In* "Metabolic Pathways", Vol. II (D. M., Greenberg, ed.). Academic Press, New York and London.
Kaplan, N. O., Colowick, S. P., and Ciotti, M. M. (1952). *J. biol. Chem.* **194**, 579.
Kidder, G. W., Dewey, V. C., and Andrews, M. B. (1949). *J. Nutr.* **37**, 521.

Knox, W. E., and Mehler, A. H. (1951). *Science*, **113**, 237.

Kornberg, A. (1950). *J. biol. Chem.* **182**, 805.

Kornberg, A. (1951). *In* "Phosphorus Metabolism", **1**, 392, (W. D. McElroy and H. B. Glass, eds.). Johns Hopkins Press, Baltimore.

Kornberg, H. L., and Beevers, H. A. (1957). *Nature, Lond.* **180**, 35.

Kornberg, A., Lieberman, I., and Simms, E. S. (1954). *J. Amer. chem. Soc.* **76**, 2027.

Kotake, Y., and Nakayama, Y. (1941). *Hoppe-Seyl. Z.* **270**, 76.

Kram, D. C., and Parks, R. E., Jr. (1960). *J. biol. Chem.* **235**, 2893.

Krehl, W. A., Sarma, P. S., and Elvehjem, C. A. (1945a). *J. biol. Chem.* **162**, 403.

Krehl, W. A., Sarma, P. S., Tepley, L. J., and Elvehjem, C. A. (1945b). *Science*, **101**, 489.

Lamborg, M., Stolzenbach, F. E., and Kaplan, N. O. (1958). *J. biol. Chem.* **231**, 685.

Langan, T. A., Jr., and Shuster, L. (1958). *Fed. Proc.* **17**, 260.

Leete, E. (1958a). *Chem. & Ind. (Rev).* 1477.

Leete, E. (1958b). *J. Amer. chem. Soc.* **80**, 2162, 4393.

Leete, E., and Leitz, F. H. B. (1957). *Chem. & Ind. (Rev.)* 1372.

Leifer, E., Roth, L. J., Hogness, D. S., and Carson, M. H. (1951). *J. biol. Chem.* **90**, 595.

Lerner, P., and Yanofsky, C. (1957). *J. Bact.* **74**, 494.

Lwoff, A., and Lwoff, A. (1937). *Proc. roy. Soc.* B, **122**, 352, 360.

Malkin, A., and Denstedt, O. F. (1956). *Canad. J. Biochem. Physiol.* **34**, 121.

Mason, H. S. (1957). *Advanc. Enzymol.* **19**, 79.

Mehler, A. H. (1956). *J. biol. Chem.* **218**, 241.

Mehler, A. H., and Knox, W. E. (1950). *J. biol. Chem.* **187**, 431.

Mehler, A. H., and May, E. L. (1956). *J. biol. Chem.* **223**, 449.

Meister, A., and Buckley, S. D. (1957). *Biochim. biophys. Acta* **23**, 202.

Meister, A., Radhakrishnan, A. N., and Buckley, S. D. (1957). *J. biol. Chem.* **229**, 789.

Melnick, I., and Buchanan, J. M. (1957). *J. biol. Chem.* **225**, 157.

Miller, I. L., and Adelberg, E. A. (1953). *J. biol. Chem.* **205**, 691.

Moline, S. Q., Walker, H. C., and Schweigert, B. S. (1959). *J. biol. Chem.* **234**, 880.

Mothes, K., Schütte, H. R., Simon, H., and Weygand, F. (1959). *Z. Naturforsch.* **14b**, 49.

Mothes, E., Gross, D., Schütte, H. R., and Mothes, K. (1961). *Naturwissenschaften*, **48**, 623.

Mudd, S. H. (1960). *Biochim. biophys. Acta* **37**, 164.

Nair, P., and Vaidyanathan, C. S. (1961). *Arch. Biochem. Biophys.* **93**, 262.

Narrod, S. A., Bonavita, V., Ehrenfeld, E. R., and Kaplan, N. O. (1961). *J. biol. Chem.* **236**, 931.

Noggle, G. R., and Wynd, F. L., (1942). *Bot. Gaz.* **104**, 455.

Nyc, J. F., Mitchell, H. K., Leifer, E., and Langham, W. H. (1949). *J. biol. Chem.* **199**, 783.

Oka, Y. (1954). *J. Biochem., Tokyo* **41**, 89, 107.

Ortega, M. V., and Brown, G. M. (1959). *J. Amer. chem. Soc.* **81**, 4437.

Ortega, M. V., and Brown, G. M. (1960). *J. biol. Chem.* **235**, 2939.

Partridge, C. W. H., Bonner, D. M., and Yanofsky, C. (1952). *J. biol. Chem.* **194**, 269.

Pitot, H. C., and Cho, Y. S. (1961). *Fed. Proc.* **20**, 224.

Porcellati, G. (1954). *G. Biochim.* **3**, 231.

Porcellati, G. (1955). *Boll. Soc. ital. Biol. sper.* **31**, 1.

Preiss, J. (1958). *Fed. Proc.* **17**, 291.

Preiss, J., and Handler, P. (1957). *J. Amer. chem. Soc.* **79,** 1514, 4246.
Preiss, J., and Handler, P. (1958). *J. biol. Chem.* **233,** 488, 493.
Price, J. B., and Dietrich, L. S. (1957). *J. biol. Chem.* **227,** 663.
Purvis, J. L. (1961). *Fed. Proc.* **20,** 46.
Quaglieriello, E. (1952). *Boll. Soc. ital. Biol. sper.* **28,** 685.
Quaglieriello, E., and Pietra, G. D. (1956). *Biochem. J.* **62,** 168.
Rajagopalan, J. V., Sundaram, T. K., and Sarma, P. S. (1958). *Nature, Lond.* **182,** 51.
Rajagopalan, K. V., Sarma, D. S. R., Sundaram, T. K., and Sarma, P. S. (1960). *Enzymologia,* **21,** 277.
Redetzki, H. M., O'Bourke, F. A., and Ruskin, A. (1961). *Fed. Proc.* **20,** 448.
Robinson, F. A. (1951). "The Vitamin B Complex". Chapman and Hall, London.
Robinson, T. (1962). *Fed. Proc.* **21,** 399.
Rowen, J. W., and Kornberg, A. (1951). *J. biol. Chem.* **193,** 497.
Saito, Y., Hayaishi, O., Rothberg, S., and Sench, S. (1957). *Fed. Proc.* **16,** 240.
Sarma, D. S. R., Rajalakshmi, S., and Sarma, P. S. (1961). *Biochem. biophys. Res. Comm.* **6,** 389.
Saran, A. (1958). *Biochem. J.* **70,** 182.
Savage, J. R., Reynolds, M. S., Linkswiler, H., and Harper, A. E. (1962). *Fed. Proc.* **21,** 469.
Schachter, D., and Taggart, J. V. (1953). *J. biol. Chem.* **203,** 925.
Schachter, D., and Taggart, J. V. (1954). *J. biol. Chem.* **208,** 263.
Schiedt, U., and Boeckh-Behrens, G. (1962). *Hoppe-Seyl. Z.* **330,** 58.
Schiedt, U., and Höss, H. G. (1962). *Hoppe-Seyl. Z.* **330,** 74.
Schlenk, F. (1937). *Naturwissenschaften,* **25,** 668.
Schlenk, F. (1943). *Arch. Biochem.* **3,** 93.
Schultz, J., and Rudkin, G. T. (1948). *Fed. Proc.* **7,** 185.
Schweet, R., Holden, J., and Lowy, P. H. (1954). *J. biol. Chem.* **226,** 181.
Scott, T. A. (1962). *Annu. Rep. chem. Soc.* **58,** 378.
Serlupi-Crescenzi, G., and Ballio, A. (1957). *Nature, Lond.* **180,** 1203.
Singal, S. A., Syndenstricker, V. P., and Littlejohn, J. (1947). *J. biol. Chem.* **141,** 203.
Snell, E. (1943). *Arch. Biochem.* **2,** 389.
Snyderman, S. E., Ketron, K. C., Carnetero, R., and Holt, L. E. (1949). *Proc. Soc. exp. Biol. N.Y.* **70,** 569.
Stollar, V., and Kaplan, N. O. (1961). *J. biol. Chem.* **236,** 1863.
Suhadolnik, R. J., Stevens, C. O., Henderson, L. M., and Hankes, L. V. (1957). *Fed. Proc.* **16** 257.
Suda, M., and Takeda, Y. (1950). *Med. J. Osaka Univ.* **2,** 37, 41.
Sundaram, T. K., Rajagopalan, K. V., and Sarma, P. S. (1958). *Biochem. J.* **70,** 196.
Sundaram, T. K., Rajagopalan, K. V., Pichappa, C. V., and Sarma, P. S. (1960). *Biochem, J.* **77,** 145.
Suskind, S. R. (1957). *J. Bact.* **74,** 308.
Suskind, S. R., Yanofsky, C., and Bonner, D. M. (1955). *Proc. nat. Acad. Sci., Wash.* **41,** 517.
Tanaka, T., and Knox, W. E. (1959). *J. biol. Chem.* **234,** 1182.
Tatum, E. L., and Bonner, D. M. (1944). *Proc. nat. Acad. Sci., Wash.* **30,** 30.
Taes, H. J., and Anderson, E. G. (1951). *Proc. nat. Acad. Sci., Wash.* **37,** 645.
Teas, H. J., and Newton, A. C. (1951). *Plant. Physiol.* **26,** 494.
Teas, H. J., Cameron, J. W., and Newton, A. C. (1952). *Agron. J.* **44,** 434.
Teas, H. J., Anderson, E. G., and Cameron, J. W. (1955). *Plant Physiol.* **30,** 334.
Terroine, T. (1948). *C. R. Soc. Biol., Paris,* **227,** 367.

Van Eys, J., Touster, O., and Darby, W. J. (1955). *J. biol. Chem.* **217,** 287.
Volcani, B. E., and Snell, E. E. (1948). *Proc. Soc. exp. Biol., N.Y.* **67,** 511.
von Euler, H., Karrer, P., and Bocker, B. (1936). *Helv. chim. acta.* **19,** 1060.
von Euler, H., Schlenk, F., and Vestrin, R. (1937). *Naturwissenschaften,* **25,** 318.
Waller, G. R., and Henderson, L. M. (1961a). *Biochem. biophys. Res. Comm.* **5,** 5.
Waller, G. R., and Henderson, L. M. (1961b). *J. biol. Chem.* **236,** 1186.
Waller, G. R., and Nakazawa, K. (1962). *Fed. Proc.* **21,** 467.
Wang, T. P., and Kaplan, N. O. (1954). *J. biol. Chem.* **236,** 1186.
Warburg, O., and Christian, W. (1935). *Biochem. Z.* **245,** 464.
Weinstein, L. H., Porter, C. A., and Laurencot, H. J. (1962). *Nature, Lond.* **194,** 204.
Wheat, R. W. (1959). *Arch. Biochem. Biophys.* **82,** 83.
Williams, J. N., Jr., Feigelson, P., Shahinian, S. S., and Elvehjem, C. A. (1951). *J biol. Chem.* **189,** 659.
Williams, R. T. (1959). "Detoxication Mechanisms". 2nd Edition. Chapman and Hall, London.
Wilson, K. S. (1947). *Amer. J. Bot.* **34,** 469.
Wilson, R. G., and Henderson, L. M. (1960). *Fed. Proc.* **19,** 416.
Wilson, R. G., and Henderson, L. M. (1961). *Fed. Proc.* **20,** 448.
Wiss, O., and Fuchs, H. (1951). *Experientia* **6,** 472.
Wiss, O., and Weber, F. (1956). *Hoppe-Seyl. Z.* **204,** 232.
Wiss, O., and Bettendorf, G. (1957). *Hoppe-Seyl. Z.* **306,** 145.
Withner, C. L. (1949). *Amer. J. Bot.* **36,** 317.
Woolley, D. W., Strong, F. M., Madden, R. J., and Elvehjem, C. A. (1938). *J. biol. Chem.* **124,** 715.
Wu, P-H. L., Griffith, T., and Byerrum, R. U. (1962). *J. biol. Chem.* **234,** 884.
Yanofsky, C. (1952). *J. biol. Chem.* **194,** 279.
Yanofsky, C. (1955). *In* "Amino Acid Metabolism", p. 930. (W. D. McElroy and B. Glass, eds.). Johns Hopkins Press, Baltimore; *J. biol. Chem.* **217,** 345.
Yanofsky, C. (1956). *J. biol. Chem.* **223,** 171.
Yanofsky, C., and Rachmeler, M. (1958). *Biochim. biophys. Acta,* **28,** 640.
Zatman, L. J. (1961). *In* "Proceedings of the 5th International Congress of Biochemistry, Moscow", p. 280. Pergamon Press, London.
Zeijlemaker, F. C. I. (1953). *Acta Botan. Nederl.* **2,** 123.

Chapter 4

PTEROYLGLUTAMIC ACID (FOLIC ACID) AND ITS DERIVATIVES

I. Introduction

It is obvious, in retrospect, that a number of preparations obtained between 1931 and 1943 contained "folic acid" as the active principle; that is, they all cured various nutritional anaemias in animals (e.g. nutritional cytopaenia in chicks) and also acted as growth factors for various micro-organisms (e.g. *Lactobacillus casei* and *Streptococcus lactis* R; see Sebrell and Harris, 1954). The first active crystalline factor was obtained from liver (Pfiffner *et al.*, 1943; Stokstad, 1943); the same compound was also later isolated from yeast (Pfiffner *et al.*, 1947). The structure of the active compound (I) was elucidated by Stokstad and his associates (Stokstad *et al.*, 1948; Mowat *et al.*, 1948). It is now generally known as pteroylglutamic acid (PGA)* or folic acid (FA) but synonyms are folacin and vitamin B_c.

(I)

Two polyglutamate derivatives of folic acid are known, pteroyldi-γ-glutamylglutamic acid (pteroyltriglutamate, teropterin) isolated from *Corynebact.* spp. (Hutchings *et al.*, 1948) and pteroylhexa-γ-glutamylglutamic acid (pteroylheptaglutamate, vitamin B_c conjugate) isolated from yeast (Pfiffner *et al.*, 1946). The triglutamate has also been detected in algae (Ericson, 1954). Both are as active as PGA for animals, but have only slight activity for micro-organisms. The reason for the occurrence of these polyglutamate forms is unknown.

* Care has to be taken in using this abbrevation because it is also used to designate phosphoglyceric acid and polygalacturonic acid.

The functional forms of folic acid are derivatives of 5,6,7,8-tetra-hydrofolic acid (FAH_4; II), and include N^5-formyl-5,6,7,8-tetra-hydrofolic acid (folinic acid, citrovorum factor, leucovorin; N^5-formyl-FAH_4; III), N^{10}-formyl-5, 6, 7, 8-tetrahydrofolic acid; N^{10}-

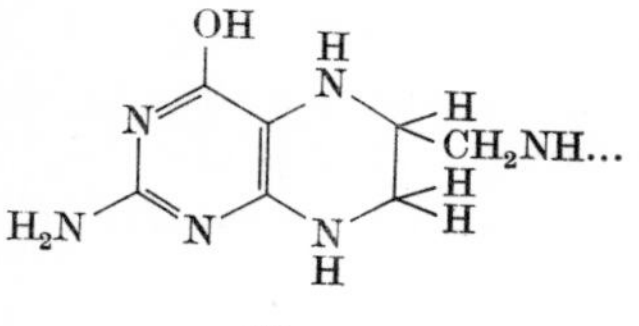

(II)

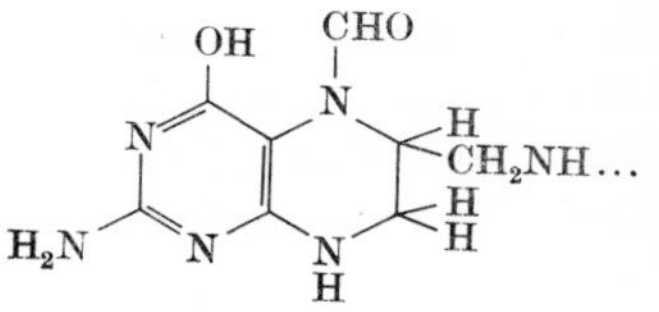

(III)

formyl-FAH_4; IV), N^5, N^{10}-methenyl 5,6,7,8-tetrahydrofolic acid

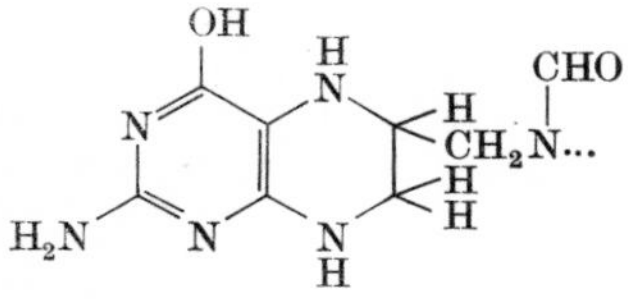

(IV)

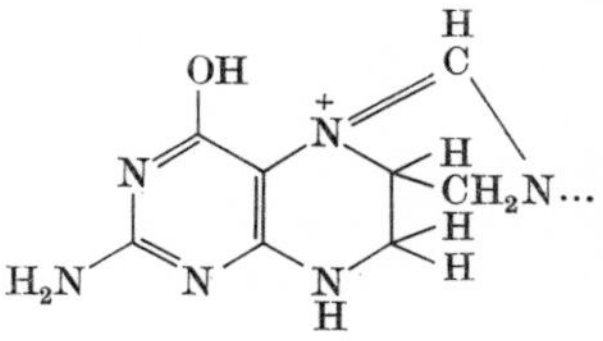

(V)

(anhydroleucovorin, isoleucovorin, N^{5-10}-formyl FAH_4; V), and N^5, N^{10}-methylenetetrahydrofolic acid ("active methylene", "active formaldehyde", N^{5-10}-hydroxymethyl-FAH_4; VI).

Pteridines other than folic acid derivatives exist naturally and are metabolically important. The origin of these will also be consi-dered in this chapter as most of them appear metabolically related to folic acid; they include N^{10}-formylpteroic acid (rhizopterin) (VII) isolated from cultures of *Rhizopus nigricans* by Keresztesy *et al.*, (1943), and biopterin (the *Crithidia* factor) which supports growth of the protozoon *Crithidia fasciculata* (Patterson *et al.*, 1956, 1958) and has the structure 2-amino-4-hydroxy-6- [1,2-di-hydroxypropyl-(L-*erythro*)]–pteridine (VIII; Patterson *et al.*, 1958). Apart from its occurrence in urine, biopterin has been isolated from royal jelly of the honey bee (Butenandt and Rembold, 1958) and, in a different optical configuration, from *Drosophila melano-*

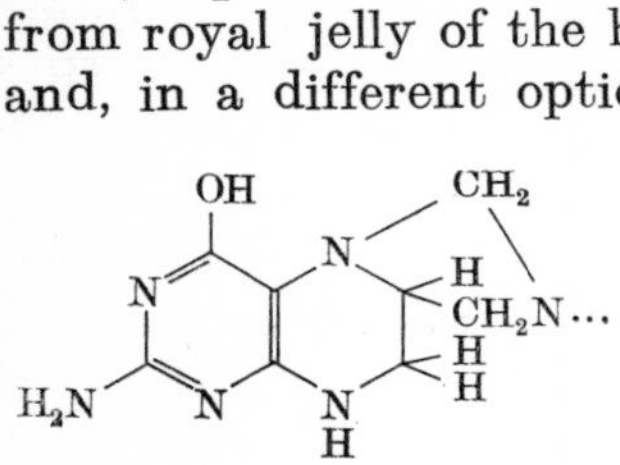

(VI)

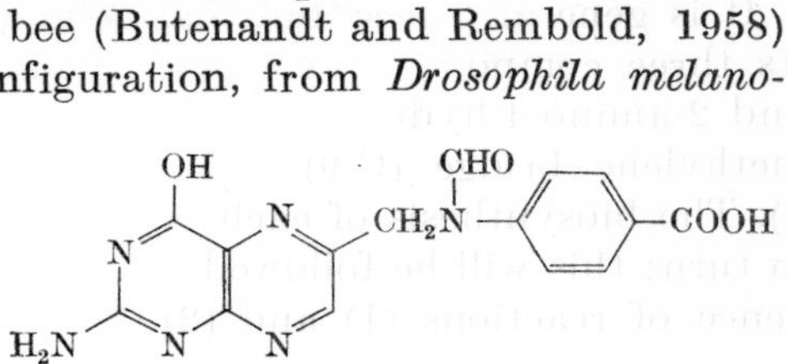

(VII)

gaster (Forrest and Mitchell, 1955). Xanthopterin (IX) and leucopterin (X), first isolated from butterfly wings in 1891 by Gowland Hopkins, were only fully characterized some twenty years ago, mainly by Wieland and his colleagues (Wieland *et al.*, 1940). These and other pteridines including 2-amino-4-hydroxypteridine (XI), 2-amino-4-hydroxypteridine-6-carboxylic acid (XII) and isoxanthopterin (XIII), are widely distributed in crustacea, insects and cold blooded vertebrates (see Fox, 1953; Ziegler-Günder, 1956, for reviews). The existence of xanthopterin in mammals is controversial (see p. 124).

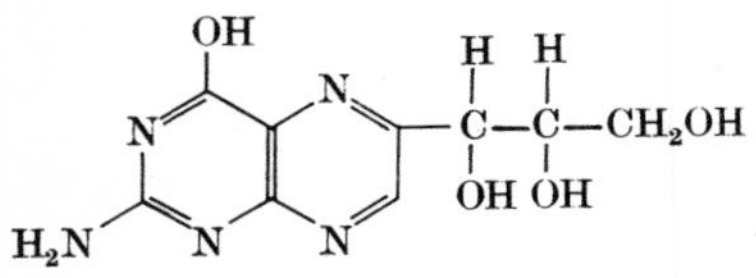

(VIII) 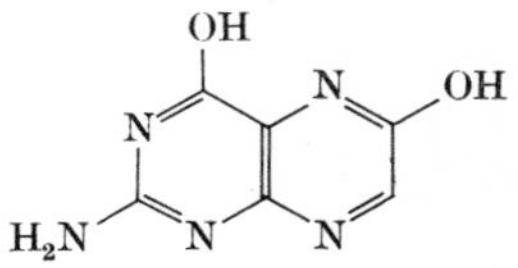   (IX)

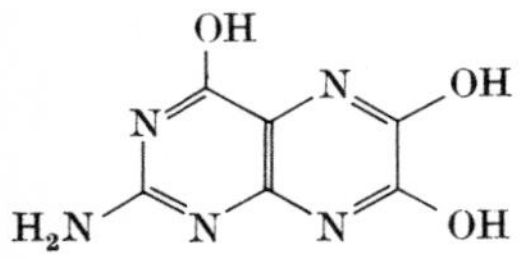

(X) 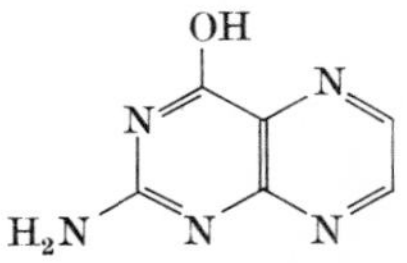   (XI)

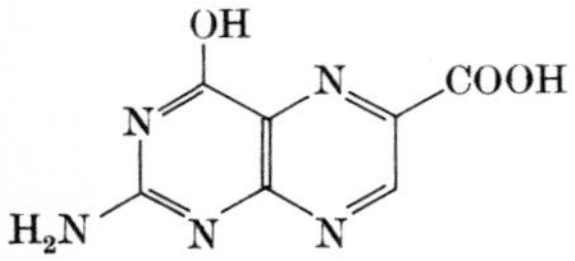

(XII) 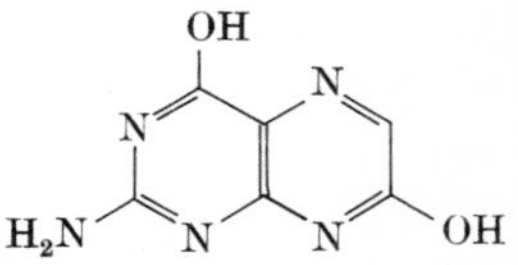   (XIII)

II. BIOSYNTHESIS OF FOLIC ACID

A. *Mechanism of Formation*

It is generally accepted that folic acid is built up stepwise from its three components, glutamic acid (A), *p*-aminobenzoic acid (B) and 2-amino-4-hydroxypteridine (C), with (B) and (C) joined by a methylene bridge (C-9). Two possibilities exist (reactions 1 and 2). The biosynthesis of each postulated unit will be first considered in turn; this will be followed by an assessment of the alleged occurrence of reactions (1) and (2).

$$\text{Pteridine} + p\text{-aminobenzoylglutamate} \rightarrow \text{FA} \qquad (1)$$

$$\text{Pteroic acid} + \text{glutamate} \rightarrow \text{FA} \qquad (2)$$

(i) *Glutamic acid*

The basic route of formation of glutamic acid, a key compound in nitrogen metabolism in both plants and animals, is by trans-amination, the amino acceptor, α-oxoglutarate being formed from carbohydrate via the tricarboxylic acid cycle (scheme 3). There are,

$$\text{Glucose} \rightarrow \text{pyruvate} \xrightarrow{\text{TCA cycle}} \alpha\text{-oxoglutarate} \xrightarrow{\text{Trans-amination}} \text{glutamate} \qquad (3)$$

AMP

PRPP
P–P

Imidazoleacetol 3-phosphate

H_2O

Imidazoleglycerol-3-phosphate

4-Aminoimidazole-5-carboxamide ribotide

Glutamine
Glutamate

L-Histidinol phosphate

P_i

L-Histidinol

NAD NADH$_2$

L-Histidinal

Glutamate
α-oxo-glutarate

NAD
NADH$_2$

L-Histidine

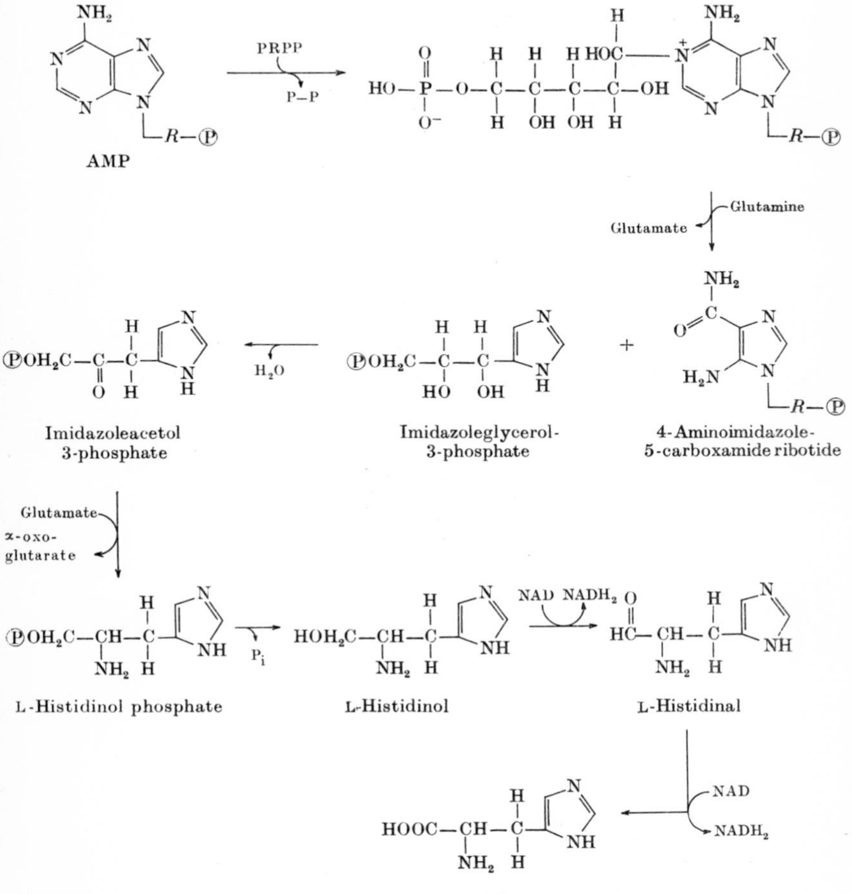

FIG. 1. The biosynthesis of L-histidine.

however, other pathways of metabolism which can also give rise to glutamic acid; these include the catabolism of histidine, the carboxylation of γ-aminobutyrate and the deamination of glutamine. With the exception of the breakdown of histidine, however, the compounds themselves are almost certainly formed originally from glutamate itself. Histidine is synthesized according to the reaction scheme set out in Fig. 1. Its degradation, with the resulting formation of glutamate, varies according to the micro-organism used

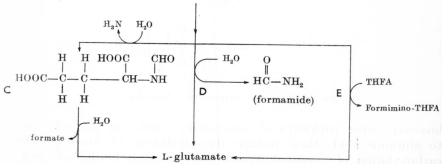

FIG. 2. The conversion of L-histidine into L-glutamic acid in various organisms.

(Fig. 2); it is also different in animals (Fig. 2), but it should be remembered that in any case animals cannot incorporate glutamate into folic acid. The first step is the deamination of histidine to urocanic acid (**A**, Fig. 2) brought about by the enzyme *histidine α-deaminase* [L-histidine ammonia lyase] (Tabor and Hayaishi, 1952; Wickremasinge and Fry, 1954); the enzyme preparations purified from guinea-pig liver and *Pseudomonas fluorescens* require pyrophosphate and a thiol for full activity (Tabor and Mehler, 1954) whilst that from rabbit liver is said to require Co^{2+} and folic acid as well as glutathione (Koizumu *et al.*, 1956). For some time imidazolone propionic acid has been postulated as the intermediate between urocanic acid and formimino-L-glutamate, but, because of its extreme instability (half life 24 min at pH 7·2; Brown and Kies, 1960) its formation (reaction **B**, Fig. 2) has only been demonstrated comparatively recently. It is an intermediate in both the animal and bacterial pathways (Feinberg and Greenberg, 1958; Rao and Greenberg, 1960; Revel and Magasanik, 1958); Coenzyme A may be involved in this transformation (Baldridge and Burket, 1960). N-Formimino-L-glutamate is then metabolized to glutamate by routes varying with the organism used. In *P. fluorescens*, ammonia is first removed hydrolytically and the resulting formyl-L-glutamate hydrolysed to formate and L-glutamate (pathway **C**, Fig. 2; Magasanik and Bowser, 1955a; Tabor and Mehler, 1954); in *Aerobacter aerogenes* (Magasanik and Bowser, 1955b) and *Clostridium tetanomorphum* (Wachsman and Barker, 1955), N-formimino-L-glutamate is directly hydrolysed to formamide and L-glutamate (pathway **D**, Fig. 2), whilst in liver L-glutamate is formed from N-formimino-L-glutamate by formimino transfer to tetrahydrofolic acid with the production of N^5-formiminotetrahydrofolic acid (pathway **E**, Fig. 2) (Miller and Waelsch, 1957; Tabor and Rabinowitz, 1956; see also p. 120).

It is possible that the reduction of the incorporation of [^{14}C] glycine into folic acid by histidine in *Corynebacterium* spp. (Sankar and Sankar, 1961) is due to the utilization of a metabolite of histidine for folic acid synthesis.

(ii) *The pteridine residue*

All available evidence points to the pathway of pteridine synthesis being similar to that involved in purine and riboflavin biosynthesis (see Chapter 2). Weygand and Waldschmidt (1955) found that [^{14}C]formate, $^{14}CO_2$ and [^{14}C]glycine were incorporated by butterflies into C-2, C-4 and C-4a+8a, respectively, of xanthopterin

(IX) and leucopterin (X). This is the same labelling pattern as that observed with purines and riboflavin. Riboflavin is synthesized via purines (p. 42) and this is also true of the pteridines; Ziegler-Günder *et al.* (1956), for example, demonstrated that injected [2-^{14}C]guanine was converted into pteridines in *Xenopus* larvae, and McNutt and Forrest (1958) and Maley and Plaut (1958) showed that adenine is converted into 6,7-dimethyl-8-ribityllumazine (XIV) in the fungus *Eremothecium ashbyii*. Only recently, however, has the incorporation of a purine into the pteridine residue of folic acid been demonstrated; Shaw and Viera (1961) have shown that [2-^{14}C]adenine is incorporated into pteroyltriglutamic acid by a *Corynebact.* spp. The reactions leading to riboflavin formation involves the removal of C-8 from adenine (McNutt and Forrest, 1958);

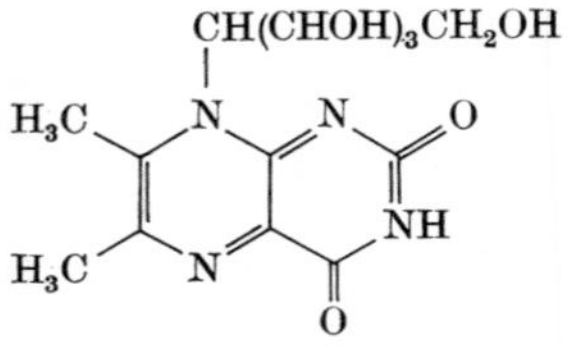

(XIV)

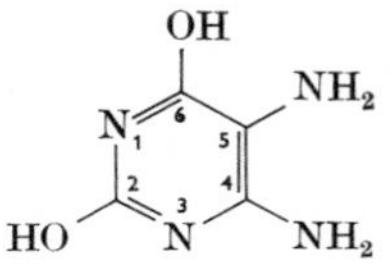

(XV)

this is also true for folic acid synthesis (Shaw and Viera, 1961) and indicates that 4,5-diaminouracil (XV) or, more likely 2,4,5-triamino-uracil (XVI) (or closely related derivatives), might be an intermediate in the conversion. Many such compounds have been examined for precursor activity, but as yet without succes. (Similar failures have been reported in studies on riboflavin biosynthesis; see Chapter 2). For example, 2,4,5-triamino-6-hydroxypyrimidine (XVI) has no effect on folic acid synthesis by washed suspensions of *Esch. coli* (Lascelles and Woods, 1952), and, in the presence of *p*-amino-

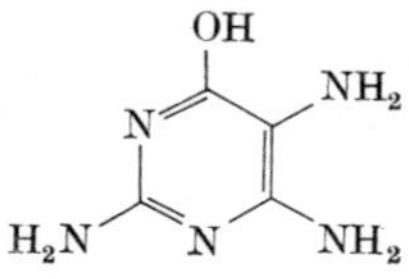

(XVI)

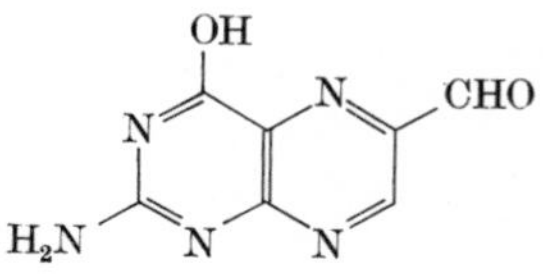

(XVII)

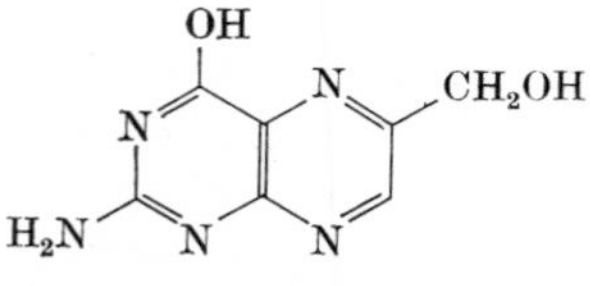

(XVIII)

benzoic acid and reductone*, would not support growth of *Strep. faecalis* R adapted to grow in the presence of 2-amino-4-hydroxy-6-pteridine aldehyde (XVII) that is, under conditions which allow the conversion of the aldehyde into folic acid (Weygand *et al.*, 1956). Furthermore, [2-¹⁴C]-2,4,5-triaminouracil (XVI) (= guanine minus C-8) is not incorporated into folic acid by *Enterococcus stei* (Weygand *et al.*, 1956); however, this does not entirely rule out (XVI) as an intermediate because the cell wall of *Ent. stei* may be impermeable to it; on the other hand, it would appear probable, on general biochemical grounds, that the purine precursor is activated in some way before C-8 is removed. The problem of the mechanism of the biosynthesis of pteridines is discussed in more detail in Chapter 2.

(iii) *The nature of the pteridine precursor*

A reasonable working hypothesis to account for the formation of the pteridine residue of folic acid would be that xanthopterin (IX) or a closely related compound, such as dihydro- or tetrahydroxanthopterin is the first pteridine formed and that a 1-C unit is transferred to C-6 to become C-9 of folic acid. 2-Amino-4-hydroxypteridine 6-aldehyde (XVII), 2-amino-4-hydroxypteridine 6-carboxylic acid (XII) and 2-amino-4-hydroxy-6-hydroxymethylpteridine (XVIII) are such compounds; on purely chemical grounds (XVII) is the compound most likely to be an intermediate in folic acid synthesis (Tschesche, 1947).

We shall first consider the fully unsaturated pteridines; xanthopterin (IX) is incorporated into folic acid by intact cells of the bacteria *Ent. stei*, *Esch. coli*, *Lact. plantarum* 105, *Strep. faecalis* R, by the fungi *Pichia membranaefaciens* and *Candida albicans*, and in cell-free extracts of *Ent. stei*, *Strep. faecalis* R, *Esch. coli* and *P. membranaefaciens* (Korte *et al.*, 1957; Korte *et al.*, 1959; Korte and Synnatschke, 1959). The incorporation was only small in all cases. One aspect of this work which should be commented on is that although *Strep. faecalis* R and *Ent. stei* require folic acid for growth, they can incorporate xanthopterin into this compound. Possibly synthesis in these organisms is not completely blocked, but is quantitatively insufficient for growth.

Cell-free preparations of *Mycobact. avium* have been obtained which will synthesize folic acid in the presence of xanthopterin, *p*-aminobenzoylglutamate, ATP, biotin and thiamine pyrophosphate

---

* Under certain conditions reductone will condense chemically with 2,4,5-triamino-6-hydroxypyrimidine and *p*-aminobenzoic acid to form pteroic acid (Angier *et al.*, 1948).

(Katunuma *et al.*, 1956, 1957; Katunuma and Shoda, 1958); however, xanthopterin was without effect on folic acid synthesis by the *p*-aminobenzoic acid *Esch. coli* auxotroph of Lascelles and Woods (1952), and is not utilized by cell-free systems from *Lact. arabinosus* (Shiota, 1959) by cell-free systems from *Lact. arabinosus* (Shiota, 1959) or *Esch. coli* (Brown, 1959).

The possibility of a 1-C transfer to xanthopterin or a related compound by carboxylation is raised by some observations of Katunuma *et al.* (1956, 1957) who found that if (XII) replaced xanthopterin in their folic acid-synthesizing system, then the requirement for biotin and thiamine pyrophosphate was abolished. However, as Plaut (1961) has pointed out, [^{14}C]formate is not incorporated into the methyl groups of 6,7-dimethyl-8-ribityllumazine, and that attached to C-6 corresponds to C-9 of folic acid (Plaut and Maley, 1959; I. Schmeltz and G.W.E. Plaut, unpublished; quoted by Plaut (1961). Furthermore, Weygand *et al.* (1961) have shown that C-6 and C-7 of leucopterin synthesized by the pupae of the cabbage white butterfly arise from C-1 and C-2 of ribose, respectively. The C-9 of folic acid also originates from ribose (Jaenicke, quoted by Jukes and Broquist, 1961). Glucose is also incorporated into C-6 and C-7 of the various pteridines synthesized by *Drosophila* as well as into the 3-C side chain of drosopterin (Brenner-Holzach and Leuthardt 1961). These observations suggest that the pteridines are first synthesized with a 3-carbon side chain which could arise formally from guanosine thus :—

There is no evidence whether the reaction takes place at the nucleoside level or the mono-, di- or triphosphate level. The product as indicated is biopterin (see p. 101) and Ziegler (1961) has shown that tetrahydrodrobiopterin, obtained from the eyes of the sepia mutant of *Drosophila*, is converted into folic acid by a yeast enzyme preparation in the presence of ATP and Mg^{2+}. Additional evidence in this direction has been recently provided by Reynolds and Brown (1962) who found that [8-^{14}C]guanosine is converted with the loss of C–8 into a pteridine compound by a cell-free extract of *Esch. coli*, and that guanosine is much more effective than guanine in stimulating folic acid synthesis in the extract by replacing 2-amino-4-hydroxy-6-hydroxymethyl-FAH_2.

Direct investigations into the folic acid activity of xanthopterin-6-aldehyde (XVII) and 6-carboxylic acid (XII) have yielded unequivocal results. Weygand *et al.* (1956) reported that [^{14}C]xanthopterin 6-aldehyde was not incorporated into folic acid by the folic acid-requiring organism *Ent. stei*, although Korte *et al.* (1959) found that xanthopterin was converted in this organism. As Weygand *et al.* (1956) used whole cells, (XVII) may have not been metabolically available.

Extracts from *Lact. arabinosus* (Shiota, 1958, 1959) and *Esch. coli* (Brown, 1959) will utilize reduced (XVII) for folic acid synthesis but utilize (XVII) itself or the corresponding hydroxymethyl derivative (XVIII) only slightly.

Nutrition experiments are equally confusing. The aldehyde (XVII) inhibits growth of *Strep. faecalis* R on a medium containing folic acid. However, after adaptation to (XVII) through seven transfers, the organism grew maximally in its presence if *p*-aminobenzoic acid or *p*-aminobenzoylglutamate was also present; quantitatively, however, (XVII) was only 0·017% as active as folic acid (Weygand *et al.*, 1949). Rather similarly, (XVII) inhibited folic acid synthesis by washed suspensions of a *p*-aminobenzoic acid-requiring mutant of *Esch. coli* (Lascelles and Woods, 1952). On the other hand in similar experiments with two strains of *Staphyloccus aureus* (which do not require *p*-aminobenzoic acid), one of which was sulphathiazole-resistant and produced ten times as much folic acid as the sulphathizole-sensitive strain, (XVII) doubled folic acid synthesis (Lascelles and Woods, 1952). An important aspect of this investigation was that the cells used were harvested after growth in the presence of sub-inhibitory amounts of sulphathiazole and thus did not already contain their maximum amounts of folic acid.

The acid (XII) is slightly effective as a folic acid precursor in some organisms. For example, a sulphathiazole-resistant strain of *Esch. coli*, which synthesized four times as much folic acid as the native, sulphathiazole-sensitive strain, utilized (XII) for folic acid synthesis in the presence of *p*-aminobenzoic acid. The sensitive strain also utilized (XII) only if the cells were grown on sub-inhibitory amounts of sulphathiazole, suggesting that the drug was producing a permanent mutation (Ishii and Sevag, 1957). However,

(XII) was inactive in the p-aminobenzoic acid-requiring mutant of Lascelles and Woods (1952).

A related compound which is active in *P. membranaefaciens* and *C. albicans* is isoxanthopterin 6-carboxylic acid (XIX), although the corresponding aldehyde (XX) is inactive; however, if (XX) is autoclaved in the presence of glucose it supports growth of these organism (Tschesche and Korte, 1953). Similar observations had previously been observed with xanthopterin (IX) and *Lact. casei* (Elion *et al.*, 1950). The mechanism of this "activation", which still leaves the pteridine some 500 times less active than folic acid itself, has not been defined, although it is assumed that a glucoside is an intermediate.

(XIX)   (XX)

(XXI)

The realization that FAH_4 is the metabolically active form of folic acid has recently led to experiments designed to discover whether or not reduced pteridines are the true folic acid precursors. In the *Lact. arabinosus* and *Esch. coli* systems just discussed the reduced 2-amino-4-hydroxy-6-hydroxymethylpteridine (XVIII) was a very effective folic acid precursor (Shiota, 1959; Brown, 1960.) Shiota (1959) believes that it is the tetrahydro derivative which is active, but in his system he could not demonstrate the reduction of (XVIII) on the addition of NADH and NADPH. Brown (1959, 1960) on the other hand, claims that the addition of NADH stimulates folic acid synthesis in the *Esch. coli* system and that this stimulation is observed if reduced (XVIII) replaces NADH. More recently Brown *et al.* (1960, 1961) concluded that the active component is the dihydro-derivative of (XVIII), and Jaenicke and Chan (1960) have obtained a soluble enzyme system from both *Esch. coli* and yeast which converts dihydro-(XVIII) into FAH_2 in the presence of ATP and Mg^{2+}. Shiota and Disraely (1961) reported the presence of a similar enzyme system in *Lactobact. plantarum* and Shiota *et al.* (1962) have synthesized 2-amino-4-hydroxy-dihydropteridinyl pyrophosphate chemically and found that it is will replace reduced (XVIII) plus ATP in their *Lact. plantarum* system.

Reduction of 2-amino-4-hydroxypteridine 6-aldehyde (XVII) increases its precursor activity in the *Lact. arabinosus* system (Shiota, 1959) but destroys its activity in the *Esch. coli* system (Brown, 1959, 1960).

These recent investigations should lead to more definitive observations in the near future.

(iv) p-*Aminobenzoic acid*

The details of the now classical microbiological investigations by B. D. Davis which led to the identification of shikimic acid as the key intermediate in the biosynthesis of the aromatic amino acids and *p*-aminobenzoic acid have frequently been discussed (see e.g. Goodwin, 1960). Enzymatic studies have now revealed most of the steps leading to the formation of shikimic acid and some of the steps leading to its conversion into phenylalanine, tyrosine, tryptophan and *p*-aminobenzoic acid via 5-phosphoshikimic acid (Fig. 3). The enzymatic conversion of 5-phosphoshikimic acid into *p*-aminobenzoic acid with glutamine as the specific amino donor has been achieved by Weiss and Srinivasan (1959) with a cell-free extract of bakers' yeast. The mechanism involved remains to be elucidated, but it is now clear that it is the amide-N of glutamine which is transferred to 5-phosphoshikimic acid (Srinivasan and Weiss, 1961).

(v) p-*Aminobenzoylglutamate*

The formation of *p*-aminobenzoylglutamate from *p*-aminobenzoic acid, glutamate, ATP, Mg^{2+} and CoA has been reported by Katunuma *et al.* (1956, 1957) with cell-free extracts of *Mycobacterium avium*. When

(4)

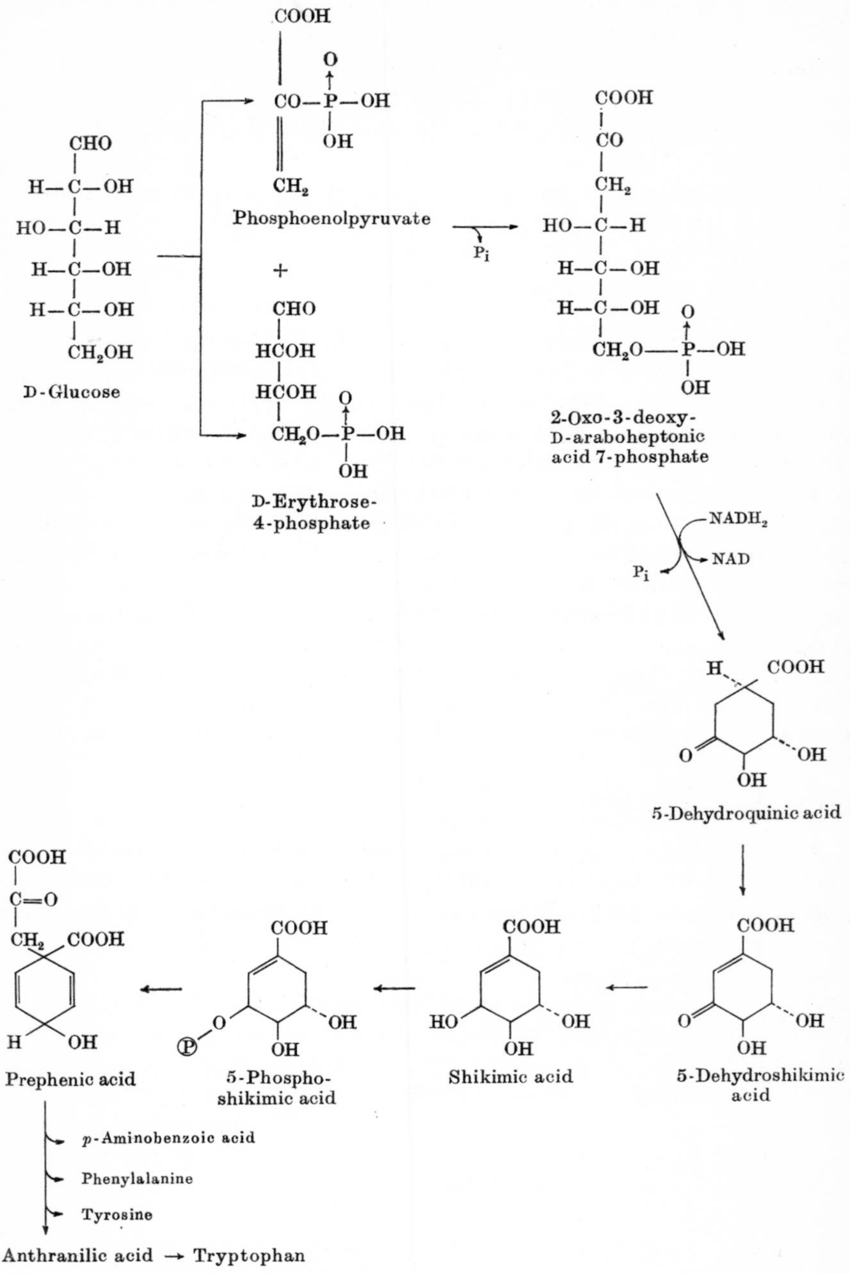

CHO
|
H—C—OH
|
HO—C—H
|
H—C—OH
|
H—C—OH
|
CH₂OH

D-Glucose

COOH
|
CO—P—OH
|| O↑ |
      OH
|
CH₂

Phosphoenolpyruvate

+

CHO
|
HCOH
|
HCOH   O↑
|
CH₂O—P—OH
        |
        OH

D-Erythrose-
4-phosphate

COOH
|
CO
|
CH₂
|
HO—C—H
|
H—C—OH
|
H—C—OH   O↑
|
CH₂O——P—OH
          |
          OH

2-Oxo-3-deoxy-
D-araboheptonic
acid 7-phosphate

P_i

NADH₂
NAD
P_i

5-Dehydroquinic acid

5-Dehydroshikimic acid

Shikimic acid

5-Phospho-shikimic acid

Prephenic acid

p-Aminobenzoic acid

Phenylalanine

Tyrosine

Anthranilic acid → Tryptophan

FIG. 3. The metabolic pathway leading to the formation of the aromatic amino acids and p-aminobenzoic acid.

glutamate was absent from the incubation mixture a positive hydroxamic reaction was obtained indicating the formation of a coenzyme A derivative of p-aminobenzoic acid. The overall reaction is considered also to involve an acyl adenylate and to take place as indicated in reaction (4).

(vi) *Formation of pteroic acids*

Although one of the first compounds of the folic acid group of vitamins to be isolated was a pteroic acid, rhizopterin (VII), virtually nothing is known about the biosynthesis of pteroic acids. Korte *et al.* (1959) and Korte and Synnatschke (1959) found [14]C– labelled N^5– formyltetrahydropteroate in the cells of all organisms which examined after addition of [8a-^{14}C]xanthopterin. Pteroic acid is also formed in folic acid-synthesizing cell-free systems of *Lac. arabinosus* and *Esch. coli* (see below) when p-aminobenzoylglutamate is replaced by p-aminobenzoate + L-glutamate and p-aminobenzoate, respectively (Shiota, 1959; Brown, 1960, 1961). Dihydropteroic acid is also formed from 2-amino-4-hydroxy-6-hydroxymethyldihydropteridine and p-aminobenzoic acid in Brown's system, and it is this step which is inhibited by sulphonamides (Brown, 1961, 1962).

(vii) *The condensation reactions*

It is still not possible to decide on the evidence currently available whether a pteridine condenses with p-aminobenzoylglutamate or whether a pteroic acid condenses with glutamate (reactions 1 and 2, p. 102). Possibly both reactions exist *in vivo*, but the confusion may be due to use of incompletely purified enzyme systems.

In support of reaction (1), its occurrence has been demonstrated in cell-free systems of *Mycobact. avium* (Katunuma *et al.*, 1957), *Lact arabinosus* (Shiota, 1959) and *Esch. coli* (Brown *et al.*, 1960, 1961). Evidence against reaction (1) includes: (a) in the *Esch. coli* system p-aminobenzoic acid is 40 times more effective as a precursor of pteroic acid than p-aminobenzoylglutamate is of folic acid (Brown, 1960) : (b) rhizopterin (VII) promotes growth of *Strep. faecalis* R (Stokes and Larsen, 1945), and (c) in only one organism, *Lact. plantarum* 105, (Aughagen, 1943) out of the numerous species examined is p-aminobenzoylglutamate better than p-aminobenzoate in reversing the growth inhibition of the sulphonamides (see Woods, 1960).

Strongest support for reaction (2) is the observation, already quoted, that p-aminobenzoate is a much more effective substrate for pteroic acid synthesis in Brown's *Esch. coli* enzyme system than is *p*-aminobenzoylglutamate for folic acid synthesis. Evidence which has accumulated against reaction (2) includes: (a) rhizopterin is inactive as a folic acid substitute in all organisms tested except *Strep. faecalis* R* (see previous paragraph), for example in *Strep. faecalis* Ralston, *L. arabinosus* and *L. plantarum*; indeed it acts as a non-competitive antagonist of folic acid in *Cl. tetanomorphum*, *Cl. acetobutylicum* and a strain of *Staph. aureus*; (Lampen and Jones, 1946, 1947; Nimmo-Smith and Woods, 1948; Möller *et al.*, 1949; Sims and Woods, 1950); (b) extracts of *Mycobact. avium* will not synthesize folic acid from pteroic acid and glutamate under conditions which allow its synthesis from other precursors (Katunuma and Shoda, 1958).

III. Synthesis of Folic Acid by Plants

Very little is known of the formation of folic acid by plants, but an investigation by Andreeva (1953) indicates that seeds lose folic acid during maturation, and on germination synthesize it more rapidly in the dark than in the light. There is a marked stimulation of synthesis following injury to plant tissues. On the other hand, Braganca *et al.* (1960) report a loss of folic acid during germination which is due to the appearance of an enzyme which splits folic acid at the C-9—N-10 linkage. This enzyme has peroxidase properties. Synthesis in shoots and roots is stimulated by *p*-aminobenzoic acid and inhibited by sulphonamides (Erismann, 1962). Some of the contradictory results reported may be connected with the report that labile precursors account for a great deal of "folic acid" activity in shoots (Erismann, 1962).

IV. Formation of Di- and Tetrahydrofolic Acids

As indicated at the beginning of this chapter, the functional forms of folic acid are all tetrahydro derivatives and, although di- and tetrahydropteridines may be intermediates in the biosynthesis of these compounds, (p. 113) enzymes are present in most tissues which convert folic acid into tetrahydrofolic acid. The overall conversion of folic acid into tetrahydrofolic acid has been demonstrated in avian liver homogenates (Reid and Couch, 1955; Futterman, 1957), pig liver homogenates (Futterman and Silverman, 1956; Silverman *et al.* 1957), in suspensions and cell-free extracts of *Strep. faecalis* (Nichol, 1954; Zakrzewski and Nichol, 1955; Lascelles and Woods, 1954)

* Rogers

and *Ent. stei* (Wacker *et al.*, 1958), and in crude extracts of soya bean leaves (Iwai and Yoshida, 1954). The reaction in liver systems is anaerobic and requires the presence of a reducing agent such as ascorbate or homocysteine; under aerobic conditions tetrahydrofolic acid is rapidly degraded to *p*-aminobenzoylglutamate and xanthopterin and other pteridines (Futterman and Silverman, 1956; Blakley, 1957).

The overall reduction of folic acid takes place in two stages with dihydrofolic acid as intermediate (reactions 5 and 6). It is generally agreed that two separate enzymes are involved, but the chicken liver enzyme of Zakrzewski (1960) appears to carry out both reactions. The enzyme involved in the first step, *dihydrofolic dehydrogenase*, [dihydrofolate:NADP oxidoreductase] has been purified from sheep liver; it requires NADPH specifically, and is inhibited non-competitively by low concentrations of aminopterin (XXI) (Peters and D.M. Greenberg, 1959). According to Kenkare and Braganca (1962) FMN or FAD is the co-factor for the sheep

$$FA + NADPH + H^+ \rightleftharpoons FAH_2 + NADP^+ \tag{5}$$

$$FAH_2 + \left. \begin{matrix} NADH \\ NADPH \end{matrix} \right\} + H^+ \rightleftharpoons FAH_4 + \left\{ \begin{matrix} NAD^+ \\ NADP^+ \end{matrix} \right. \tag{6}$$

liver enzyme. The formation of dihydrofolic acid has also been demonstrated in extracts of *Cl. sticklandii* in the presence of co-enzyme A and substrates such as pyruvate and α-oxobutyrate, which presumably provide a continuous source of NADPH (Wright and Anderson, 1957; Wright *et al.*, 1958). The enzyme concerned with the second stage (reaction 6), *tetrahydrofolic dehydrogenase*, [dihydrofolic reductase, 5, 6, 7, 8-tetrahydrofolate: NAD(P) oxidoreductase] has been purified from chicken liver (Osborn and Huennekens, 1957), guinea pig liver (Bertino 1962), sheep liver (Peters and D.M. Greenberg, 1958a) and calf thymus (Nath and D.M. Greenberg, 1961), and also from *Strep. faecalis* R (Blakley and McDougall, 1961). The avian bovine and bacterial enzymes preferentially utilize NADPH whereas NADH is the active hydrogen donor in the sheep enzyme. K_m values of 5×10^{-7}M, $1 \cdot 0 \times 10^{-5}$M and $4 \cdot 0 \times 10^{-6}$M have been reported for the chicken, sheep and bacterial enzymes respectively (Huennekens and Osborn, 1960; Peters and D.M. Greenberg, 1958b). The chicken enzyme exhibits pH optima at 4·5 and 7.5 (Mathews and Huennekens, 1961). In the purified chicken enzyme NADH and folic acid can replace NADPH and FAH_2. The exact structure of the dihydrofolic acid concerned in these reactions is still not settled, and, indeed, it appears that different tautomers function in different systems. For example, the dihydrofolate formed by the *Cl. sticklandii* enzyme is a much poorer substrate for liver tetrahydrofolic dehydrogenase than is that synthesized chemically, whilst both are equally active for the thymus enzyme (Nath and D.M. Greenberg, 1961).

The anti-leukaemia drugs aminopterin (XXI) and amethopterin (XXII) inhibit dihydrofolic dehydrogenase, according to Werkheiser (1961), who considers this the primary site of action for these inhibitors; furthermore, the development of increased resistance to aminopterin by Sarcoma–180 cells in tissue culture parallels their increased levels of dihydrofolic dehydrogenase (Hakala *et al.*, 1961). On the other hand these drugs inhibit the chicken enzyme non-competitively at very low concentrations, the respective K_i values being 1×10^{-9}M and $2 \cdot 3 \times 10^{-9}$M, respectively (Huennekens and Osborn, 1960). No indication that the reaction was reversible was observed with the *Strep. faecalis* enzyme (Blakley and McDougall, 1961), The K_i for aminopterin in the bacterial enzyme is $2 \cdot 4 \times 10^{-9}$M (Blakley and McDougall, 1961). It also inhibits the sheep enzyme (Kenkare and Braganca, 1962). The enzyme from *Cl. sticklandii* differs from that from animal sources in that aminopterin and amethopterin are substrates for the bacterial enzyme (Wright *et al.*, 1958). Braganca and Kenkare (1959) claim that the conversion of folate into FAH_4 by a sheep liver enzyme, requires FMN as well as NADPH, but this was found not to be so with the *Strep. faecalis* enzyme (Blakley and McDougall, 1961). Enzyme preparations from a number of sources, including a highly purified preparation from guinea pig liver, were stimulated by monovalent and divalent cations (Bertino, 1962).

V. FORMYLTETRAHYDROFOLIC ACID

Two isomers of formyltetrahydrofolic acid exist, one with the formyl residue attached to N^5 (III) and the other with the residue attached to N^{10} (IV). It is the N^{10} isomer which is effective as "active formate" in most systems, but the N^5 isomer is specifically required in one reaction (see below). The formate-activating enzyme, *formyltetrahydrofolate synthetase* [formate: tetrahydrofolate ligase ATP], has been purified from *Micrococcus aerogenes* (Whiteley *et al.*, 1958a), from pigeon liver (Jaenicke, 1958) developing chick embryo (Silber *et al.*, 1962), and from leaves of higher plants (Byers *et al.*, 1961); it has been obtained crystalline from *Cl. cylindrosporum* (Rabinowitz and Pricer, 1957a, 1962, Himes and Rabinowitz, 1962). The overall mechanism of the reaction (7) is ATP-dependent, as first indicated by G. R. Greenberg (1954) and G. R. Greenberg and Jaenicke (1957).

$$HCOOH + FAH_4 + ATP \xrightleftharpoons{Mg^{2+}} N^{10}\text{-formyl-}FAH_4 + ADP + P_i \qquad (7)$$

The reaction has now been resolved into two steps (8 and 9) by

$$FAH_4 + ATP \rightleftharpoons pFAH_4 + ADP \qquad (8)$$
$$pFAH_4 + HCOOH \rightleftharpoons N^{10}\text{-formyl-}FAH_4 + P_i \qquad (9)$$

using the purified *M. aerogenes* enzyme. In the absence of formate the production of ADP was demonstrated by coupling the reaction with the pyruvate kinase-lactate dehydrogenase system (Whiteley *et al.*, 1958b). The availability of ADP allows reactions (10) and (11) to pro-

$$\text{phosphoenol pyruvate} + ADP \rightleftharpoons \text{pyruvate} + ATP \qquad (10)$$
$$\text{pyruvate} + NADH + H^+ \rightleftharpoons \text{lactate} + NAD^+ \qquad (11)$$

ceed with the oxidation of NADH, which can be measured spectrophotometrically. The existence of a phosphorylated derivate of tetrahydrofolic acid ($pFAH_4$) was demonstrated on chromatography of the products of the reaction carried out in the presence of [^{32}P]-ATP. Furthermore, chemical phosphorylation of tetrahydrofolic acid yielded a compound, chromatographically identical with the enzymatically synthesized compound, which would take part in reaction (9) and stimulate ATP synthesis by reaction (8) (Whiteley, *et al.*, 1958b). A somewhat similar conclusion has been arrived at for the mechanism of the formate-activating system from pigeon and sheep liver (Jaenicke, 1958; Jaenicke and Brode, 1961) although these authors consider that the first step is the formation of an enzyme phosphate, by reaction of the enzyme with ATP, and that this reacts with FAH_4 to form enzyme-bound $pFAH_4$. However, with the crystalline *Cl. cylindrosporum* enzyme Himes and Rabinowitz (1960) could obtain no evidence for an initial phosphorylation of tetrahydrofolic acid or formate. For example, the rate of ADP formation from ATP in the presence of either substrate alone was negligible compared with the rate observed in the presence of both substrates. This and other observations have led Rabinowitz and Himes (1960) to suggest the mechanism outlined in Fig. 4. The first step is the binding of ATP to the enzyme and the bound ATP then undergoes a concerted reaction in the presence of formic acid and FAH_4. The reaction is initiated by nucleophilic attack of the nitrogen atom on the formic acid. (See also Himes and Rabinowitz, 1962.)

A *N^{10}-formyltetrahydrofolic acid deformylase* [10-formyltetrahydrofolate amidohydrolase] is present in beef liver (Osborn *et al.*, 1957).

This allows the regeneration of tetrahydrofolic acid in the absence
of a formyl acceptor. A fully documented account of the various
reactions involving activated one carbon units has been prepared
by Huennekens and Osborn (1959).

N^5-Formyltetrahydrofolic acid is, up to the time of writing, the
coenzyme for only one well-authenticated reaction, that involving
the formation of α-N-formyl-L-glutamate (12). The reaction, the
equilibrium of which is far to the left, does not require ATP (Sil-

$$N^5\text{-Formyl-FAH}_4 + \text{L-glutamate} \rightleftarrows \alpha\text{-N-formyl-L-glutamate} + \text{FAH}_4 \quad (12)$$

verman *et al.*, 1957). N^5-Formyltetrahydrofolic acid can also be converted into the N^{10}-isomer and the mechanism of the isomerization may

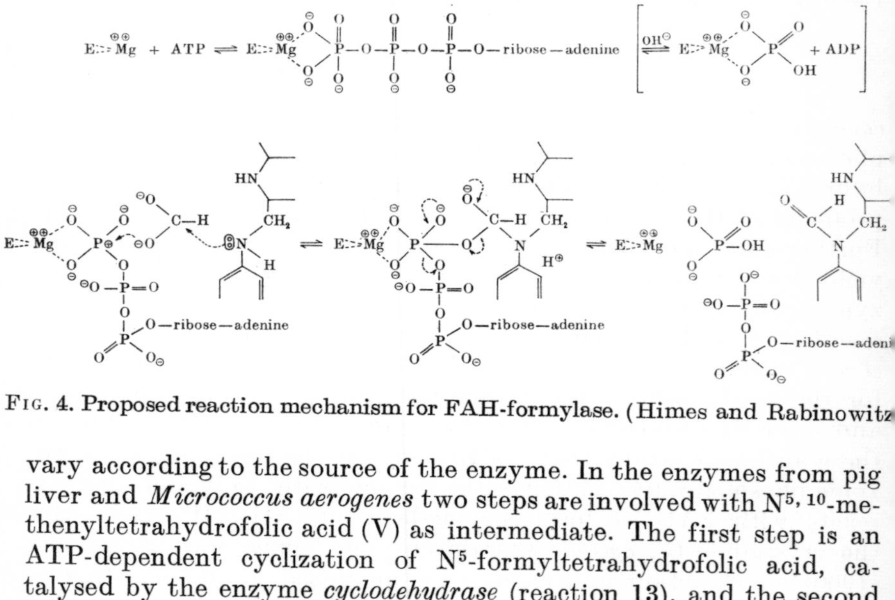

FIG. 4. Proposed reaction mechanism for FAH-formylase. (Himes and Rabinowitz

vary according to the source of the enzyme. In the enzymes from pig
liver and *Micrococcus aerogenes* two steps are involved with $N^{5, 10}$-me-
thenyltetrahydrofolic acid (V) as intermediate. The first step is an
ATP-dependent cyclization of N^5-formyltetrahydrofolic acid, catalysed by the enzyme *cyclodehydrase* (reaction 13), and the second
step is a hydrolysis of the intermediate involving the enzyme *cyclohydrolase* (reaction 14; Peters and D.M. Greenberg, 1958a; Kay
et al., 1960). It is important to note that the compound produced
by sheep liver cyclodehydrase is similar to but not identical with
$N^{5,10}$-methenyltetrahydrofolic acid. Although reaction (14) is a reversible reaction (13) is not, so these reactions do not constitute a

$$N^5\text{-formyl-FAH}_4 + \text{ATP} \xrightarrow{\text{Mg}^{2+}} N^{5,10}\text{-methenyl-FAH}_4 + \text{ADP} + P_i \quad (13)$$
$$N^{5,10}\text{-methenyl-FAH}_4 + \text{H}_2\text{O} \rightleftarrows N^{10}\text{-formyl-FAH}_4 + \text{H}^+ \quad (14)$$

route for the generation of N^5-formyltetrahydrofolic acid. However,
its formation enzymatically from N^{10}-formyltetrahydrofolic acid has

been indicated from experiments of Silverman and Keresztesy (1953) and G.R. Greenberg and Jaenicke (1957).

Buchanan and Hartman (1959) have shown that the cyclized intermediate $N^{5,10}$-methenyltetrahydrofolic acid, is specifically the cofactor for the enzyme *glycinamide ribotide transformylase* which catalyses the transfer of the 1-C unit to glycinamide ribotide to form α-N-formylglycinamide ribotide (reaction 15). This is a key reaction in purine biosynthesis. The other step in purine biosynthesis which also involves 1-C transfer, the conversion of 5-amino-4-imidazolecarboxamide ribotide into inosinic acid via 5-formamido-4-imidazole carboxamide ribotide (16), specifically requires N^{10}-formyltetrahydrofolic acid.

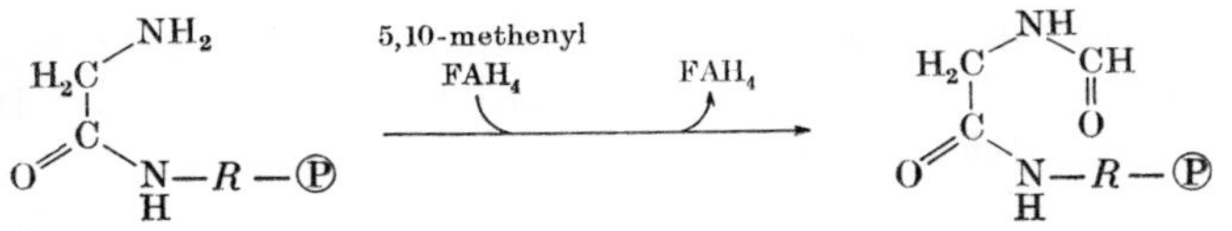

(15)

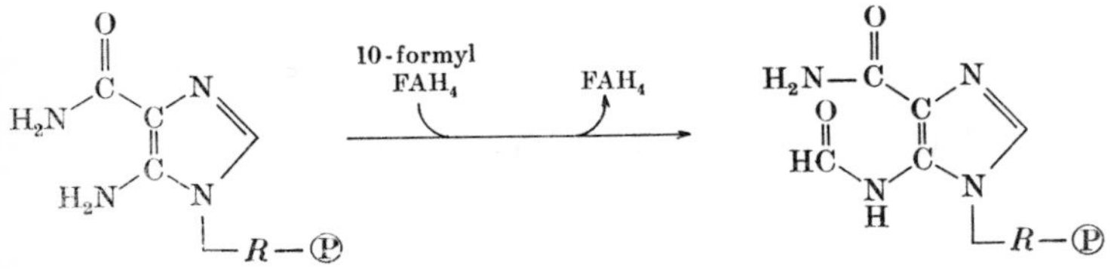

(16)

The cyclodehydrase purified from chick liver does not appear to involve the intermediation of $N^{5,10}$-methenyl-FAH_4 and also differs from the pig liver enzyme in that its pH optimum is 7 whilst that of the latter enzyme is 4 (Kay *et al.*, 1960).

VI. $N^{5,\ 10}$-METHYLENETETRAHYDROFOLIC ACID ("ACTIVE FORMALDEHYDE")

It has been known for some time from tracer studies that formate can be incorporated into various compounds at the oxidation levels of formate (in purines) and of formaldehyde (into the β-carbon atom of serine). Blakley (1954), Kisliuk and Sakami (1954) and G.R. Greenberg and Jaenicke (1958) first reported a NADP-dependent enzyme, *hydroxymethyltetrahydrofolic dehydrogenase* [10-hydroxymethyltetrahydrofolate: NADP oxidoreductase] catalysing the interconversion of N^{10}-formyltetrahydrofolic acid and hydroxymethyltetrahydrofolic acid (reaction 17). Later work with an enzyme purified from chicken liver so that it was free from cyclohydrolase

$$\text{Hydroxymethyl-FAH}_4 + \text{NADP} + \rightleftharpoons \text{N}^{10}\text{-formyl FAH}_4 + \text{NADPH} + \text{H}^+ \quad (17)$$

(reaction 14) revealed that the true substrates were the cyclic compounds $N^{5,10}$-methylene and $N^{5,10}$-methenyltetrahydrofolic acid (reaction 18) (Osborn and Huennekens, 1957; Osborn and Talbert, 1957,

$$\text{N}^{5,10}\text{-Methylene-FaH}_4 + \text{NADP}^+ \rightleftharpoons \text{N}^{5,10}\text{-methenyl-FAH}_4 + \text{NADPH} + \text{H}^+ \quad (18)$$

1958; Silber *et al.*, 1962). The equilibrium position of reaction (18) lies to the left ($K_m = 1{\cdot}7 \times 10^{-2}$ M; Huennekens and Osborn, 1959). Scrimgeour and Huennekens (1960) have reported the existence of a NAD-dependent enzyme which also catalyses reaction 18. The enzyme has also been purified from bakers' yeast; K_m for DL-$N^{5,\,10}$-methylene FAH_4 is $6{\cdot}9 \times 10^{-4}$M and for NADP is $3{\cdot}7 \times 10^{-5}$M (Ramasastri and Blakley, 1962).

The various reactions involving "active formaldehyde" have been discussed by Huennekens and Osborn (1959).

VII. FORMIMINOTETRAHYDROFOLIC ACID

The anaerobe *Cl. cylindrosporum* can utilize purines for growth, and one of the steps in the fermentation of the purines (see Fig. 5) involves

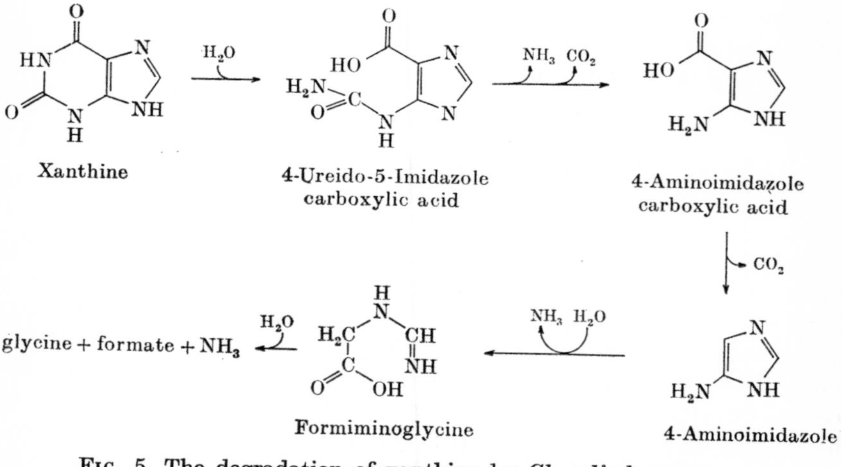

FIG. 5. The degradation of xanthine by *Cl. cylindrosporum*.

the transfer of a formimino group $(HC=NH)$ from formiminoglycine to tetrahydrofolic acid with the liberation of glycine. The reaction (19) is catalysed by the enzyme *glycine formiminotransferase* [N-formiminoglycine: tetrahydrofolate 5-formiminotransferase] and, with an equilibrium constant near unity, is readily reversible. A second enzyme, *formiminotetrahydrofolic cyclodeaminase* [5-formiminotetrahydrofolate ammonia-lyase (cyclizing)] irreversibly deaminates N^5-formiminotetrahydrofolic acid forming $N^{5,\,10}$-methenyltetrahydrofolic acid (reaction 20) (Rabinowitz and Pricer, 1956, 1957b). The enzyme cyclohydrolase (reaction 14) converts $N^{5,\,10}$-

$$\text{N-Formiminoglycine} + \text{FAH}_4 \rightleftharpoons N^5\text{-formimino-FAH}_4 + \text{glycine} \qquad (19)$$

$$N^5\text{-Formimino FAH}_4 \rightarrow N^{5,10}\text{-methenyl FAH}_4 + \text{NH}_3 \qquad (20)$$

methenyl tetrahydrofolic acid into N^{10}-formyltetrahydrofolic acid and this, in the presence of tetrahydrofolic formylase (reaction 7) which represents about 3% of the total cellular protein of *Cl. cylindrosporum* (J. C. Rabinowitz, quoted by Huennekens and Osborn, 1959), is deformylated with the production of ATP. Although the equilibrium of reaction (4) is well over to the right, the overall reaction just described probably represents an important source of ATP for the purine-fermenting anaerobes.

Formiminotetrahydrofolic acid can also be generated during the degradation of histidine by animals (Fig. 2). One of the intermediates is formimino-L-glutamate and an enzyme, *glutamate formiminotransferase*, [N-formimino-L-glutamate:tetrahydrofolate 5-formiminotransferase] which has been obtained from calf (Miller and Waelsch, 1954, 1955, 1956, 1957) and pig liver (Tabor and Rabinowitz, 1956; Tabor and Wyngarden, 1959), transfers the formimino group to N^5 of tetrahydrofolic acid. This compound is then converted into N^{10}-formyltetrahydrofolic acid in the same manner as in the bacterial systems just described. Formimino-L-glutamate is not however a substrate for the bacterial enzyme, glycine formiminotransferase, and furthermore, formiminoglycine is not a substrate for the mammalian formiminotransferase.

It has already been noted (p. 104) that in the bacterial degradation of histidine, formimino-L-glutamate can be hydrolysed with the liberation of formamide as in *A. aerogenes* (Magasanik and Bowser, 1955b) and *Cl. tetanomorphum* (Wachsman and Barker, 1955), or as with *Pseudomonas fluorescens*, glutamate and formate are the resultants with N-formylglutamate an intermediate (Tabor and Mehler, 1954). In both cases the pathway is different from that observed in liver.

VIII. Prefolic Acid, 5-Methyltetrahydrofolate

Donaldson and Keresztesy (1959, 1961) partly purified from un-autolysed liver a material which develops folic acid activity for *Strep. faecalis* R. and *Leuconostoc citrovorum* 8081 only after in-cubation with an enzyme preparation from pig liver. This compound which has been termed prefolic acid, is very probably 5-methyltetrahydrofolate (XXIII), the immediate 1-C donor in methionine biosynthesis (Stevens and Sakami, 1959; Larrabee and Buchanan, 1961; Jaenicke, 1961).

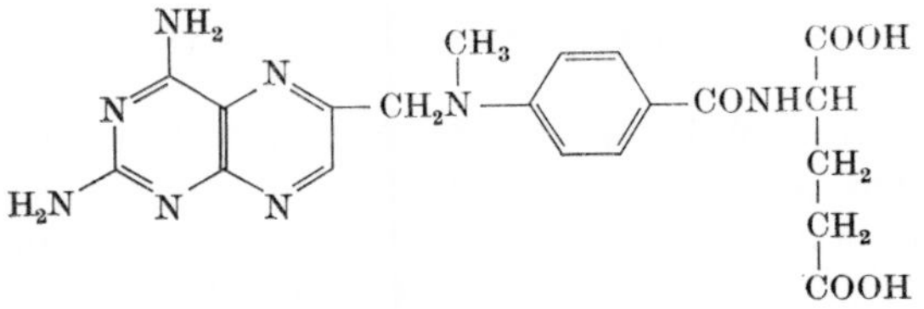

(XXII)

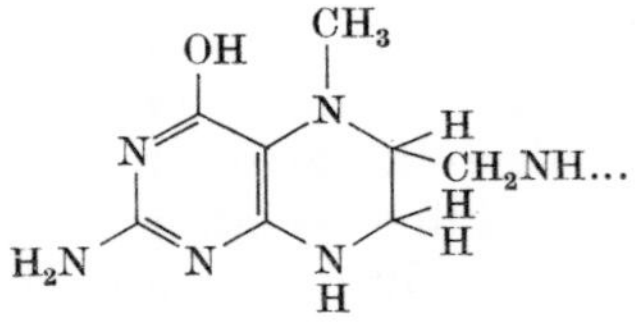

(XXIII)

Prefolic acid, which has been synthesized chemically from FAH_4 and formaldehyde (Keresztesy and Donaldson, 1961), is converted enzymatically into FAH_4 and formate under anaerobic conditions by a FAD-dependent system which also requires menadione as electron acceptor (Donaldson and Keresztesy, 1961). The formation of prefolic acid from $N^{5,10}$-methylene FAH_4 can also be a-chieved with an enzyme preparation from pig liver under anaerobic conditions and in the presence of NADH (Donaldson and Keresztesy, 1961; Jaenicke, 1961).

The discovery of prefolic acid in unautolysed liver may have some connection with an early observation that the growth-promoting effect for *Strep. faecalis* R and *Leuconostoc citrovorum* 8081 of a hot water extract of fresh horse liver was only 2% of that of a similar extract of autolysed liver (Chang, 1953).

IX. Vitamin B_{12} and Folic Acid Interconversions

A variety of investigations over the past few years has implicated vitamin B_{12} in the biosynthesis of 1-C units (see e.g. Hutner *et al.*, 1959) but only recently has the locus of action been pinpointed. Dinning *et al.* (1958) followed up the observation of Deibel *et al.* (1956) that thymidine replaced folic acid and vitamin B_{12} in the nutrition of *Lactobacillus leishmannii*, and found that vitamin B_{12} increased the incorporation of [^{14}C]formate into DNA-thymine fivefold, whilst the degree of incorporation of [3-^{14}C]serine, [2-^{14}C]glycine or [^{14}C-methyl]methionine was unaffected. Similar results were obtained with bone marrow cells, and the observations were extended to show that the incorporation of formaldehyde was not stimulated by the addition of vitamin B_{12} (Dinning and Young, 1959). All these results indicated that vitamin B_{12} was concerned with the reduction of "active formate" to "active formaldehyde", that is, it appeared to act as a co-factor for hydroxymethyltetrahydrofolic dehydrogenase (see p.) Roberts and Nichol (1962) could not confirm this in *Lact. leishmannii*, but support for Dinning's conclusion comes from the observations that the activity of this enzyme is reduced in the bone marrow and liver of vitamin B_{12}-deficient chicks and that addition of vitamin B_{12} to the bone marrow enzyme stimulated its activity Dinning and Hogan, 1960). Addition of vitamin B_{12} to the partly purified liver enzyme from which most of the vitamin B_{12} had been removed stimulated activity (Henderson and Dinning, 1962). The observations by Guest *et al.* (1960) and Guest and Woods (1961) on *Esch. coli* strain 121/176 that a vitamin B_{12} coenzyme is concerned with the formation of methionine from folic acid and a 1-C precursor, have been confirmed and extended by Larrabee and Buchanan (1961) and Hatch *et al.* (1961) using *Esch. coli* strain 205-2. They found that the B_{12} coenzyme is not required by hydroxymethyltetrahydrofolic dehydrogenase, but by an enzyme which transfers the 1-C group from, presumably, N^5-methyltetrahydrofolic acid to a methionine precursor (see also p. 189).

X. Folic Acid Synthesis by Viruses

In 1958 Colon and Moulder found that the psittacosis group of viruses (mouse pneumonitis and meningopneumonitis) was susceptible to the sulphonamide group of drugs, which suggested that the viruses contained enzymes requiring or synthesizing folic acid coenzymes. Later Colon (1959) showed that these organisms synthesize folic acid derivatives when incubated at $37°$ in the allantoic fluid of chick embryos, and he has provided good evidence that they were synthesized by constituent enzymes of the viruses and not of the growth medium.

XI. Pteridines Related to Folic Acid

As noted at the beginning of this Chapter, xanthopterin (IX) and isoxanthopterin (XIII) are widely distributed in the lower animals; they have also been isolated from mammalian urine. However, the presence of the former in urine is now considered to be an artefact. Floystrup et al. (1949) and Slavik et al. (1957) for example, could not find xanthopterin in urine, but did find a colourless, non-fluorescent material which gave rise to xanthopterin on atmospheric oxidation; furthermore, Blair (1958a) found no xanthopterin in normal kidney tissue, and xanthopterin injected into hamsters was converted into leucopterin (X) which is not found in human urine. As Blakley (1957) demonstrated the spontaneous formation of xanthopterin from tetrahydrofolic acid and Slavik and Slavikova (1958) found xanthopterin in the urine of rats fed tetrahydrofolic acid, Blair concluded that urinary xanthopterin is an artefact. Support for this view comes from work on the action of xanthine oxidase on various pteridines; Bergmann and Kwietny (1958) foundthat oxidation of the parent pteridine, 2,-4-, and 7-monohydroxypteridines and 2,4-dihydroxypteridine resulted in the formation of 2,3,7-trihydroxypteridine in every case; no 6-hydroxy (xanthopterin) derivative was ever formed, and 6-hydroxypteridine was not attacked by the enzyme. It would appear that the 6-hydroxy function of xanthopterin could not arise by the action of xanthine oxidase on appropriate precursors. These observations also indicate that leucopterin formed from xanthopterin by xanthine oxidase is a terminal metabolite of pteridine metabolism and corresponds to uric acid in purine metabolism. The pathway of the formation of these compounds is visualized in reaction (21).

Folic acid →

→tetrahydrofolicacid $\xrightarrow{\text{spontaneously}}$ xanthopterin $\xrightarrow{\text{xanthine oxidase}}$ leucopterin (21)

All evidence available indicates that isoxanthopterin (XIII) arises via a different route, with 2-amino-4-hydroxpteridine (XI) as the immediate precursor. For example, (a) 2-amino-4-hydroxypteridine accumulates in the maroon mutant of Drosophila which lacks xanthine oxidase (Glassman et al., 1958); (b) 2-amino-4-hydroxypteridine is converted into isoxanthopterin by xanthine oxidase obtained from both cream and wild type *Drosophila* (Forrest *et al.*, 1956); (c) the *white-apricot* mutant of *Drosophila,* which normally lacks 2-amino-4-hydroxypteridine but contains xanthine oxidase, will produce isoxanthopterin when fed 2-amino-4-hydroxypteridine

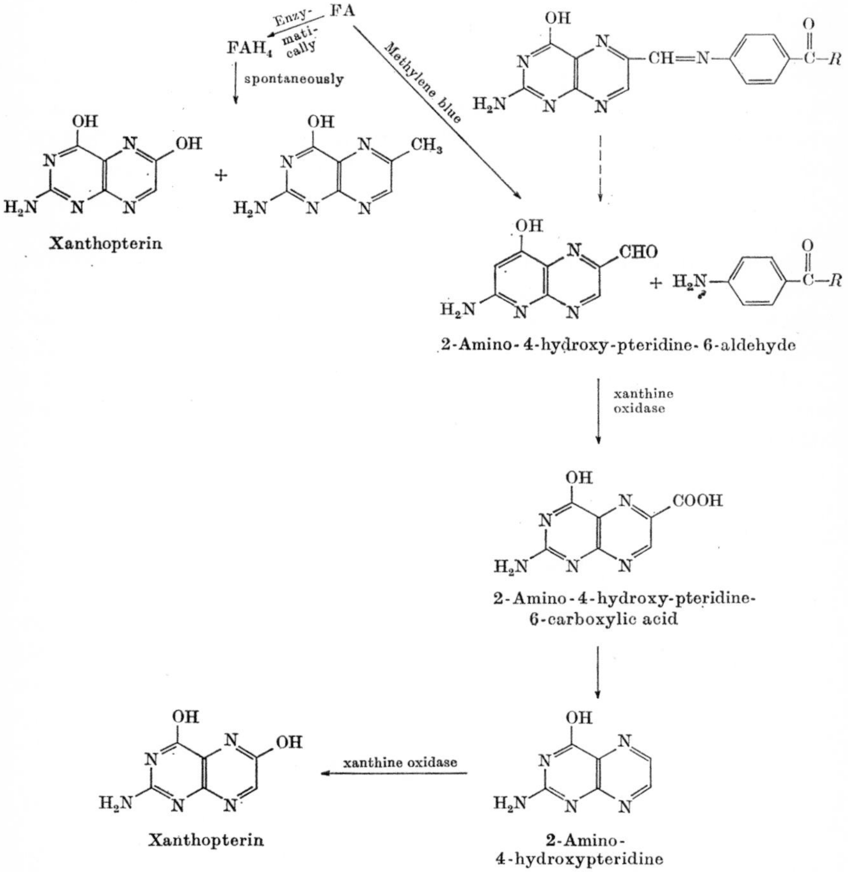

FIG. 6. Possible route of conversion of folic acid into xanthopterin. Dotted lines indicate hypothetical steps.

(Forrest *et al.*, 1956). The steps between folic acid and 2-amino-4-hydroxypteridine are not completely clear but Blair (1958b) has proposed the scheme illustrated in Fig. 6. Folic acid is itself not attacked by xanthine oxidase but, if incubated with the enzyme and methylene blue, 2-amino-4-hydroxypteridine-6-carboxylic acid (XII) is formed. This is the result of methylene blue converting folic acid into 2-amino-4-hydroxypteridine-6-aldehyde

(XVI), which is then acted upon by xanthine oxidase (Blair, 1957a). A biological agent carrying out the first step has not yet been described. 2-Amino-4-hydroxypteridine-6-aldehyde has also not yet been found in nature, and although it is apparently a substrate for xanthine oxidase when used in very low concentrations, it is also the most potent inhibitor of xanthine oxidase known (De Renso, 1956). 2-Amino-4-hydroxypteridine-6-carboxylic acid is present, *inter alia* in the skin of the green mamba *Dendroaspis viridis* (Blair, 1957b) but not in human urine (Blair, 1958b); its enzymatic decarboxylation has not yet been observed, although it can easily be achieved by heat and ultraviolet irradiation.

It should be pointed out that folic acid is not necessarily the source of all the pteridines which occur naturally (see p.   ).

The biosynthetic route to biopterin (VIII) with its three additional carbon atoms at C-6, has already been discussed on p. 108. It is sufficient here to report the recent isolation from *Esch. coli* of small amounts of (2-amino-4 hydroxy-6-pteridinyl) glycerol phosphate (XXIV; Goto and Forrest, 1961); this is biopterin phosphate and, by analogy with biopterin, which arises from guanosine, could arise from guanylic acid.

(XXIV)

REFERENCES

Andreeva, N. A. (1953). *Biochemistry, Lening.* **18,** 675.
Angier, R. B., Stokstad, E. R. L., Mowat, J. H., Hutchings, B. L., Boothe, J. H., Waller, C. W., Semb, J., Subba Row, Y., Cosulich, D. B., Fahrenback, M. J., Hultquist, M. E., Kuhn, E., Northey, E. H., Seeger, E. R., Sickels, J. P., and Smith, J. M. (1948). *J. Amer. chem. Soc.* **70,** 25.
Aughagen, E. (1943). *Hoppe-Seyl. Z.* **70,** 25.
Baldridge, R. C., and Burket, R. (1960). *Fed. Proc.* **19,** 4.
Bergmann, F., and Kwietny, H. (1958). *Biochim. biophys. Acta* **28,** 613.
Bertino, J. R. (1962). *Biochim. biophys. Acta* **58,** 377.
Blair, J. A. (1957a). *Biochem. J.* **65,** 209.
Blair, J. A. (1957b). *Nature, Lond.* **180,** 1371.
Blair, J. A. (1958a). *Nature, Lond.* **181,** 996.
Blair, J. A. (1958b). *Biochem. J.* **68,** 385.
Blair, J. A. (1961). *Nature, Lond.* **192,** 757.
Blakley, R. L. (1954). *Biochem. J.* **58,** 448.

Blakley, R. L. (1957). *Biochem. J.* **65,** 331.
Blakley, R. L., and McDougall, B. M. (1961). *J. biol. Chem.* **236,** 1163.
Braganca, B. M., and Kenkare, U. W. (1959). *Nature, Lond.* **184,** 1488.
Braganca, B. M., Krishnamurthi, V., and Ghanekar, D. S. (1960). *In* "Proceedings of the 4th International Congress of Biochemistry, Vienna" XI, 109. Pergamon Press, London.
Brown, D. D., and Kies, M. W. (1960). *J. biol. Chem.* **234,** 3182, 3188.
Brenner – Holzach, O. and Leuthardt, F. (1961) *Helv. chim. Acta* **44,** 1480.
Brown, G. M. (1959). *Fed. Proc.* **18,** 19; *Int. Congr. Chem.* **17,** Vol. 2, 28.
Brown, G. M. (1960). *Physiol. Rev.* **40,** 331.
Brown, G. M. (1961). "Abstract of the 5th International Congress of Biochemistry Moscow", p. 101. Pergamon Press, London.
Brown, G. M., (1962). *J. biol. Chem.* **237,** 536.
Brown, G. M., Weisman, R. A., and Molnar, D. (1960). "Abstract of the 5th International Congress of Nutrition", p. 44.
Brown, G. M., Weisman, R. A., and Molnar, D. (1961). *J. biol. Chem.* **236,** 2534.
Buchanan, J. M., and Hartman, S. C. (1959). *Advanc. Enzymol.* **21,** 200.
Butenandt, A., and Rembold, H. (1958). *Hoppe-Seyl. Z.* **311,** 79.
Byers, E. H., Stewart, J., and Bond, T. J. (1961). *Nature, Lond.* **191,** 179.
Chang, S. C. (1953). *J. biol. Chem.* **200,** 827.
Colon, J. I. (1959). *J. Bact.* **79,** 741.
Colon, J. I., and Moulder, J. W. (1958). *J. infect. Dis.* **103,** 109.
Deibel, R. H., Dowing, M., Niven, C. F., Jr., and Schweigert, B. S. (1956). *J. Bact.* **71,** 255.
De Renzo, E. C. (1956). *Advanc. Enzymol.* **17,** 293.
Dinning, J. S., and Young, R. S. (1959). *J. biol. Chem.* **234,** 1199, 3241.
Dinning, J. S., and Hogan, R. (1960). *Fed. Proc.* **19,** 418.
Dinning, J. S., Allen, B. K., Young, R. S., and Day, P. L. (1958). *J. biol. Chem.* **233,** 674.
Donaldson, K. O., and Keresztesy, J. C. (1959). *J. biol. Chem.* **234,** 3235.
Donaldson, K. O., and Keresztesy, J. C. (1961). *Fed. Proc.* **20,** 453; *Biochem. biophys. Res. Comm.* **5,** 289.
Elion, G. B., Hitchings, G. H., Sherwood, M. B., and Van der Werff, H. (1950). *Arch. Biochem. Biophys.* **26,** 337.
Ericson, L. E. (1954). *Ark. Kemi.* **6,** 503.
Erismann, K. H. (1962). *Intern. Z. Vitaminforsch.* **32,** 36.
Feinberg, R. H., and Greenberg, D. M. (1958). *Nature, Lond.* **181,** 897.
Floystrup, T., Schou, M. A., and Kalckar, H. (1949). *Acta. chem. scand.* **3,** 985.
Forrest, H. S. (1960). *Int. Congr. Chem.* **17,** Vol. 2, 40.
Forrest, H. S., and Mitchell, H. K. (1955). *J. Amer. chem. Soc.* **77,** 4865.
Forrest, H. S., Glassman, E., and Mitchell, H. K. (1956). *Science,* **124,** 725.
Fox, D. L., (1953). "Animal Biochromes and Structural Colours". Cambridge University Press, London.
Futterman, S. (1957). *J. biol. Chem.* **228,** 1031.
Futterman, S., and Silverman, M. (1956). *J. biol. Chem.* **224,** 31.
Glassman, E., Hubby, J. L., and Mitchell, H. K. (1958). *In* "Proceedings of the 10th Inst. Congress of Genetics" p. 98.
Goodwin, T. W. (1960). "Recent Advances in Biochemistry". Churchill, London.
Goto, M., and Forrest, H. S. (1961). *Biochem. biophys. Res. Comm.* **6,** 180.
Greenberg, G. R. (1954). *J. Amer. chem. Soc.* **76,** 1458.
Greenberg, G. R., and Jaenicke, L. (1957). *In* "The Chemistry and Biology of Purines", p. 204. (G. E. W. Wolstenholme, and C. M. O'Connor, eds). Churchill, London.

Guest, J. R., Helleiner, C. W., Cross, M. J., and Woods, D. D. (1960) *Biochem. J.* **76**, 396.

Guest, J. R., and Woods, D. D. (1961) "International Symposium on Vitamin B_{12} and Intrinsic Factor." Hamburg. 2nd Meeting.

Hakala, M. T., Zakrzewski, S. F., and Nichol, C. A. (1961). *J. biol. Chem.* **236**, 952.

Hatch, F. T., Larrabee, A. R., Cathou, R. E., and Buchanan, J. M. (1961) *J. biol. Chem.* **236**, 1095.

Henderson, R. F., and Dinning, J. S. (1962). *Fed. Proc.* **21**, 471.

Himes, R. H., and Rabinowitz, J. C. (1960). *Fed. Proc.* **19**, 47.

Himes, R. H., and Rabinowitz, J. C. (1962). *J. biol. Chem.* **237**, 2903, 2915.

Huennekens, F. M., and Osborn, M. J. (1959). *Advanc. Enzymol.* **21**, 369.

Huennekens, F. M., and Osborn, M. J. (1960). *In* "Proceedings of the 4th International Congress of Biochemistry, Vienna", XI, 112. Pergamon Press, London.

Hutchings, B. L., Stokstad, E. L. R., Bokonos, N., Sloane, N. H., and Subba Row, Y. (1948). *J. Amer. chem. Soc.* **70**, 1.

Hutner, S. H., Nathan, H. A., and Baker. H. (1959). *Vitam. & Horm.* **17**, 1.

Ishii, K., and Sevag, M. G. (1957). *Bact. Proc.* 71.

Iwai, K. and Yoshida, T. (1954). *Bull. Res. Inst. Food. Sci., Kyoto Univ.* **15**, 115

Jaenicke, L. (1958). "Abstracts of the 4th International Congress of Biochemistry, Vienna", p. 47. Pergamon Press, London.

Jaenicke, L. (1961). *Angew. Chem.* **73**, 449; *Hoppe-Seyl. Z.* **326**, 168.

Jaenicke, L. and Brode, E. (1961) *Biochem. Z.* **334**, 108, 342.

Jaenicke, L., and Chan, P. C. (1960). *Angew. Chem.* **72**, 752.

Jukes, T. H., and Broquist, H. P. (1961). *In* "Metabolic Pathways", **2**, 713. (D. M. Greenberg, ed.) Academic Press, New York and London.

Katunuma, N., and Shoda, T. (1958). *Chem. Abstr.* **52**, 6488.

Katunuma, N., Shoda, T., and Noda, H. (1956). *Vitamins (Kyoto)*, **11**, 322.

Katunuma, N., Shoda, T., and Noda, H. (1957). *J. Vitaminol. (Osaka)*, **3**, 77.

Kay, L. D., Osborn, M. J., Hatefi, Y., and Huennekens, F. M. (1960). *J. biol. Chem.* **235**, 195.

Kenkare, U. W., and Braganca, B. M. (1962). *Biochem. J.* **86**, 160.

Keresztesy, J. C., and Donaldson, K. O. (1961). *Biochem. biophys. Res. Comm.* **5**, 286.

Keresztesy, J. C., Rickes, E. L., and Stokes, J. L. (1943). *Science*, **97**, 465.

Kisliuk, R. L., and Sakami, W. (1954). *J. Amer. chem. Soc.* **76**, 1456.

Koizumu, T., Uchida, M., and Ichihara, K. (1956). *J. Biochem., Tokyo*, **43**, 345.

Korte, F., and Synnatschke, G. (1959). *Liebigs Ann.* **628**, 153.

Korte, F., Weitkamp, H., and Schicke, H. G. (1957). *Ber. dtsch. chem. Ges.* **90**, 1100.

Korte, F., Barkemeyer, H., and Synnatschke, G. (1959). *Hoppe-Seyl. Z.* **314**, 106.

Lampen, J. O., and Jones, M. J. (1946). *J. biol. Chem.* **166**, 435.

Lampen, J. O., and Jones, M. J. (1947). *J. biol. Chem.* **170**, 133.

Larrabee, A. R., and Buchanan, J. M. (1961). *Fed. Proc.* **20**, 9.

Lascelles, J., and Woods, D. D. (1952). *Brit. J. exp. Path.* **33**, 288.

Lascelles, J., and Woods, D. D. (1954). *Biochem. J.* **58**, 486.

Magasanik, B., and Bowser, H. R. (1955a). *In* "Amino Acid Metabolism", p. 398. (W.D. McElroy and H. B. Glass, eds.) John Hopkins Press, Baltimore.

Magasanik, B., and Bowser, H. R. (1955b). *J. biol. Chem.* **213**, 571.

Maley, G. F., and Plaut, G. W. E. (1958). *Fed. Proc.* **17**, 268.

Mathews, C. K., and Huennekens, F. M. (1961). *Fed. Proc.* **20**, 453.

McNutt, W. S., and Forrest, H. S., (1958). *J. Amer. chem. Soc.* **80**, 951.

Miller, A., and Waelsch, H. (1954). *J. Amer. chem. Soc.* **76,** 6195.
Miller, A., and Waelsch, H. (1955). *Biochim. biophys. Acta,* **17,** 278.
Miller, A., and Waelsch, H. (1956). *Arch. Biochem. Biophys.* **63,** 263.
Miller, A., and Waelsch, H. (1957). *J. biol. Chem.* **228,** 383, 397.
Möller, E. F., Weygand, F., and Wacker, A. (1949). *Z. Naturforsch.* **46,** 100.
Mowat, J. H., Boothe, J. H., Hutchings, B. L., Stokstad, E. L. R., Waller, C. W., Angier, R. B., Semb J., Cosulich, D. B., and Subba Row, Y. (1948). *J. Amer. chem. Soc.* **70,** 14.
Nath, R., and Greenberg, D. M. (1962). *Biochemistry* **1,** 435.
Nichol, C. A. (1954). *J. biol. Chem.* **207,** 725.
Nimmo-Smith, R. H., and Woods, D. D. (1948). *J. gen. Microbiol.* **2,** x.
Osborn, M. J., and Huennekens, F. M. (1957). *Biochim. biophys. Acta* **26,** 646.
Osborn, M. J., and Talbert, P. T. (1957). *Fed. Proc.* **16,** 230.
Osborn, M. J., and Talbert, P. T. (1958). *J. biol. Chem.* **233,** 989.
Osborn, M. J., Hatefi, Y., Kay, L. D., and Huennekens, F. M. (1957). *Biochim. biophys. Acta* **26,** 208.
Patterson, E. L., Milstrey, R., and Stokstad, E. L. R. (1956). *J. Amer. chem. Soc.* **78,** 5868.
Patterson, E. L., Milstrey, R., and Stokstad, E. L. R. (1958). *J. Amer. chem. Soc.* **80,** 2018.
Peters, J. M., and Greenberg, D. M. (1958a). *J. Amer. chem. Soc.* **80,** 6679.
Peters, J. M., and Greenberg, D. M. (1958b). *Nature, Lond.* **181,** 1669.
Peters, J. M., and Greenberg, D. M. (1959). *Biochim. biophys. Acta* **32,** 273.
Pfiffner, J. J., Binkley, S. B., Bloom, E. S., Brown, R. A., Bird, O. D., Emmett, A. D., Hogan, A. G., and O'Dell, B. L. (1943). *Science* **94,** 404.
Pfiffner, J. J., Catkins, D. G., Bloom, E. S., and O'Dell, B. L. (1946). *J. Amer. chem. Soc.* **68,** 1392.
Pfiffner, J. J., Binkley, S. B., Bloom, E. S., and O'Dell, B. L. (1947). *J. Amer. chem. Soc.* **69,** 1476.
Plaut, G. W. E. (1961). *Annu. Rev. Biochem.* **30,** 409.
Plaut, G. W. E., and Maley, G. F. (1959). *Arch. Biochem. Biophys.* **80,** 219.
Rabinowitz, J. C., and Pricer, W. E., Jr. (1956). *J. Amer. chem. Soc.* **78,** 5702.
Rabinowitz, J. C., and Pricer, W. E., Jr. (1957a). *J. biol. Chem.* **229,** 321.
Rabinowitz, J. C., and Pricer, W. E., Jr. (1957b). *Fed. Proc.* **16,** 236.
Rabinowitz, J. C., and Pricer, W. E., Jr. (1962). *J. biol. Chem.* **237,** 2898.
Rabinowitz, J. C., and Himes, R. H. (1960). *Fed. Proc.* **19,** 963.
Ramasastri, B. V., and Blakley, R. L. (1962). *J. biol. Chem.* **237,** 1982.
Rao, D. R., and Greenberg, D. M. (1960). *Biochem. biophys. Res. Comm.* **2,** 264.
Reid, B. L., and Couch, J. R. (1955). *Arch. Biochem. Biophys.* **56,** 388.
Revel, H. R. B., and Magasanik, B. (1958). *J. biol. Chem.* **233,** 930.
Reynolds, J. .J., and Brown, G. M. (1962). *J. biol. Chem.* **237,** PC 2713.
Roberts, DeW., and Nichol, C. A. (1962). *Fed. Proc.* **21,** 470.
Sankar, D. B., and Sankar, D. V. S. (1961). "Proceedings of the 5th International Congress of Biochemistry, Moscow," p. 296. Pergamon Press, London.
Scrimgeour, K. G., and Huennekens, F. M. (1960). *Biochem. biophys. Res. Comm.* **2,** 230.
Sebrell, W. H., Jr., and Harris, R. S. (1954). "The Vitamins", Vol. III. Academic Press, New York.
Shaw, E., and Viera, E. (1961). *Fed. Proc.* **20,** 454; *J. biol. Chem.* **236,** 2507.
Shiota, T. (1958). *Bact. Proc.* 113.
Shiota, T. (1959). *Arch. Biochem. Biophys.* **80,** 155.
Shiota, T., and Disraely, M. N. (1961). *Biochim. biophys. Acta* **52,** 467.

Shiota, T., Disraely, M.N., and McCann, P. (1962). *Biochem. biophys. Res. Comm.* **7,** 194.
Silber, R., Huennekens, F. N., and Gabrio, B. W. (1962). *Arch. Biochem. Biophys.* **99,** 328.
Silverman, M., and Keresztesy, J. C., (1953). *Fed. Proc.* **12,** 268.
Silverman, M., Keresztesy, J. C., Koval, G. J., and Gardiner, R. C. (1957). *J. biol. Chem.* **226,** 83.
Sims, K. A., and Woods, D. D. (1950). *J. gen. Microbiol.* **4,** ii.
Slavik, K., and Slavikova, V. (1958). "Abstract of the Proceedings of the 4th International Congress of Biochemistry, Vienna", p. 95. Pergamon Press, London.
Slavik, K., Dvorakova, A., and Slavikova, V. (1957). *Chem. Listy* **51,** 1536.
Stevens, A., and Sakami, W. (1959). *J. biol. Chem.* **234,** 2063.
Stokes, J. L., and Larsen, A. (1945). *J. Bact.* **50,** 219.
Srinivasan, P. R., and Weiss, B. (1961). *Biochim. biophys. Acta* **51,** 597.
Stokstad, E. L. R. (1943). *J. biol. Chem.* **149,** 573.
Stokstad, E. L. R., Hutchings, B. L., Mowat, J. H., Boothe, J. H., Waller, C. W., Angier, R. B., Semb, J., and Subba Row, Y. (1948). *J. Amer. chem. Soc.* **70,** 5.
Tabor, H., and Mehler, A. H. (1954). *J. biol. Chem.* **210,** 559.
Tabor, H., and Hayaishi, O. (1952). *J. biol. Chem.* **194,** 171.
Tabor, H., and Rabinowitz, J. C. (1956). *J. Amer. chem. Soc.* **78,** 5705.
Tabor, H., and Wyngarden, L. (1959). *J. biol. Chem.* **234,** 1830.
Tschesche, R. (1947). *Z. Naturforsch.* **2**b, 10. .
Tschesche, R., and Korte, F. (1953). *Z. Naturforsch.* 8b, 87.
Wachsman, J. T., and Barker, H. A. (1955). *J. Bact.* **69,** 83.
Wacker, A., Ebert, M., and Kolm, H. (1958). *Z. Naturforsch.* **13**b, 141.
Weiss, **B., and Srinivasan, P. R.** (1959). *Proc. nat. Acad. Sci., Wash.* 1491.
Werkheiser, W. C. (1961). *J. biol. Chem.,* **236,** 888.
Weygand, F., and Waldschmidt, M. (1955). *Angew. Chem.* **67,** 327.
Weygand, F., Möller, E. F., and Wacker, A. (1949). *Z. Naturforsch.* 4b, 269.
Weygand, F., Wacker, A., Trebst, A., and Swoboda, O. P. (1956). *Z. Naturforsch.* **11b,** 689.
Weygand, F., Simon, H., Dahms, G., Waldschmidt, M., Schliep, H. J., and Wacker, A. (1961). *Angew. Chem.* **73,** 402.
Whiteley, H. R., Osborn, M. J., and Huennekens, F. M. (1958a). *J. Amer. chem. Soc.* **80,** 757.
Whiteley, H. R., Osborn, M. J., Talbert, P. T., and Huennekens, F. M. (1958b). *Fed. Proc.* **17,** 334.
Wickremasinghe, R. L., and Fry B. A. (1954). *Biochem. J.* **58,** 268.
Wieland, H., Tartter, A., and Purrmann, R. (1940). *Liebigs Ann.* **545,** 209.
Woods, D. D. (1960). *In* "Proceedings of the 4th International Congress of Biochemistry Vienna". XI, 89. Pergamon Press, London.
Wright, B. E., and Anderson, M. L. (1957). *J. Amer. chem. Soc.* **79,** 2027.
Wright, B. E., Anderson, M. L., and Herman, E. C. (1958). *J. biol. Chem.* **230,** 271.
Zakrzewski, S. F. (1960). *J. biol. Chem.* **235,** 1776, 1780.
Zakrezwski, S. F., and Nichol, C. A. (1955). *J. biol. Chem.* **213,** 697.
Ziegler, I. (1961). *Naturwissenschaften* **48,** 458.
Ziegler-Günder, I. (1956). *Biol. Rev.* **31,** 313.
Ziegler Günder, I., Simon, H., and Wacker, A. (1956). *Z. Naturforsch.* **11b,** 82.

CHAPTER 5

PANTOTHENIC ACID AND COENZYME A

I. INTRODUCTION

As with nearly all the water-soluble vitamins, the history of the isolation and identification of pantothenic acid as a *bona fide* vitamin is characterized by considerable confusion; this has been well described by Robinson (1951) and by Lepkovsky (1954).

The fact that R. J. Williams managed to determine the chemical structure of pantothenic acid under these circumstances merely emphasizes his great achievement. The first clue to the structure of pantothenic acid, which Williams had isolated from liver and found to be widely distributed in plants and animals, came when Weinstock *et al.* (1939) reported the isolation of β-alanine from alkali-inactivated pantothenic acid. This also indicated that the chick anti-dermatitis factor previously isolated from liver by Elvehjem and Koehn (1935) and Lepkovsky and Jukes (1936) was probably identical with pantothenic acid, because Woolley *et al.* (1939) had found that β-alanine could be isolated from the factor following alkali-treatment.

The nature of the other cleavage product was finally shown by Williams and Major (1940) to be the lactone of αγ-dihydroxy-ββ-dimethylbutyric acid (pantoic acid) (I); this compound when condensed with β-alanine yielded racemic pantothenic acid (II).

$$CH_3$$
$$CH_2OHCCH(OH)COOH$$
$$CH_3$$
(I)

$$CH_3$$
$$CH_2OHCCH(OH)CONHCH_2CH_2COOH$$
$$CH_3$$
(II)

The realization that pantothenic acid itself was not the functional form of the vitamin began with the observation of Lipmann in 1945 (see Lipmann 1954) that a coenzyme (coenzyme A) was involved in the acetylation of sulphonamides by cell-free systems from pigeon liver, and that this coenzyme contained "bound" pantothenic acid (Lipmann *et al.* 1947). A turning point in the structural studies on coenzyme A was the discovery by Lynen *et al.* (1951) that "active acetate" was an acyl mercaptan. By 1952 almost pure coenzyme A had been obtained and it was clear that it contained 1 mole of adenine, 3 moles of phosphate, of which one mole was a phosphomonoester, and one atom of sulphur (Gregory *et al.*, 1952). A combination of enzymatic degradations and enzymatic syntheses carried out mainly by Novelli and Kaplan and their colleagues (see e.g. Novelli, 1953) eventually revealed the structure of coenzyme A as indicated in formula (III). The fact that some of the biosynthetic steps as originally formulated in deducing the structure are now known to be incorrect in detail (see p. 139) does not

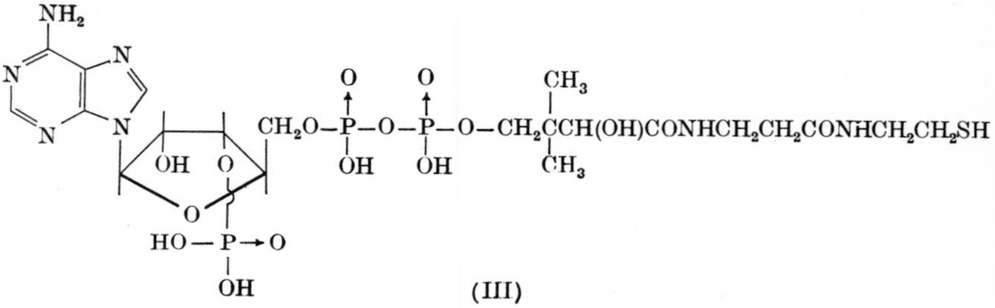

$$CH_2O-P-O-P-O-CH_2CCH(OH)CONHCH_2CH_2CONHCH_2CH_2SH$$

(III)

$$CH_2OHCCH(OH)CONHCH_2CH_2CONHCH_2CH_2SH$$

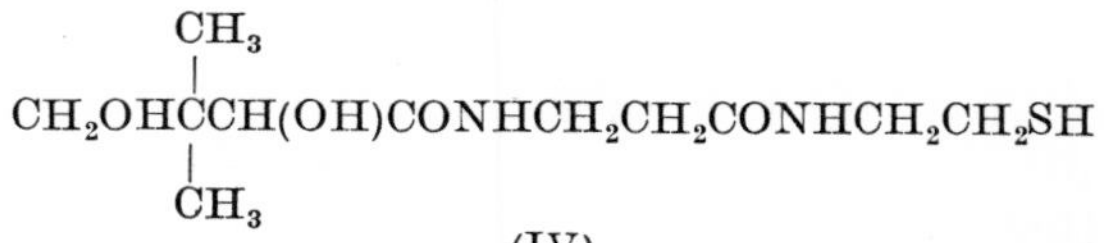

(IV)

alter the conclusions drawn nor detract from the elegance of the approach. The same conclusions were also reached by Lynen *et al.* (1951). The sulphur-containing residue which remains after removal of the nucleotide is N-pantothenyl-thioethylamine (pantetheine, IV; Snell *et al.*, 1950).

II. BIOSYNTHETIC PATHWAYS

A. *Pantothenic acid*

The three specific reactions leading to the formation of pantothenic acid are indicated in Fig. 1. The experiments which originally revealed this pathway were mainly nutritional in which pantothenic acid-requiring mutants of *Escherichia coli* and *Neursopora crassa* were used. The suggestion that the final step was the condensation of β-alanine and pantoic acid was first put on a firm

basis by Maas and Davis (1950) who obtained a series of pantothenate auxotrophs of *Esch. coli* which fell into three main groups;

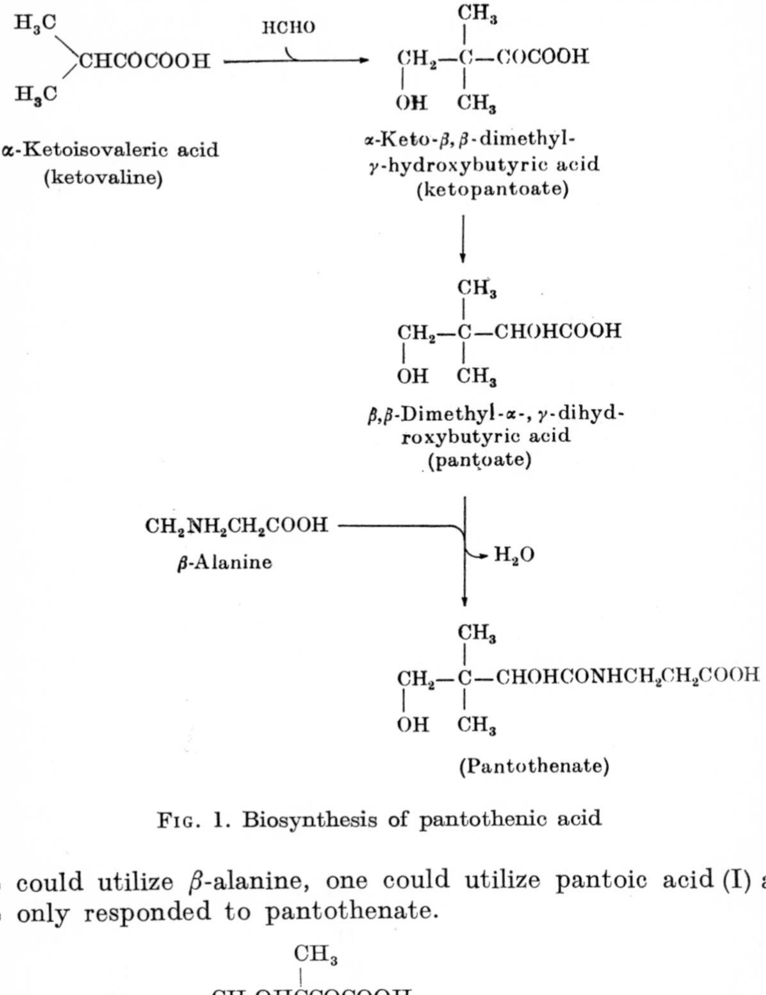

$$\begin{array}{c} H_3C \\ \\ H_3C \end{array}\!\!\!> CHCOCOOH \xrightarrow{\ \ HCHO\ \ } \begin{array}{c} CH_3 \\ | \\ CH_2-C-COCOOH \\ | \qquad | \\ OH \quad CH_3 \end{array}$$

α-Ketoisovaleric acid
(ketovaline)

α-Keto-β,β-dimethyl-
γ-hydroxybutyric acid
(ketopantoate)

$$\begin{array}{c} CH_3 \\ | \\ CH_2-C-CHOHCOOH \\ | \qquad | \\ OH \quad CH_3 \end{array}$$

β,β-Dimethyl-α-,γ-dihyd-
roxybutyric acid
(pantoate)

CH$_2$NH$_2$CH$_2$COOH ⎯⎯⎯

β-Alanine

H$_2$O

$$\begin{array}{c} CH_3 \\ | \\ CH_2-C-CHOHCONHCH_2CH_2COOH \\ | \qquad | \\ OH \quad CH_3 \end{array}$$

(Pantothenate)

Fig. 1. Biosynthesis of pantothenic acid

one could utilize β-alanine, one could utilize pantoic acid (I) and
one only responded to pantothenate.

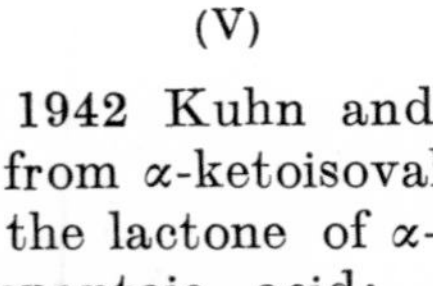

$$\begin{array}{c} CH_3 \\ | \\ CH_2OHCCOCOOH \\ | \\ CH_3 \end{array}$$

(V)

As long ago as 1942 Kuhn and Wieland synthesized pantoyl
lactone chemically from α-ketoisovaleric acid (ketovaline, dimethyl
pyruvic acid) via the lactone of α-keto- β, β-dimethyl-γ-hydroxy-
butyric acid (ketopantoic acid; V) and showed that yeast
could convert the lactone of ketopantoic acid into the lactone of

pantoic acid (I). They suggested that valine was the precursor of pantoate; this is true in the sense that if valine is present in the culture medium it can be converted into pantoate; but the endogenous source of both pantoate and valine is α-ketoisovaleric acid.
This was first demonstrated by Maas (1952) who extended an earlier observation of Ivanovics (1942) that salicylate in low concentrations inhibits the growth of bacteria which are capable of synthesizing their own pantothenic acid, whilst it has no effect on those
which require exogenous pantothenate for growth. Maas found
that salicylate inhibition is reversed non-competitively by pantothenate, pantoate or ketopantoate; valine and α-ketoisovaleric acid
are also active but only at higher concentrations; furthermore salicylate does not inhibit the growth of a pantoate auxotroph of
E. coli. The conclusions drawn from these observations were (a)
salicylate inhibited the biosynthesis of pantoate, and (b) α-keto-
isovaleric acid and ketopantoate were concerned in the synthesis
of pantoate (Fig. 1). Further studies with pantothenate auxotrophs
set these conclusions on firmer foundations (Maas and Vogel, 1953).
Wild type cells and cells of a mutant blocked between valine and
α-ketoisovaleric acid could form pantoate from glucose. On the other hand, a mutant blocked in the synthesis of α-ketoisovaleric
acid required either this compound, or ketopantoate, or high concentrations of valine, thus indicating that α-ketoisovaleric acid
is the primary precursor and that valine is active only in so far as
it can be deaminated to α-ketoisovaleric acid. Finally, Maas and
Vogel described a mutant which required ketopantoate or pantoate
for growth and which would not respond to any compound preceding ketopantoate in the biosynthetic scheme illustrated in Fig. 1.

The conclusion that the step from α-ketoisovaleric acid to ketopantoate involves a 1-C transfer was first reached with nutritional
experiments with mutants, and then confirmed in cell-free extracts.
Purko et al. (1953) examined a strain of Bacterium linens which required either pantothenate or p-aminobenzoic acid (PABA) for growth,
and found that the pantothenate requirement could be satisfied
by pantoate or ketopantoate, but not by α-ketoisovaleric acid.
This suggested that 1-C transfer could not take place because of
the absence of the appropriate form of folic acid caused, presumably,
by the inability of the bacterium to synthesize p-aminobenzoic
acid. The same group (McIntosh et al., 1957) proceeded to isolate
an enzyme system from Esch. coli which, after 36-fold purification,
carried out the 1-C transfer reaction in the presence of formaldehyde as the obligatory 1-C donor and Co^{2+} or Mn^{2+}; surprisingly, a
folic acid derivative was not required. To reconcile this with the
nutritional findings, is must be assumed that a folic acid cofactor

is required for the production of formaldehyde from, for example, serine or methionine but not, in this case, for the transfer of formaldehyde (see Chapter 4). Similar cell-free system have also been obtained from *Esch. coli* by Matsuyama (1955).

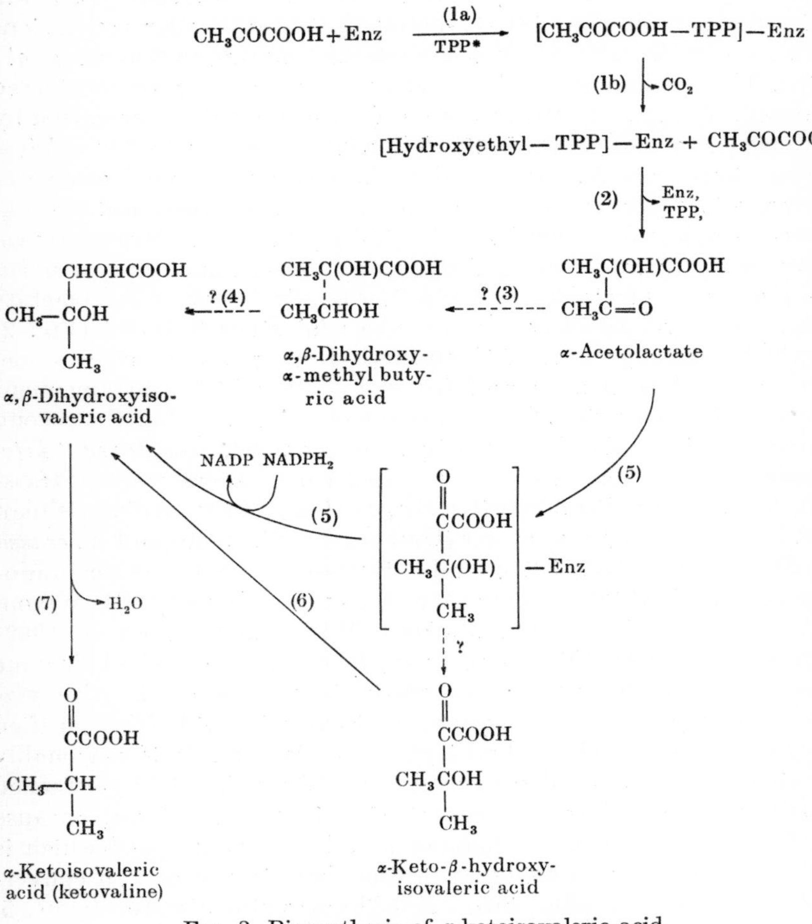

$$CH_3COCOOH + Enz \xrightarrow[TPP^*]{(1a)} [CH_3COCOOH-TPP]-Enz$$

$$(1b) \downarrow CO_2$$

$$[Hydroxyethyl-TPP]-Enz + CH_3COCOOH$$

$$(2) \downarrow \begin{array}{l} Enz, \\ TPP, \end{array}$$

FIG. 2. Biosynthesis of α-ketoisovaleric acid.

The formation of α-ketoisovaleric acid (ketovaline) has still to be considered. The probable pathway involved is indicated in Fig. 2. Experiments with [14C]pyruvate indicated that α-ketoisovaleric acid arose from two molecules of pyruvate (Strassman *et al.*, 1958), but the pattern of labelling indicated that

* TPP = Thiamine pyrophosphate

a pinacol-type rearrangement had to occur (step 3, Fig. 2) following the intermediate production of α-acetolactate (steps 1 and 2, Fig. 2). Lewis and Weinhouse (1938) were amongst the first to show that yeast will form α-acetolactate from pyruvate, and Strassman et al. (1958) were the first to show that yeast will convert α-acetolactate into α-ketoisovalerate; similar conclusions were reached from a study of *Neurospora* mutants (Wagner et al., 1958). The mechanism of the reaction has recently been considered in detail. The mechanism envisaged for α-acetolactate formation by Radhakrishan and Snell (1960), following their work with cell-free preparations from *N. crassa* and *Esch. coli*, is that one molecule of pyruvate is decarboxylated on the enzyme concerned and the enzyme-acetaldehyde complex [Enz-(2-hydroxyethylthiamine pyrophosphate)] transfers acetaldehyde to a second molecule of pyruvate to form α-acetolactate (step 2, Fig. 2). From α-acetolactate two alternative pathways are possible: (a) steps 3 and 4 (Fig. 2) in which rearrangement of the α-methyl group occurs after reduction of the keto group; and (b) step 5 in which rearrangement occurs before reduction. The consensus of opinion is that the second alternative is generally operative. An enzyme, *α-hydroxy-β-ketoreductoisomerase*, has now been purified from bakers' yeast (Strassman et al., 1960), *Esch. coli* (Umbarger et al., 1960: Radhakrishnan et al. 1960), *Aerobacter aerogenes* (Umbarger et al., 1960) and *N. crassa* (Radhakrishnan et al., 1960), and it is present in many other microorganisms and in higher plants (Armstrong and Wagner, 1961; Wixom and Hudson, 1961; Wixom et al., 1961; Wixom and Kanamori, 1962; Satayanarayana and Radhakrishnan, 1962). The microbial enzyme does not rearrange either of the spatial isomers of α,β-dihydroxy-α-methylbutyric acid to α,β-dihydroxyisovaleric acid. The purified enzyme requires NADPH and Mg^{2+} as co-factors. It is reasonably certain that α-keto-β-hydroxyisovalerate, if formed, is tightly attached to the enzyme surface and never exists in the free form, because the free acid is reduced either not at all or with a speed which is not consistent with its being an intermediate in the overall conversion of α-acetolactate into α,β-dihydroxyisovalerate (step 5, Fig. 2). Furthermore, Radhakrishnan et al. (1960) have isolated an enzyme *α-keto-β-hydroxyvaleric acid reductase*, which is quite different from the reductoisomerase, and which, in the presence of NADPH, reduces α-keto-β-hydroxyisovaleric acid to α,β-dihydroxyisovaleric acid (reaction 6, Fig. 2). A number of α-keto-β-hydroxy acid reductases with different substrate specificities are present in *Salmonella typhimurium* (Armstrong and Wagner, 1961).

In bakers' yeast, the reductoisomerase (reaction 5, Fig. 2) is a soluble enzyme, whilst that carrying out the final step in the reaction, the dehydration of α,β-dihydroxyisovaleric acid (reaction 7, Fig. 2) *(dihydroxyacid dehydrase)*, is particulate; it has a pH optimum between 7·2 and 7·4 and requires Mg^{2+} but no organic cofactors for activity (Wixom *et al.*, 1960; Wixom, 1962). The dehydrase from higher plants does not appear to be particulate and has been purified 120-fold. Its pH optimum is 8·0–8·2 and its divalent cation requirement is best met by Mg^{2+}; it does not require cysteine for activation (Kanamori *et al.*, 1961; Wixom and Kanamori, 1962). The enzyme from *Esch. coli*, on the other hand, requires cysteine and ferrous ions for activation (Myers, 1961). The substrate specificities of the dihydroxy acid dehydrases isolated from a number of microbial and plant sources were similar; each enzyme catalysed keto acid production from DL-β-dihydroxy– isovalerate at a greater rate than from DL-β-dihydroxybutyrate, and the *threo* isomer of DL-α,β-dihydroxybutyrate was dehydrated faster than than the *erythro* isomer (Wixom *et al.*, 1962).

B. *The Formation of β- Alanine*

There are various reactions which lead to the formation of β-alanine: (a) decarboxylation of aspartate, which was first demonstrated in *Rhizobium trifolii* (Virtanen and Laine, 1937) and later in numerous micro-organisms (Billen and Lichstein, 1949; Mardeshev and Etingof, 1948); (b) from propionate via acrylyl-CoA (reaction 1) in *Clostridium propionicum* (Stadtman, 1955). The last step, which

$$CH_3CH_2COOH{\rightarrow}CH_2{=}CHCOSCoA \xleftarrow{NH_3} CH_2NH_2CH_2COSCoA \quad (1)$$

is freely reversible, is carried out by a purified enzyme system in which NH_3 is the obligatory amino donor (Vagelos *et al.*, 1959), although it should be noted that Goldfine and Stadtman (1960) find that pyruvate will accept the amino group from β-alanine during its catabolism; (c) transamination (i) in animal tissues, between malonic semialdehyde (formylacetic acid), again arising from propionate, and glutamate (Kupiecki and Coon, 1957, reaction 2), and (ii) in a *Pseudomonas* species in a pyruvate-β-alanine transaminase system (Nishizuka *et al.*, 1959); (d) by the degradation of pyrimidines by the pathway outlined in reaction (3) which is

$$CH_3CH_2COOH{\rightarrow}CHOCH_2COOH \xrightarrow[\alpha\text{-ketoglutarate}]{\text{glutamate}} CH_2(NH_2)CH_2COOH \quad (2)$$

well established in animals (Fink *et al.*, 1953), and in one microorganism, *Clostridium uracilicum* (Campbell, 1957, 1960). The pathway may, however be widespread in bacteria, because the metabolic lesion in a mutant of *Esch. coli* which would respond to dihydro-

(3)

uracil, was eventually traced to a requirement for β-alanine which was being produced from dihydrouracil (Slotnick and Weinfeld, 1957). Isolated embryos of pine seedlings and sterile pine callus tissue also synthesize β-alanine via route (3) (Barnes and Naylor, 1961, 1962).

C. *Coupling of β-Alanine and Pantoic Acid*

The enzymatic formation of pantothenic acid from β-alanine and pantoic acid (Fig. 1) was first achieved in 1941 by Wieland and Möller (1941) using yeast macerates. The enzyme responsible, *pantothenate synthetase*, [L-pantoate: β-alanine ligase (AMP)] has been studied in detail by Maas (1952). The purified enzyme requires ATP, K^+ or NH_4^+, and Mg^{2+}, and during the reaction AMP and inorganic pyrophosphate are formed (Maas and Novelli, 1953). The reaction mechanism proposed (reactions 4 and 5) has the following

$$\text{Enz} + \text{ATP} + \text{Pantoate} \xrightleftharpoons{\text{K}+, \text{Mg}^{2+}} \text{Enz-pantoyl adenylate} + \text{P-P} \quad (4)$$

$$\text{Enz-pantoyl adenylate} + \beta\text{-alanine} \rightarrow \text{Pantothenate} + \text{AMP} + \text{Enz} \quad (5)$$

experimental support (Maas, 1956, 1959): (a) if β-alanine is removed from the complete enzyme system then $[^{32}P]$pyrophosphate but not $[^{32}P]$-AMP is incorporated into ATP; (b) if β-alanine is removed from the complete system and a high concentration (1 M) of hydroxylamine added, equimolar amounts of pantoylhydroxamic acid and inorganic pyrophosphate are formed, indicating the formation of a pantoyl intermediate; (c) the transfer of one atom of ^{18}O from the carboxyl group of pantoate to the phosphate group of AMP during the synthesis of pantothenic acid indicates that the pantoyl intermediate is pantoyl adenylate (reactions 6 and 7); the pantoyl adenylate is assumed to remain bound to the enzyme (reactions 4 and 5)

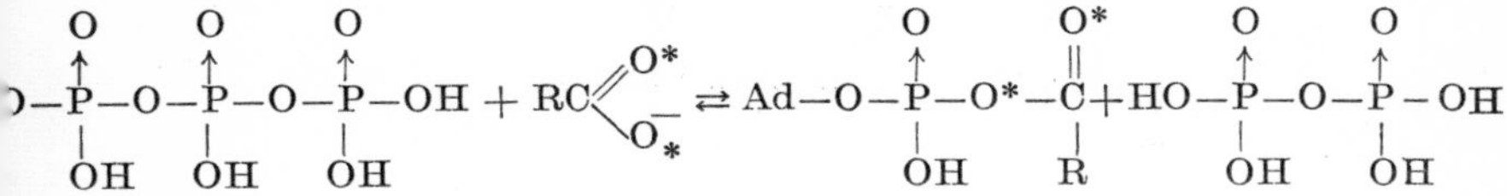

$$)-\overset{O}{\underset{OH}{P}}-O-\overset{O}{\underset{OH}{P}}-O-\overset{O}{\underset{OH}{P}}-OH + RC\overset{O*}{\underset{O*}{\diagdown}} \rightleftarrows Ad-O-\overset{O}{\underset{OH}{P}}-O*-\overset{O*}{\underset{R}{C}}+HO-\overset{O}{\underset{OH}{P}}-O-\overset{O}{\underset{OH}{P}}-OH \quad (6)$$

$$)-\overset{O}{\underset{OH}{P}}-O*-\overset{O*}{\underset{R}{C}}+H_2NCH_2CH_2COOH \rightleftarrows Ad-O-\overset{O}{\underset{OH}{P}}-O*H+R\overset{O*}{C}NHCH_2CH_2COOH \quad (7)$$

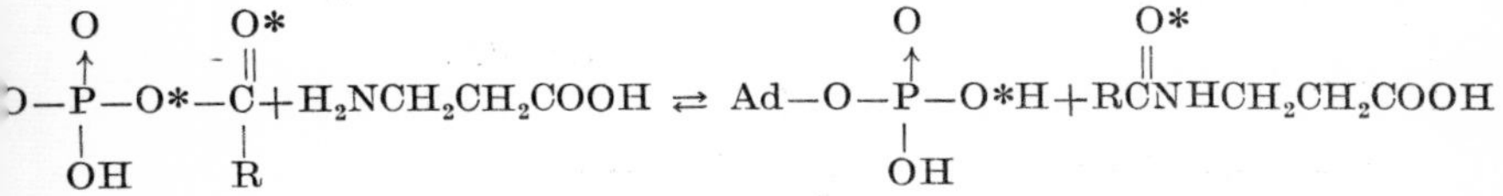

because the formation of the free adenylate has not been demonstrated. It should be noted that this reaction results in the formation of a peptide bond.

D. *Formation of Coenzyme A*

The main pathway for the conversion of pantothenic acid into coenzyme A has been recently elucidated by G. M. Brown (1959; Fig. 3).

The first step (Fig. 3), the formation of 4′-phosphopantothenate, is catalysed by *pantothenate kinase* [ATP: pantothenate 4′-phosphotransferase] which has been purified from animal and bacterial sources and from yeast. The formation of 4′-phosphopantothenate is assayed microbiologically, using *Saccharomyces carlsbergensis* strain 4228 which responds to 4′-phosphopantothenate but not to pantothenate itself (King and Strong, 1951). The assay is carried out on the test material before and after treatment with intestinal phosphatase.

The next reaction involves the coupling of 4′-phosphopantothenate and cysteine to yield 4′-phosphopantothenylcysteine (reaction 2, Fig. 3). The coupling enzyme concerned, *(phosphopantothenoylcysteine synthetase)* has been purified from mammalian and bacterial sources (Brown, 1959). CTP is obligatory in the bacterial enzymes examined *(Esch. coli, Proteus morganii)* but other nucleoside triphosphates can substitute for CTP in animal systems (rat liver and kidney). The course of the reaction is followed microbiologically, after treatment of the reaction mixture with intestinal phosphatase, with the help of *Lactobacillus helveticus* strain 80 (Craig and Snell, 1951), which responds to pantothenylcysteine and pantetheine.

Phosphopantothenoylcysteine decarboxylase, which has not yet been fully purified, has been detected in yeast and *Neurospora crassa*

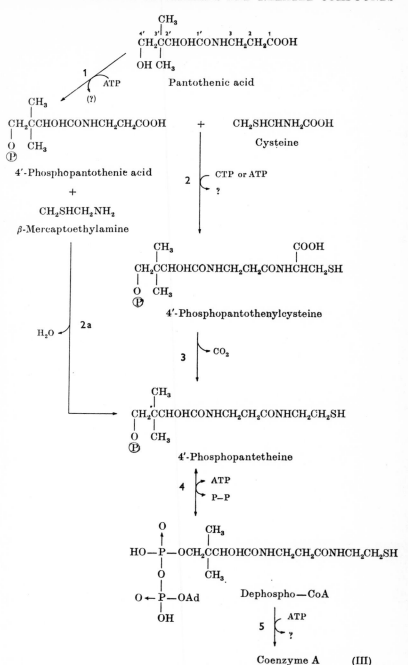

FIG. 3. Formation of coenzyme A from pantothenic acid.

and carries out the step which converts 4′-phosphopantothenoyl-cysteine into 4′-phosphopantetheine (step 3, Fig. 3; Brown, 1959). The enzyme has no action on pantothenoylcysteine. After treatment with intestinal phosphatase the reaction mixture is assayed micro-biologically for pantetheine using *Lac. helveticus* strain 80. 4′-Phospho-pantetheine then condenses with ATP to form dephospho-CoA with the liberation of inorganic pyrophosphate (step 4, Fig. 3). This is the only reversible reaction in the biosynthesis of coenzyme A, and is catalysed by *dephospho-CoA pyrophosphorylase* [ATP: pantetheine 4′-phosphate adenylyltransferase]. The enzyme has not yet been obtained free from *dephospho-CoA kinase* [ATP: dephospho-CoA 3′-phosphotransferase] which brings about the final step (5, Fig. 3) in the biosynthesis of coenzyme A. This enzyme requires ATP specifically as phosphate donor, requires cysteine for maximum activity and is not inhibited by adenosine, adenosine 2′, 3′ or 5′-phosphates (Brown, 1959).

The observation that the coupling enzyme will utilize β-mercapto-ethylamine in place of cysteine indicates that reaction (2a) (Fig. 3) can occur, and thus the decarboxylase enzyme (step 3) can be bypassed. It has previously been reported that in neither rat liver (Hoagland and Novelli, 1954), washed suspension of *Lactobacillus arbinosus* Pierpoint and Hughes, 1952) nor *Proteus morganii* (Brown, 1959) could β-mercaptoethylamine replace cysteine for coenzyme A synthesis. The probable reason for this is that as β-mercapto-ethylamine is much less effective than cysteine as substrate for the enzyme, insufficient was used in the earlier experiments just quoted. Cellular impermeability may also have played some part in these observations.

According to Brown (1959) the pathway outlined in Fig. 3 also functions in animal tissues. This is contrary to the view of Novelli (1959) who postulates a pathway (reaction 8) in which phosphory-lation does not occur until pantetheine is formed. Brown makes the following criticisms of this scheme: (a) the analytical methods used for pantetheine assay would also measure 4′-phosphopantetheine:

$$\text{antothenate} \rightarrow \text{pantothenoylcysteine} \rightarrow \text{pantetheine} \rightarrow 4'\text{-phosphopantetheine} \rightarrow \text{CoA} \quad (8)$$

(b) the enzymes used were not sufficiently pure to exclude the possi-bility that they contained pantothenate kinase: (c) purified 4′-panto-thenoylcysteine decarboxylase will not, in his hands, decarboxylate pantothenoy cysteine: (d) nutritional work by Thompson and Bird (1954) indicated that pantothenoylcysteine could not replace coenzy-me A for growth of chicks. However, there is no doubt that pante-theine itself can be channelled into coenzyme A synthesis: it was active in the nutrition experiments of Thompson and Bird (1954) and kinases exist in animal tissues (Levintow and Novelli, 1954) and in micro-organisms (Ward *et al.*, 1955) which convert it into 4'-phospho-pantetheine. Its origin is, however, probably from coenzyme A itself, for it is found in largest quantities in autolysed materials (Williams *et al.*, 1949), and Novelli *et al.* (1954) have prepared a nucleotide pyrophosphatase from potatoes and from snake venom which splits coenzyme A into 4'-phosphopantetheine and 3',5'-diphosphoadenosine. The nucleotide pyrophosphatase obtained from potato by Kornberg and Pricer (1950) has a similar action on coenzyme A. A phosphatase could then convert 4'-phosphopantetheine into pantetheine. Another route to pantetheine involves firstly the removal of the 3'-phosphate from coenzyme A by a phosphomono-

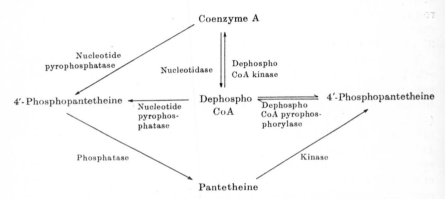

Fig. 4. Inter-relationships between pantetheine and coenzyme A.

esterase such as that obtained from human prostate gland (Novelli, 1953); this is followed by the removal of adenosine 5'-phosphate by the nucleotide pyrophosphatase just discussed, and the 4'-phosphate by phosphatase. Pantetheine can then re-enter the coenzyme A pathway by being phosphorylated by the kinases mentioned previously. The known interconversions of CoA and pantetheine are indicated in Fig. 4.

The outstanding difference between the results of Brown and those of Novelli which has yet no adequate explanation is the fact that Novelli finds in animal tissues a decarboxylase which will use pantothenoylcysteine, and not 4'-phosphopantothenoylcysteine, as substrate. However, the route envisaged by Novelli (reaction 8) may function in one bacterium, *Lactobacillus helveticus*. Evidence for this includes (a) pantothenoylcysteine decarboxylase is present (Brown, 1959); (b) this organism when supplied with large amounts of pantothenate will not accumulate 4'-phosphopantothenate (Brown,

1959);(c) mutant strains of *Lact. helveticus* can use pantothenoyl cysteine as a growth factor (Brown, 1957). Two other organisms-*Lact. bulgaricus* and *Acetobacter suboxydans*, which can also utilize pantothenoylcysteine possibly also follow Novelli's pathway (Brown, 1957).

REFERENCES

Armstrong, F. B., and Wagner, R. P. (1961). *J. biol. Chem.* **236**, 3252.
Barnes, R. L., and Naylor, A. W. (1961). *Plant Physiol.* Proc. xviii.
Barnes, R. L., and Naylor, A. W. (1962). *Plant Physiol.*, **34**, 171.
Billen, D., and Lichstein, H. C. (1949). *J. Bact.* **58**, 215.
Brown, G. M. (1957). *J. biol. Chem.* **226**, 651.
Brown, G. M. (1959). *J. biol. Chem.* **234**, 370, 379.
Campbell, L. L. (1957). *J. Bact.* **73**, 220.
Campbell, L. L. (1960). *J. biol. Chem.* **235**, 2375.
Craig, J. A., and Snell, E. E. (1951). *J. Bact.* **61**, 283.
Elvehjem, C. A., and Koehn, C. J. (1935). *J. biol. Chem.* **108**, 709.
Fink, R. M., Fink, K., and Henderson, R. B. (1953). *J. biol. Chem.* **201**, 349.
Goldfine, H., and Stadtman, E. R. (1960). *J. biol. Chem.* **235**, 2238.
Gregory, J. D., Novelli, G. D., and Lipmann, F. (1952). *J. Amer. chem. Soc.* **74**, 854.
Hoagland, M. B., and Novelli, G. D. (1954). *J. biol. Chem.* **207**, 767.
Ivanovics, G. (1942). *Hoppe-Seyl. Z.* **276**, 33.
Kanamori, M., Sherwood, T., and Blankenship, J. W. (1961). *Fed. Proc.* **20**, 11.
King, T. E., and Strong, F. M. (1951). *J. biol. Chem.* **189**, 315.
Kornberg, A., and Pricer, W. E., Jr. (1950). *J. biol. Chem.* **182**, 763.
Kuhn, R., and Wieland, T. (1942). *Ber. dtsch. chem. Ges.* **75B**, 121.
Kupiecki, F. P., and Coon, M. J. (1957). *J. biol. Chem.* **229**, 743.
Lepkovsky, S. (1954). *In* "The Vitamins", Vol. II, p. 591. (W. H. Sebrell and R. S. Harris, eds). Academic Press, New York.
Lepkovsky, S., and Jukes, T. H. (1936). *J. biol. Chem.* **114**, 109.
Levintow, L., and Novelli, G. D. (1954). *J. biol Chem.* **207**, 761.
Lewis, K. F., and Weinhouse, S. (1958). *J. Amer. chem. Soc.* **80**, 4913.
Lipmann, F. (1954). *In* "The Vitamins", Vol., II, p. 598. (W. H. Sebrell and R. S. Harris, eds.) Academic Press, New York.
Lipmann, F., Kaplan, N. O., Novelli, G. D., Tuttle, L. C., and Guirard, B. M. (1947). *J. biol. Chem.* **167**, 869.
Lynen, F., Reichert, E., and Rueff, L. (1951). *Liebigs Ann.* **574**, 1.
Maas, W. K. (1952). *J. biol. Chem.* **198**, 23.
Maas, W. K. (1956). *Fed. Proc.* **15**, 315.
Maas, W. K. (1959). *In* "Proceedings of the 4th International Congress of Biochemistry Vienna", XI, 161, Pergamon Press, London.
Maas, W. K., and Davis, B. D. (1950). *J. Bact.* **60**, 733.
Maas, W. K., and Novelli, G. D. (1953). *Arch. Biochem. Biophys.* **43**, 236.
Maas, W. K., and Vogel, H. J. (1953). *J. Bact.* **65**, 388.
Mardeshev, S. R., and Etingof, R. N. (1948). *Biochemistry Leningr.* **13**, 402.
Matsuyama, A. (1955). *J. agric. chem. Soc. Japan* **29**, 973.
McIntosh, E. N., Purko, M., and Wood, W. A. (1957). *J. biol. Chem.* **228**, 499.
Myers, J. W. (1961). *J. biol. Chem.* **236**, 141.
Nishizuka, Y., Takeshita, M., Kuno, S., and Hayaishi, O. (1959). *Biochim. biophys. Acta* **33**, 591.

Novelli, G. D. (1953). *Fed. Proc.* **12,** 675; *J. cell. comp. Physiol.* **41,** Suppl. 1, 67.

Novelli, G. D. (1959). *In* "Proceedings of the 4th International Congress of Biochemistry, Vienna", XI, 169. Pergamon Press, London.

Novelli, G. D., Schmetz, F. J., Jr., and Kaplan, N. O. (1954). *J. biol. Chem.* **206,** 533.

Pfleiderer, G., Kreiling, A., and Wieland, T. (1960). *Biochem. Z.* **333,** 308.

Pierpoint, W. S., and Hughes, D. E. (1952). "Abstracts of the 2nd International Congress of Biochemistry, Paris".

Purko, M., Nelson, W. O., and Wood, W. A. (1953). *J. Bact.* **66,** 561.

Radhakrishnan, A. N., and Snell, E. E. (1960). *J. biol. Chem.* **235,** 2316.

Radhakrishnan, A. N., Wagner, R. P., and Snell, E. E. (1960). *J. biol. Chem.* **235,** 2322.

Robinson, F. A. (1951). "The Vitamin B Complex". Chapman and Hall, London.

Satayanarayana, T., and Radhakrishnan, A. N. (1962). *Biochim. biophys. Acta,* **56,** 197.

Slotnick, I. J., and Weinfeld, H. (1957). *J. Bact.* **74,** 122.

Snell, E. E., Brown, G. M., Peters, V. J., Craig, J. A., Wittle, E L., Moore, J. A., McGlohon, V. M., and Bird, O. D., (1950). *J. Amer. chem Soc.* **74,** 854.

Stadtman, E. R. (1955). *J Amer. chem. Soc.* **77,** 5765.

Strassman, M., Shatton, J. B., Corsey, M. E., and Weinhouse, S. (1958). *J. Amer. chem. Soc.* **80,** 1771.

Strassman, M., Shatton, J. B., and Weinhouse, S. (1960). *J. biol. Chem.* **235,** 700.

Thompson, R. Q., and Bird, O. D. (1954). *Science* **120,** 763.

Umbarger, H. E., Brown, B., and Eyring, E. J. (1960). *J. biol. Chem.* **235,** 1425.

Vagelos, P. R., Earl, J. M., and Stadtman, E. R. (1959). *J. biol. Chem.* **234,** 490.

Virtanen, A. I., and Laine, T. (1937). *Enzymologia,* **3,** 266.

Wagner, R. P., Radhakrishnan, A. N., and Snell, E. E. (1958). *Proc. nat. Acad. Sci., Wash.* **44,** 1047.

Ward, G. B., Brown, G. M., and Snell, E. E. (1955). *J. biol. Chem.* **213,** 869.

Weinstock, H. N., Jr., Mitchell, H. K., Pratt, E. F., and Williams, R. J. (1939). *J. Amer. chem. Soc.* **61,** 1421.

Wieland, T. and Möller, E. F. (1941). *Hoppe-Seyl. Z.* **269,** 227.

Wieland, T., Kreiling, A., Buck, W., and Pfleiderer, G. (1960). *Biochem.Z.* **333,** 311.

Williams, R. J., and Major, R. T. (1940). *Science* **91,** 246.

Williams, W. L., Hoff-Jorgensen, E., and Snell, E. E. (1949). *J. biol. Chem.* **177,** 933.

Wixom, R. L. (1962). *Biochem. J.* **84,** 46P.

Wixom, R. L., and Hudson, R. J. (1961). *Plant Physiol.* **36,** 598.

Wixom, R. L., and Kanamori, M. (1962). *Biochem. J.* **83,** 90.

Wixom, R. L., Stratton, J. B., and Strassman, M. (1960). *J. biol. Chem.* **235,** 128.

Wixom, R. L., Wickman, J. H., and Howell, G. B. (1961). *J. biol. Chem.* **236,** 3259.

Wixom, R. L., Kanamori, M., and Blankenship, J. W. (1962). *Biochem. J.* **84,** 41P.

Woolley, D. W., Aisman, H. A., and Elvehjem, C. A. (1939). *J. Amer. chem. Soc.* **61,** 977.

CHAPTER 6

BIOTIN

I. INTRODUCTION

The complex nature of "Bios", the material necessary for the growth of certain yeasts (Wildiers, 1901), was first fully investigated by Miller (1924) who resolved it into three factors. The third of these, "Bios IIB", was shown to be identical with biotin isolated from egg yolk by Kögl and Tönnis (1936). After considerable efforts du Vigneaud *et al.* (1942c), working with biotin isolated from liver, elucidated its structure as 2'-oxo-3,4-imidazolido-2-tetrahydro-thiophene-*n*-valeric acid (I). This structure has been confirmed by

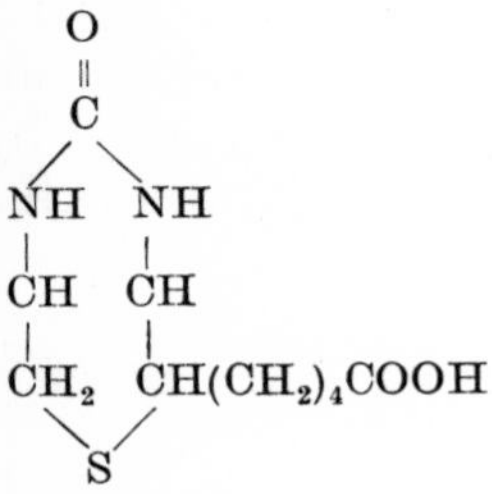

$$
\begin{array}{c}
O \\
\parallel \\
C \\
\diagup \diagdown \\
NH \quad NH \\
| \qquad | \\
CH \quad CH \\
| \qquad | \\
CH_2 \quad CH(CH_2)_4COOH \\
\diagdown \diagup \\
S
\end{array}
$$

(I)

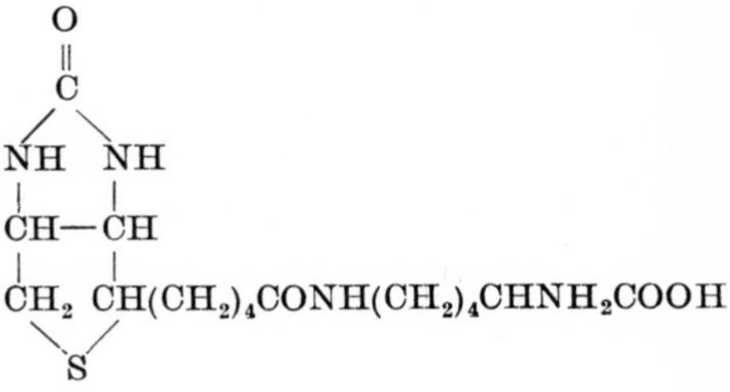

$$
\begin{array}{c}
O \\
\parallel \\
C \\
\diagup \diagdown \\
NH \quad NH \\
| \qquad | \\
CH—CH \\
| \qquad | \\
CH_2 \quad CH(CH_2)_4CONH(CH_2)_4CHNH_2COOH \\
\diagdown \diagup \\
S
\end{array}
$$

(II)

$$
\begin{array}{c}
O \\
\parallel \\
C \\
\diagup \diagdown \\
NH \quad NH \\
| \qquad | \\
CH—CH \\
| \qquad | \\
CH_2 \quad CH(CH_2)_4COOH \\
\diagdown \diagup \\
S \\
\downarrow \\
O
\end{array}
$$

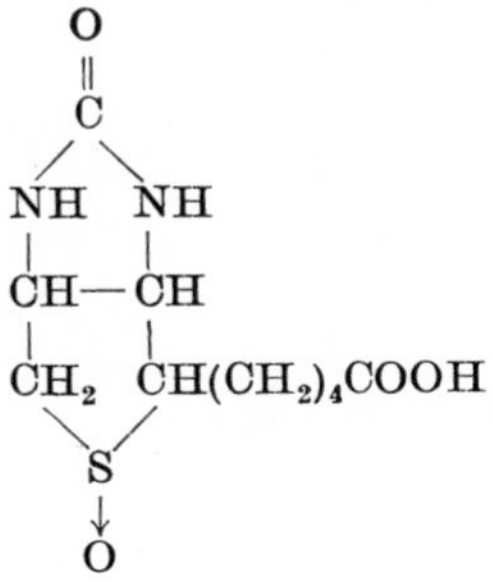

(III)

complete chemical synthesis. Kögl and Borg (1944) considered that egg yolk biotin (α-biotin) is structurally slightly different from liver biotin(β-biotin); but this is not now generally accepted [see e.g. Sebrell and Harris (1954) for a full discussion].

Two naturally occurring derivatives of biotin are known, biocytin (II) and biotin sulphoxide (III). Biocytin, a growth factor for a number of organisms, is ε-N-biotinyllysine (Wright *et al.*, 1951); D-biotin-L-sulphoxide (III) was isolated from cultures of *Aspergillius niger* and identified as the AN factor which possesses biotin activity for *Neurospora crassa* (Wright and Cresson, 1954; Wright *et al.*, 1954a); it also occurs in *Phycomyces blakesleeanus* (Eisenberg, 1962). The diastereoisomer, D-biotin-D-sulphoxide, has been isolated from milk as its methyl ester (Melville, 1954).

An unidentified biotin derivative has recently been reported in *P. blakesleeanus* (Eisenberg, 1962).

A. *Functional Form of Biotin*

Although for some years past there have been various suggestions that biotin was implicated in CO_2 metabolism, it is only recently that these ideas have been substantiated at the enzyme level. Firstly, the enzyme *acetyl-CoA carboxylase*, [acetyl-CoA: CO_2 ligase (ADP)] which catalyses a key reaction in the biosynthesis of fatty acids (reaction 1), was found to be rich in biotin and to be inhibited by avidin, the biotin – binding factor from raw egg white (Wakil *et al.*, 1958; Wakil and Gibson, 1960).

$$CH_3COSCoA + CO_2 + ATP \longleftrightarrow \underset{\underset{COOH}{|}}{CH_2COSCoA} + ADP + P_i \tag{1}$$

The same situation was found to exist with β-*methylcrotonyl-CoA carboxylase* [β-methylcrotonyl-CoA: CO_2 ligase (ADP)] (reaction 2) (Lynen *et al.*, 1959), *propionyl-CoA carboxylase* [propionyl-CoA: CO_2 ligase (ADP)] (reaction 3) (Kaziro *et al.*, 1960), *transcarboxylase* (reaction 4) (Swick and Wood, 1960; Wood and Stjernholm, 1961), and with an ATP-dependent *pyruvate carboxylase* [pyruvate: CO_2 ligase (ADP)] (reaction 5) (Utter and Keech, 1960). Lynen *et al.*

$$\underset{CH_3}{\overset{CH_3}{\diagdown}} C=CHCOSCoA + CO_2 + ATP \rightleftarrows \underset{CH_2COOH}{\overset{CH_3}{\diagdown}} C=CHCOSCoA + ADP + P_i \tag{2}$$

$$CH_3CH_2COSCoA + CO_2 + ATP \rightleftarrows \underset{\underset{COOH}{|}}{CH_3CHCOSCoA} + ADP + P_i \tag{3}$$

$$\underset{\underset{COOH}{|}}{CH_3CHCOSCoA} + CH_3CO.COOH \rightleftarrows CH_3CH_2COSCoA + \underset{\underset{COOH}{|}}{CH_2COCOOH} \tag{4}$$

(1959) found that when D-biotin was incubated with β-methylcrotonyl carboxylase it was carboxylated; L-biotin, on the other hand was not

$$CH_3COCOOH + CO_2 + ATP \rightleftharpoons CH_2COCOOH + ADP + P_i \qquad (5)$$
$$\underset{\displaystyle COOH}{|}$$

carboxylated. The structure of the carboxylated biotin which is a highly unstable molecule was shown to be (IV) (Lynen *et al.*, 1959;

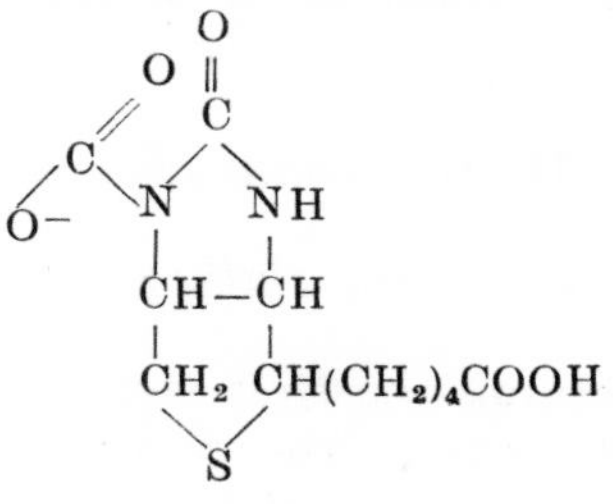

(IV)

Knappe *et al.*, 1961, 1962). It is designated as biotin$\sim CO_2$, because the linkage is a "high energy bond". As biotin is bound covalently to its apoenzymes (Kaziro *et al.*, 1960), it was reasonable to assume that as biocytin is a naturally occurring product, biotin is enzyme-bound through the ε-amino group of lysine, and that (V) represents the carboxylated enzyme. This has recently been proved for propionyl-CoA carboxylase (Kosow and Lane, 1962).

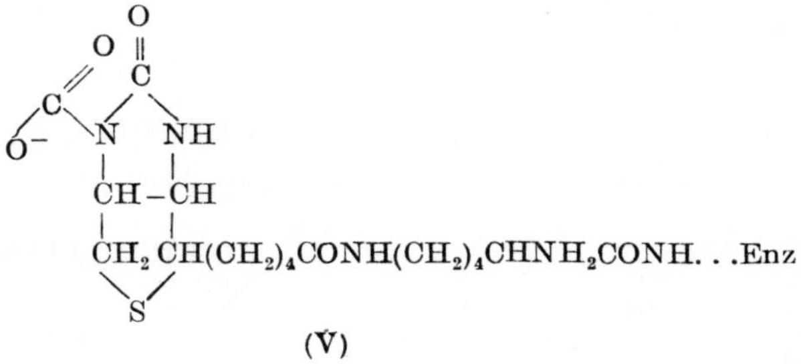

(V)

The situation with acetyl CoA carboxylase appears to be different. Wakil and Waite (1962) report experiments which indicate that it is the ureido-carbon of enzyme-bound biotin which is the "active carbon" of biotin. They found, for example, that (a) one mole of $^{14}CO_2$ is incorporated into the enzyme for every one mole of biotin present; (b) hydrolysis of the labelled enzyme yields biotin containing more than 80% of the original activity; (b) ^{14}C is located exclusively in the ureido-carbon of the biotin; (c) if the enzyme is incubated in the presence of acetyl-CoA or $ADP + P_i$, and then hydrolysed, not biotin but a compound probably "diamino biotin"

(VII, below) is formed; (d) the "diamino biotin"-enzyme can be converted back to the biotin-enzyme only in the presence of HCO_3^-, ATP and Mn^{2+}; and (e) when *Lact. arabinosus* is grown on limiting amounts of [ureido-^{14}C]biotin the biotin recovered from the cells contains very little label.

It is interesting in this connection to point out that, as will be shown in the next section, "diamino biotin" cannot be considered as a normal biosynthetic precursor of biotin.

II. BIOSYNTHESIS

A. *General Pathway*

Little is known concerning the first steps in the biosynthesis of biotin; this is probably because of the very small amounts produced by biotin-synthesizing organisms and because of the lack of simple chemical methods of detection and quantitative determination. There is, however, a considerable amount of information from nutritional experiments and from experiments with biotin-requiring mutants concerning the last stages of the synthesis in micro-organisms. Rather surprisingly, few isotope experiments have yet been reported.

Two possibilities exist for the final step: (a) the insertion of the sulphur atom into desthiobiotin (VI); or (b) the insertion of the ureido carbon atom into *cis*-3,4-diamino-2-tetrahydrothiophene-n-valeric acid (VII).

Tatum (1945) examined two biotin-requiring mutants of *Penicillium chrysogenum* and found that one would respond to both desthiobiotin and biotin, and that the other accumulated desthiobiotin but could not convert it into biotin.

A number of naturally occurring organisms which require biotin will also respond equally well to desthiobiotin; for example, amongst the fungi, *Saccharomyces cerevisiae*, *Blastomyces dermatitidis*, *Neurospora crassa*, *Ceratostomella ips*, *Aspergillus niger* (Lilly and Leonian, 1944; Dittmer *et al.*, 1944; Wright and Driscoll, 1954; Halliday and McCoy, 1955), and amongst the bacteria, *Escherichia coli* (Tatum,

1945), *Clostridium* spp. (Perlman, 1948), *Bacillus coagulans* and *B. stearothermophilus* (Campbell and Williams, 1953).

It is clear that in these organisms desthiobiotin is converted into biotin and not utilized *per se*; the substance formed after incubating the cells with desthiobiotin is active in stimulating growth in those bacteria which will respond only to biotin (Leonian and Lilly, 1945; Stokes and Gunness, 1945; Wright and Driscoll, 1954).

With regard to alternative (b), (VII) has been shown to be either inactive (Chu and Williams, 1944) or only slightly active (10% that of biotin) in *S. cerevisiae* (du Vigneaud *et al.*, 1941, 1942b), and very slightly active (1·8–3·6% that of biotin) in *Lactobacillus* spp. (Stokes and Gunness, 1945). Thus it would appear that reaction (6) represents the last stage in biotin synthesis. There are, however, a number of biotin-requiring fungi, *Ceratostomella pini* and *Sordaria fimicola*, for example, (Lilly and Leonian, 1944; Leonian and Lilly,

$$\text{Desthiobiotin} + \text{``Sulphur''} \rightarrow \text{Biotin} \qquad (6)$$

1945), and bacteria, *Lactobacillus helveticus* (Melville *et al.*, 1943; Stokes and Gunness, 1945) and *Rhizobium trifolii* (Leonian and Lilly 1945), which do not respond to desthiobiotin. This inability probably is due to a single metabolic lesion caused by the absence of the enzyme (s) carrying out reaction (6).

B. *The Source of Sulphur in Biotin*

There is as yet no direct indication of the immediate source of the sulphur atom in biotin. Stokes and Gunness (1945) found that methionine and SO_4^{2-} were more effective than cystine in stimulating the conversion of desthiobiotin into biotin in yeasts. In *Aspergillus niger*, which synthesizes biotin sulphoxide (III) as well as biotin, the combined synthesis of biotin and biotin sulphoxide is not affected by the presence of cysteine in the medium; the amount of biotin relative to that of the sulphoxide was, however, increased (Wright and Driscoll, 1954; Wright *et al.*, 1955). Probably the presence of the cysteine reduced the amount of biotin oxidized to the sulphoxide.

C. *The Precursors of Desthiobiotin*

It seems clear that pimelic acid (VIII), or a very closely related compound, is a precursor of desthiobiotin. Eakin and Eakin (1942)

$$\underset{\text{(VIII)}}{HOOC(CH_2)_5COOH} \qquad \underset{\text{(IX)}}{HOOC(CH_2)_7COOH} \qquad \underset{\text{(X)}}{HOOC(CH_2)_6COOH}$$

were first to demonstrate that pimelic acid stimulated biotin synthesis; they used *Aspergillus niger*. Thioctic acid plus pimelic acid increases the biotin level three times compared with pimelic acid alone, although thioctic acid itself is not stimulatory (Elford and Wright, 1962). First indications that pimelic acid was a precursor of desthiobiotin in bacteria came in an interesting but roundabout way. It had been shown in the late 1930s that pimelic acid stimulated the growth of various strains of *Corynebact. diphtheriae* (Mueller, 1937; Evans *et al.*, 1939), but it was du Vigneaud *et al.* (1942a) who found that pimelic acid could replace biotin as a growth factor in these organisms. Tatum (1945) later showed that, in his mutant of *Penicillium chrysogenum* which accumulated desthiobiotin, the addition of pimelic acid to the medium enhanced this accumulation. The precursor activity of pimelic acid was also indicated in the experiments of Campbell and Williams (1953) who used the thermophilic *Bacillus coagulans* and *B. stearothermophilus* and in those of Eisenberg (1962) who used *P. blakesleeanus*. Recently direct proof of the utilization of pimelic acid for biotin synthesis has been obtained in *A. niger;* after addition of [1,7-^{14}C]pimelic acid [^{14}C]biotin sulphone was isolated (Elford and Wright, 1962). Similar results were obtained with *P. blakesleeanus* (Eisenberg, 1962).

Azelaic acid (IX), but not suberic acid (X) or sebacic acid (XI), is as effective as pimelic acid in *A. niger* (Wright *et al.*, 1955), but oleic acid (XII), which in the laboratory yields azelaic acid as one

$$HOOC(CH_2)_8COOH \qquad CH_3(CH_2)_7CH=CH(CH_2)_7COOH$$
$$(XI) \qquad\qquad\qquad (XII)$$

product of oxidative scission, was ineffective. The stimulatory effect of oleic acid on biotin synthesis in other micro-organisms (see p. 151) is also probably not due to its activity as a precursor. It is generally assumed that azelaic acid is active because it is first degraded to pimelic acid (Wright *et al.*, 1955). There is yet no indication of the primary source of pimelic acid. It is not unexpected that a number of biotin-requiring fungi and bacteria could not utilize pimelic acid in place of biotin (Robbins and Ma, 1942; Wright, 1942).

A possible intermediate between pimelic acid and desthiobiotin is ζ, η-diaminopelargonic acid (XIII). However, (XIII) has only one

$$
\begin{array}{cc}
NH_2 & NH_2 \\
| & | \\
CH — & CH(CH_2)_4COOH \\
| & | \\
CH_3 & CH_3
\end{array}
$$
$$(XIII)$$

tenth the activity of desthiobiotin as a source of biotin in yeast (du Vigneaud *et al.*, 1942b; Winnick, *et al.*, 1945). It is also inactive in the biotin heterotrophe *Lactobacillus casei* (Dittmer and du Vigneaud, 1944); however, its possible conversion into biotin by bacteria which can synthesize biotin has not been investigated.

The results with yeast would suggest that (XIII) is not on the direct pathway of biotin synthesis, but definitive experiments with isotopes are required finally to decide this problem.

D. *The Role of Oleic Acid*

Many experiments have been reported which clearly demonstrate that under certain conditions oleic acid dispersed with a Tween (e.g. Tween 80, a polyoxyethylene derivative of sorbitan mono-oleate) spares biotin for various biotin-requiring bacteria such as *Lactobacillus* spp., *Clostridium butyricum* (Williams and Fieger, 1946; Broquist and Snell, 1951, 1953), *Leuconostoc* spp. (Carlson *et al.*, 1950) certain strains of *Bacillus coagulans* and *B. stearothermophilus* (Campbell and Williams, 1953), and a number of staphylococci (Gretler *et al.*, 1955). The reasonable conclusion from this was that biotin is concerned with the biosynthesis of oleic acid, rather than that oleic acid can be converted into precursors of biotin. This view received strong support from the finding of Broquist and Snell (1953) that, in the presence of avidin, added biotin but not oleic acid will support growth. Further indirect proof was apparently forthcoming when Wakil (1958) discovered the malonyl coenzyme A system for fatty acid synthesis (reaction 7), in which a key enzyme is the

$$CH_3COSCoA + n\overset{\displaystyle COOH}{\underset{\displaystyle |}{C}}H_2COSCoA + 2nNADPH + 2nH^+ \rightarrow$$
$$CH_3(CH_2CH_2)_nCOSCoA + nCO_2 + nCoASH + 2nNADP^+ \qquad (7)$$

biotin-dependent acetyl-CoA carboxylase (reaction 1, p. 146). With a purified "fatty acid synthetase" from yeast stearyl-CoA is formed via (7) (Lynen, 1961)*. It was generally assumed that in the absence of biotin added oleic acid was reduced to stearic acid which could then be converted into other saturated fatty acids. However, the recent work of Bloch *et al.* (1961) has revealed a more complicated situation. Experiments with [14C]acetate have shown that in the absence of biotin the lactobacilli can synthesize either saturated or unsaturated fatty acids; furthermore although these acids are synthesized by cells grown in the presence of oleic acid, experiments with [1-14C]oleic acid have demonstrated the inability of the cells to reduce oleic acid;

---

* Palmityl-CoA is apparently the main product of the enzyme isolated from animal sources (see Mercer, 1962).

the main metabolic route in lactobacilli is methylation of the central double bond of oleic acid to form cyclopropane acids such as lacto-bacilli acid (XIV) (Hofmann and Lucas, 1950; Hofmann and Sax, 1953; Hofmann and Panos, 1955; O'Leary, 1959).

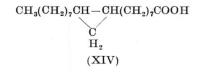

(XIV)

The failure to reduce oleic acid has also been noted in yeast (Yuan and Bloch, 1961) and in animal tissues (Bernhard *et al.*, 1958); it is ascribed to the fact that the centres of unsaturation at C-9 and C-10 are too remote from the activating carboxyl group to allow polarization of the double bond, which is probably a prerequisite for attack by a hydride ion (Bloch *et al.*, 1961).

The source of the saturated fatty acids in the lactobacilli grown in the absence of biotin but in the presence of oleic acid must therefore be exogenous. The Tweens would appear to be the most probable sources, especially as other types of detergent will not replace the Tweens in biotin-deficient, oleate-supplemented media, but the situation remains obscure (Bloch *et al.*, 1961).

Cl. butyricum, which responds similarly to oleic acid in the absence of biotin, will synthesize saturated fatty acids when grown on a biotin-less medium containing oleic acid, but will not convert oleic acid into saturated acids. Because the acids are synthesized it is concluded that endogenous biotin synthesis in this organism is not completely absent (Goldfine and Bloch, 1961).

E. *The Role of Aspartate*

It is well established that aspartate (or asparagine) spares biotin in many bacteria, for example, *Lactobacillus arabinosus* (Broquist and Snell, 1951), and fungi, *Torula cremoris* (Koser *et al.*, 1942) *Memnoniella echinata* and *Stachbobrys atra* (Perlman, 1948). The recent demonstration (p. 146) that biotin is an essential cofactor for pyruvic carboxylase, provides an explanation of the sparing of biotin. Oxaloacetate is synthesized from pyruvate and CO_2 (reaction 3) and then transaminated in the usual manner. The overall reaction can then be represented by reaction (8).

$$CH_3COCOOH + CO_2 \rightarrow HOOCCH_2COCOOH \xrightarrow[\text{amination}]{\text{trans-}} HOOCCH_2CHNH_2COOH \quad ($$

The observations that in the absence of aspartate, threonine, lysine and uracil will spare biotin (Woods *et al.*, 1954) probably means that they can be metabolized to oxaloacetate, but this has yet to be demonstrated.

III. General Factors Controlling Synthesis

A. *Higher Plants*

Biotin is synthesized in germinating seedlings (Burkholder, 1943) and in leaves (Filippov, 1950). Leaves of *Lappa major* and *Helianthus annuus* produce more biotin in light than in darkness; synthesis continues after illuminated plants are placed in the dark owing to the utilization of precursors formed by photosynthesis (Filippov, 1950).

It is assumed that biotin formed in the leaves is translocated to the roots of plants, from whence it may be excreted. The excreted biotin may be utilized either to stimulate root growth and/or the growth of the soil micro-flora (Went and Thimann, 1937). Isolated tissues of *Daucus carota*, *Vitis vinifera* (normal and tumourous) and *Parthenocissus tricuspidata* cultured *in vitro* synthesize biotin (Czosnowski, 1952).

B. *Micro-organisms*

a. Temperature. A strain of *Bacillus coagulans* will utilize desthiobiotin only at 36° but not at either 45° or 55°, whilst all other strains, and those of *B. stearothermophilus*, will utilize this precursor at any incubation temperature (Campbell and Williams, 1953). Increasing the culture temperature from 18° to 25° doubles the biotin production by *Phycomyces blakesleeanus* without affecting growth (Schopfer, 1943); this effect has recently been confirmed (Eisenberg, 1962).

b. Trace elements. The addition of a mixture of Cu, B, Fe^{3+}, Ga, Mn, Zn and Mo ions increases biotin production by *Phycomyces blakesleeanus* (Schopfer, 1943).

C. *Partial Synthesis by Animals*

The rat cannot insert the sulphur atom into desthiobiotin to any significant extent; the biological activity of *dl*-desthiobiotin is only 0·01-0·1% of that of biotin (Rubin *et al.*, 1945).

In both rats and chickens the specific effects of biotin deficiency can be cured by oxybiotin (XV), although in chickens it is claimed that the effect is only observed after parenteral administration of oxybiotin (Winnick *et al.*, 1945). The activity of oxybiotin in micro-organisms and animals is some 5–30% that of biotin itself (Hofmann *et al.* 1945; Axelrod *et al.*, 1947; Rubin *et al.*, 1945; McCoy *et al.*, 1946). In chickens, oxybiotin appears to be effective *per se* and not by virtue of its conversion into biotin. Biotin-deficient chickens were cured by oxybiotin without the biotin levels in the tissues increasing above the deficiency values (McCoy *et al.*, 1948).

$$\begin{array}{c} \overset{\displaystyle O}{\overset{\displaystyle \|}{C}} \\ \diagup\;\diagdown \\ NH\quad NH \\ |\qquad | \\ CH-CH \\ |\qquad | \\ CH_2\quad CH(CH_2)_4COOH \\ \diagdown\;\diagup \\ O \end{array}$$

(XV)

On the other hand, oxybiotin was found in the tissues in increasing amounts (McCoy *et al.*, 1948). This observation would fall in line with that of Axelrod *et al.* (1947) who found that the biotin activity of oxybiotin for *Saccharomyces cerevisiae* is an inherent property of the molecule; that is, it is active *per se* and not by virtue of its conversion into biotin.

IV. BIOCYTIN

Virtually nothing is known of the formation of biocytin. It is as active as biotin for native *Neurospora crassa*, for a biotin-requiring mutant of *Penicillium chrysogenum* (Wright *et al.*, 1952), and for a number of staphylococci (Gretler *et al.*, 1955). Wright *et al.* (1954b) noted an enzyme, *biocytinase*, in human blood which hydrolyses biocytin to L-lysine and *d*-biotin; a similar enzyme has been partly purified from pig liver (Thoma and Peterson, 1954). It is not known whether either of these enzymes has any synthetic activity.

V. BIOTIN SULPHOXIDE

It is known that biotin sulphoxide is synthesized from biotin by *Aspergillus niger* (Wright and Driscoll, 1954) but the mechanism of the reaction remains unelucidated.

VI. Biotin-CO$_2$

It has already been indicated that one metabolically active form of biotin is (IV) bound to the appropriate enzyme probably through lysine (p. 147). The mechanism of the formation of the energy rich enzyme biotin-CO$_2$ complex has been made clear by the experiments of Boyer (quoted by Ochoa and Kaziro, 1961). He found that with crystalline propionyl-CoA carboxylase incubated with propionyl-CoA and [^{18}O]HCO$_3'$, one ^{18}O atom appeared in orthophosphate and two atoms in methylmalonyl-CoA; when [^{18}O]H$_2$O was used there was no incorporation of isotope into orthophosphate or methyl-malonyl-CoA. This leads to the conclusion that the carboxylation of the bound biotin is a concerted reaction which involves nucleophilic attack of the biotin nitrogen on the bicarbonate carbon, followed by attack of the bicarbonate oxygen on the terminal phosphate of ATP (reaction 9). Thus, the activation of CO$_2$ by carboxylases is a one-step reaction which can be summarized in reaction (10). This mechanism may not hold for acetyl-CoA carboxylase (see p. 147).

$$(9)$$

$$\text{ATP} + \text{``CO}_2\text{''} + \text{Enzyme} \underset{}{\overset{\text{Mg}^{2+}}{\rightleftharpoons}} \text{ADP} + \text{P}_i + \text{Enz-``CO}_2\text{''} \qquad (10)$$

VII. Incorporation of Biotin into Enzymes

An enzyme preparation can be obtained from pig liver which in the presence of d-biotin, ATP, Mg^{2+} and a thiol activates apo-propionyl-CoA carboxylase present in extracts of liver from biotin-deficient rats (Foote $et\ al.$, 1962). The pig liver preparation contains a biotin-activating enzyme as evidenced by the production of biotin hydroxamate in the presence of ATP, CoA and Mg^{2+}. A similar

156 THE BIOSYNTHESIS OF VITAMINS AND RELATED COMPOUNDS

activating enzyme has been observed in bacteria (Christner *et al.*, 1961; Coon *et al.*, 1961).

Rather similar results with biotin-deficient rats have also been obtained by Kosow and Lane (1962). The mechanism of the linkage of biotin to the enzyme, which probably occurs on a lysine residue (see p. 147), remains to be elucidated.

REFERENCES

Andrews, E. A., and Williams, V. R. (1951). *J. biol. Chem.* **193,** 11.
Axelrod, A. E. Flinn, B. C., and Hofmann, K. (1947). *J. biol. Chem.* **169,** 195.
Bernhard, K., Rothlin, M., Vuilleumier, J. P., and Wyss, R. (1958). *Helv. chim. acta* **41,** 117.
Bloch, K., Baronowsky, P., Goldfine, H., Lennarz, W. J., Light, R., Norris, A. T., and Scheuerbrandt, G. (1961). *Fed. Proc.* **20,** 921.
Broquist, H. P., and Snell, E. E. (1951). *J. biol. Chem.* **188,** 431.
Broquist, H. P., and Snell, E. E. (1953). *Arch. Biochem. Biophys.* **46,** 432.
Burkholder, P. R. (1943). *Science* **97,** 562.
Campbell, L. L., and Williams, O. B. (1953). *J. Bact.* **65,** 146.
Carlson, W. W., Whiteside-Carlson, V., and Kospetos, K. (1950). *Fed. Proc.* **9,** 159.
Christner, J. E., Foote, J. L. and Coon, M. J. (1961). *Fed. Proc.* **20,** 271.
Chu, E. H. J., and Williams, R. J. (1944). *J. Amer. chem. Soc.* **66,** 1678.
Coon, M. J., Foote, J. L., and Christner, J. E. (1961). *In* "Proceedings of the 5th International Congress of Biochemistry, Moscow" **5,** in press. Pergamon Press, London.
Czosnowski, J. (1952). *Poznam ace Komisji Biol.* **13,** 1.
Dittmer, K., and du Vigneaud, V. (1944). *Science* **100,** 129.
Dittmer, K., Melville, D. B., and du Vigneaud, V. (1944). *Science* **99,** 203.
du Vigneaud, V., Hofmann, K., Melville, D. B., and Rachele, J. R. (1941). *J. biol. Chem.* **140,** 763.
du Vigneaud, V., Dittmer, K., Hague, E., and Long, B. (1942a). *Science* **96,** 186.
du Vigneaud, V., Dittmer, K., Hofmann, K., and Melville, D. B. (1942b). *Proc. Soc. exp. Biol., N. Y.* **50,** 374.
du Vigneaud, V., Melville, D. B., Folkers, K., Wolf, D. E., Mozingto, R., Keresztesy, J. C., and Harris, S. A. (1942c). *J. biol. Chem.* **146,** 475.
Eakin, R. E., and Eakin, E. A. (1942). *Science* **96,** 187.
Eisenberg, M. A. (1962). *Fed. Proc.* **21,** 467; *Biochem. biophys. Res. Commun.* **8,** 437.
Elford, H. L., and Wright, L. D. (1962). *Fed. Proc.* **21,** 467.
Evans, W. C., Happold, F. C., and Handley, W. H. C. (1939). *Brit. J. exp. Path.* **20,** 41.
Filippov, V. V. (1950). *Trud. Inst. Fiziol. Rast. Timiryazeva,* **7,** 232.
Foote, J. L., Christner, J. E., and Coon, M. J. (1962). *Fed. Proc.* **21,** 239.
Goldfine, H., and Bloch, K. (1961). *J. biol. Chem.* **236,** 2596.
Gretler, A. C., Mucciolo, P., Evans, J. B., and Niven, C. F. (1955). *J. Bact.* **70,** 44.
Halliday, W. J., and McCoy, E. (1955). *J. Bact.* **70,** 464.
Hofmann, K., and Lucas, R. A. (1950). *J. Amer. chem. Soc.* **72,** 4328.
Hofmann, K., and Sax, S. M. (1953). *J. biol. Chem.* **205,** 55.
Hofmann, K., and Panos, C. (1955). *J. biol. Chem.* **210,** 687.

Hofmann, K., McCoy, R. H., Felton, J. R., Axelrod, A. E., and Pilgrim, F. J. (1945). *Arch. Biochem.* **7,** 393.

Kaziro, Y. E., Leone, E., and Ochoa, S. (1960). *Proc. nat. Acad. Sci., Wash.* **46,** 1319.

Knappe, J., Biederbick, K. and Brümmer, W. (1962). *Angew. Chem. (Int. Ed.),* **1,** 401.

Knappe, J., Ringelmann, E., and Lynen, F. (1961). *Biochem. Z.* **335,** 168.

Kögl, F., and Tönnis, B. (1936). *Hoppe-Seyl. Z.* **242,** 43.

Kögl, F., and Borg, W. A. J. (1944). *Hoppe-Seyl. Z.* **281,** 65.

Koser, S. A., Wright, M. H., and Dorfman, A. (1942). *Proc. Soc. exp. Biol., N. Y.* **51,** 204.

Kosow, D. P., and Lane, M. D. (1962a). *Biochem. biophys. Res. Comm.* **7,** 439.

Kosow, D. P., and Lane, M. D. (1962). *Fed. Proc.* **21,** 286.

Leonian, L. H., and Lilly, V. G. (1945). *J. Bact.* **49,** 291.

Lilly, V. G., and Leonian, L. H. (1944). *Science,* **99,** 205.

Lynen, F. (1961). *Fed. Proc.* **20,** 941.

Lynen, F., Knappe, J., Lorch, E., Jütting, G., and Ringelmann, E. (1959). *Angew. Chem.* **71,** 481.

Lynen, F., Knappe, J., Lorch, E., Jütting, G., and Ringelman, E. (1961). *Biochem. Z.* **335,** 123.

McCoy, R. H., Felton, J. P., and Hofmann, K. (1946). *Arch. Biochem.* **9,** 141.

McCoy, R. H., McKibben, J. R., Axelrod, A. E., and Hofmann, K. (1948). *J. biol. Chem.* **176,** 1319, 1327.

Melville, D. B. (1954). *J. biol. Chem.* **208,** 495.

Melville, D. B., Dittmer, K., Brown, G. B., and du Vigneaud, V. (1943). *Science* **98,** 497.

Mercer, E. I. (1962). *Annu. Rep. Chem. Soc.* **58,** 353.

Miller, W. L. (1924). *Science* **59,** 197.

Mueller, J. H. (1937). *Science* **85,** 502.

Ochoa, S., and Kaziro, Y. (1961). *Fed. Proc.* **20,** 982.

O'Leary, W. M. (1959). *J. Bact.* **78,** 709.

Perlman, D. (1948). *Amer. J. Bot.* **35,** 36.

Robbins, W. J., and Ma, R. (1942). *Science,* **96,** 406.

Robinson, F. A. (1951). "The Vitamin B Complex." Chapman and Hall, London.

Rubin, S. H., Flower, D., Rosen, F., and Drekter, L. (1945). *Arch. Biochem.* **8,** 79.

Schopfer, W. H. (1943). "Plants and Vitamins". Chronica Botanica Co., Waltham, Mass.

Sebrell, W. H., and Harris, R. S. (1954). "The Vitamins", Vol. 1. Academic Press, New York.

Stokes, J. L., and Gunness, M. (1945). *J. biol. Chem.* **157,** 121.

Swick, R. W., and Wood, H. G. (1960). *Proc. nat. Acad. Sci., Wash.* **46,** 28.

Tatum, E. L. (1945). *J. biol. Chem.* **160,** 455.

Thoma, R. W., and Peterson, W. H. (1954). *J. biol. Chem.* **210,** 569.

Utter, M. F., and Keech, D. B. (1960). *J. biol. Chem.* **235,** PC17.

Wakil, S. J. (1958). *J. Amer. chem. Soc.* **80,** 6465.

Wakil, S. J., and Gibson, D. M. (1960). *Biochim. biophys. Acta,* **41,** 122.

Wakil, S. J., Tichener, E. B., and Gibson, D. M. (1958). *Biochim. biophys. Acta,* **29,** 225.

Wakil, S. J., and Waite, M. (1962). *Biochem. biophys. Res. Comm.* **9,** 18.

Went, F. W., and Thimann, K. V. (1937). "Phytohormones". Macmillan, London.

Wildiers, E. (1901). *Cellule* **18,** 313.

Williams, V. R., and Fieger, E. A. (1946). *J. biol. Chem.* **166,** 335.

Winnick, T., Hofmann, K., Pilgrim, F. J., and Axelrod, A. E. (1945). *J. biol. Chem.* **161**, 405.

Wood, H. G., and Stjernholm, R. (1961). *Proc. nat. Acad. Sci.*, *Wash.* **47**, 289.

Woods, L., Ravel, J. M., and Shive, W. (1954). *J. biol. Chem.* **209**, 559.

Wright, L. D. (1942). *Proc. Soc. exp. Biol.*, *N. Y.* **51**, 27.

Wright, L. D., and Cresson, E. L. (1954). *J. Amer. chem. Soc.* **76**, 4156.

Wright, L. D., and Driscoll, C. A. (1954). *J. Amer. chem. Soc.* **76**, 4999.

Wright, L. D., Cresson, E. L., Skeggs, H. R., Peck, R. L., Wolk, D. E., Wood, T.R., Valiant, J., and Folkers, K. (1951). *Science* **114**, 635.

Wright, L. D., Cresson, E. L., Liebert, K. V., and Skeggs, H. R. (1952). *J. Amer. chem. Soc.* **74**, 2002.

Wright, L. D., Cresson, E. L., Valiant, J., Wolf, D. E., and Folkers, K. (1954a). *J. Amer. chem. Soc.* **76**, 4160, 4163.

Wright, L. D., Driscoll, C. A., and Bodger, W. P. (1954b). *Proc. Soc. exp. Biol.*, *N. Y.* **86**, 335-337.

Wright, L. D., Cresson, E. L., and Driscoll, C. A. (1955). *Proc. Soc. exp. Biol.*, *N. Y.* **89**, 234.

Yuan, C., and Bloch, K. (1961). *J. biol. Chem.* **236**, 1277.

Chapter 7

VITAMIN B₆ (PYRIDOXINE) AND RELATED COMPOUNDS

I. Introduction

The identification of vitamin B_6, the component of the "vitamin B_2 complex" which cured acrodynia (a pellagra-like dermatitis) in rats, with various other factors which cured deficiency dermatites in other animals, followed the tortuous route characteristic of the early work on most water-soluble vitamins (see Robinson, 1951). However, the work of Chick *et al.* (1940a, b) eventually clarified the position.

The material responsible for these biological responses was obtained crystalline almost simultaneously in a number of laboratories. For example, Keresztesy and Stevens (1938) isolated it from rice whilst György (1938) and Kuhn and Wendt (1938) obtained it from yeast. The structure of vitamin B_6 (I) (3-hydroxy-4,5-dihydroxy-methyl-2-methylpyridine), which was eventually given the trivial name pyridoxine, was worked out by Kuhn and his colleagues (Kuhn *et al.*, 1939a, b) in Germany and by Stiller *et al.* (1939) in the United States.

Snell *et al.* (1942) discovered two closely related compounds during their work on the role of pyridoxine in microbial nutrition; these were the corresponding aldehyde, pyridoxal (II) and amine, pyri-

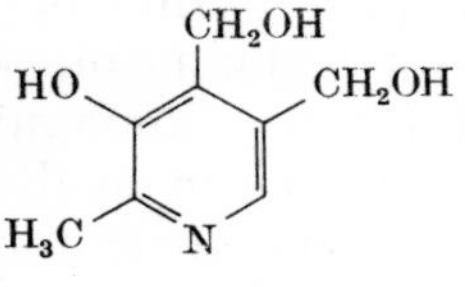

(I)

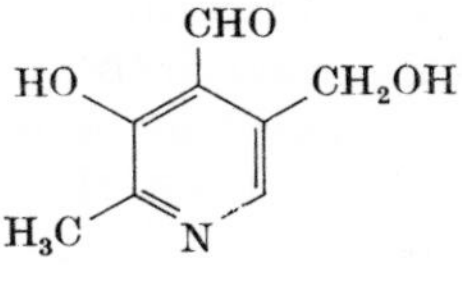

(II)

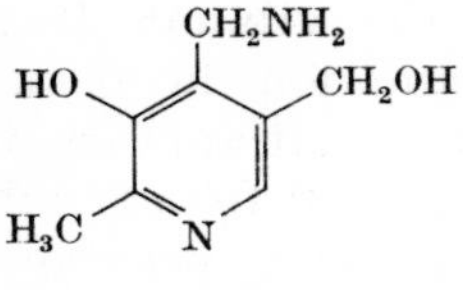

(III)

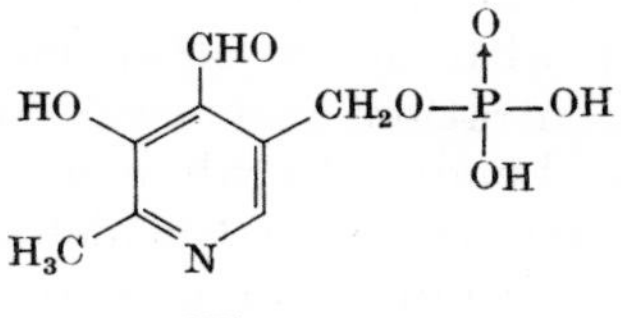

(IV)

doxamine (III). It is now known from later work by Snell's group that the main metabolically active form of these compounds is pyridoxal phosphate (IV), which is a coenzyme for, *inter alia*, amino acid decarboxylases, transaminases and racemases. Pyridoxamine phosphate (Rabinowitz and Snell, 1947) can, however, act as the coenzyme for transaminases (see Snell, 1960).

II. Biosynthesis

A. *General*

This section will be extremely short, for the comment of Snell in 1960, "although twenty years have elapsed since pyridoxine was first isolated and characterized, nothing is yet known of the biosynthetic precursors from which this or related forms of the vitamin arise naturally", still holds at the time of writing.

It was considered for some time that D-alanine, which will replace pyridoxine in the nutrition of certain *Lactobacilli*, might be a precursor of the vitamin (Snell and Guirard, 1943), but it was later shown that the reason for these observations was that pyridoxine is concerned with the synthesis of D-alanine which is an essential component of the cell wall of many bacteria (Holden *et al.*, 1949; Holden and Snell, 1951). It still remains possible that alanine is concerned in pyridoxine biosynthesis but there is now no evidence to support this view.

According to Nurmikko and Raunio (1961) the formation of vitamin B_6 by *Esch. coli* increases during the lag phase, reaches a maximum during the acceleration phase and decreases during exponential growth; excretion of vitamin B_6 into the medium does not occur.

Certain mutants of *Neurospora crassa* require pyridoxine only at low pH; this is not related to the problem of pyridoxine biosynthesis. Apparently *N. crassa* has a requirement for free ammonia when pyridoxine is absent from the medium, and thus in media of low pH, insufficient ammonia is present to satisfy their nutritional requirements (Strauss, 1951).

Little is known about pyridoxine synthesis in higher plants, but in common with many other members of the vitamin B complex, its concentration increases during germination in oats, wheat, barley and maize (Burkholder, 1943). However, it appears that light is necessary, for while Cheldelin and Lane (1943) found substantial increases within 36 hr of germinating black-eyed peas and cotton seeds in the light, Burkholder and McVeigh (1945), on the other hand, found no synthesis in soya and mung beans germinated in the

dark. The distribution of vitamin B$_6$ in tomato plants is very similar
to that of the other B vitamins (Bonner and Dorland, 1943).

From the list compiled by Bonner and Bonner (1948), it can be
seen that isolated roots of some tissues can grow without pyridoxine,
so it must be assumed that they have the ability to synthesize this
factor. An early report that glycine could replace pyridoxine in the
nutrition of isolated tomato roots (White, 1939) has now been discounted (Robbins and Schmidt, 1939; White, 1943; Bonner, 1943).

The only structural variation which the isolated tomato root can
tolerate, apart from the acetylation of the hydroxyl groups is the
substitution of ethyl for methyl at C-2 (I). Replacement of the
hydroxymethyl groups on positions 4 and 5, either singly or together,
destroys biological activity (Robbins, 1942; Table 1). It is interesting
to find that the root cannot oxidize a methyl group on C-4 to hydroxymethyl, although it presumably can oxidize the latter to formyl to
form pyridoxal.

TABLE 1. Effect of Alteration of the Side Chains
of Pyridoxine on its Activity as a Growth Factor
for Isolated Tomato Roots. The Medium Contained Sucrose, Salts and Thiamine*

| \multicolumn{4}{c}{Substituents in position} | Activity |
2	3	4	5	
CH$_3$	OH	CH$_2$OH	CH$_2$OH	+
C$_2$H$_5$	OH	CH$_2$OH	CH$_2$OH	+
CH$_3$	CH$_2$COO$^-$	CH$_2$CH$_2$COO$^-$	CH$_2$CH$_2$COO$^-$	+
CH$_3$	OCH$_3$	CH$_2$OH	CH$_2$OH	—
CH$_3$	OH	CH$_2$	CH$_2$OH	—
CH$_3$	OH	CH$_2$OC$_2$H$_5$	CH$_2$OH	—

* From Robbins (1942) and Bonner and Bonner (1948).

III. PHOSPHORYLATION OF PYRIDOXINE, PYRIDOXAL AND PYRIDOXAMINE

The enzyme which catalyses the phophorylation of pyridoxal,
pyridoxal phosphokinase [ATP: pyridoxal 5-phosphotransferase]
has been demonstrated in *Streptococcus faecalis* (Bellamy *et al.*,
1945), *Escherichia coli* and yeast (Hurwitz, 1953, 1955), liver (Trufanov and Kirsanova, 1946; Binkley and Christensen, 1951; McCormick and Snell, 1960), brain (Roberts and Frankel, 1957; McCormick
and Snell, 1959), kidney and muscle (McCormick *et al.*, 1961).

It was first purified from yeast by Hurwitz (1955) but recently McCormick *et al.* (1961) have developed a method for producing active enzymes of high purity from a number of animal and microbial sources. All the enzymes carry out the same reaction (equation 1)

$$\text{Pyridoxal} + \text{ATP} \xrightarrow{\text{Mg}^{2+}} \text{Pyridoxal phosphate} + \text{ADP} \qquad (1)$$

but they differ amongst themselves in a number of important respects. For example, (a) Zn^{2+} is a more effective activator than Mn^{2+} or Mg^{2+} for the yeast and animal kinases, whilst Mg^{2+} is superior to Zn^{2+} in all bacterial kinases so far examined; (b) the pH optimum varies between 4·5 for the *Lactobacillus bulgaricus* enzyme and 6·8 for the yeast enzyme, and (c) the individual enzymes differ in their stability towards heat. All the kinases phosphorylate pyridoxal, pyridoxamine and pyridoxine but there are important differences in their affinities for these substrates (Table 2). Although the affinities for pyridoxal and for ATP vary independently with pH they became equal at the optimum pH.

McCormick and Snell (1961) have reported in detail on the effect

TABLE 2. The Affinites of Pyridoxal Phosphokinases from Various Sources for Pyridoxal, Pyridoxamine and Pyridoxine (McCormick *et al.*, 1961). [Apparent K Values (moles/l. x10^4)]

Source of enzyme	Pyridoxal	Pyridox- ine	Pyridox- amine
L. casei	0·3	40	50
S. faecalis	0·15	15	25
Yeast (brewers')	4·0	0·25	0·15
Rat liver	0·15	0·25	1·5

of two groups of inhibitors (structural analogues and pyridoxal condensation products with aldehyde reagents) on the pyridoxal phosphokinases obtained from five different sources. The structural analogues which retained a formyl group on position 4, as in pyridoxal, had K_s values similar to pyridoxal; those which lacked this grouping had K_s values similar to pyridoxine. ω-Methylpyridoxal is only phosphorylated slowly by the kinase from *S. faecalis*, although its phosphate is as active as pyridoxal phosphate as co-enzyme for tyrosine decarboxylase isolated from the same source. The condensation products of pyridoxal with O-substituted hydroxylamines, hydrazine and substituted hydrazines were invariably potent inhibitors of all the enzyme preparations; in some cases the affinity of the inhibitor for the enzyme was 100–1000 times greater than that of pyridoxal. On the other hand the corresponding derivatives of pyridoxal phosphate were not inhibitory and the free reagents were also ineffective.

IV. Interconversion of Pyridoxal, Pyridoxamine and Pyridoxine

As animals respond to all three vitamers [there are, however, some quantitative differences in, for example, chicks (Luckey et al., 1945)], and as the same situation exists in many fungi (including yeasts) and bacteria which require vitamin B₆ (Snell and Rannefeld, 1945; Melnick et al., 1945), there must exist mechanisms for interconverting the three derivatives. Satisfactory evidence regarding these interconversions has only recently become available. Fig. 1 summarizes the transformations known to occur in animal tissues. It is probable that the main pathway of interconversion involves the phosphorylated derivatives (Wada et al., 1959; Snell, 1960). As pointed out in the previous section pyridoxine, pyridoxal and pyridoxamine are all equally rapidly phosphorylated by pyridoxal kinase. Pyridoxine phosphate and pyridoxamine phosphate are then rapidly oxidized to pyridoxal phosphate by *pyridoxine oxidase* [pyridoxamine: O₂ oxidoreductase (deaminating)] (Pogell, 1957; Wada and Snell, 1961). The conversion of pyridoxine and pyridoxamine into pyridoxal does occur in animal tissues (Braunstein and Bukin, 1956; Wada and Snell, 1961), but the reaction is very much slower than the reaction between the phosphorylated derivatives (Wada et al., 1959) and can assume metabolic importance only at very high substrate concentrations. An alternative route for the conversion of pyridoxamine into pyridoxal is by transamination with oxaloacetate as amino acceptor (Wada and Snell, 1961). Again, this pathway can only become important at high substrate concentrations. The analogous reaction, the conversion of pyridoxamine phosphate into pyridoxal phosphate by transamination does not occur in animal tissues (Wada and Snell, 1961). An earlier claim that this reaction did occur in *Esch. coli* (Beechey and Happold, 1957) has been discounted (Turner and Happold, 1961; Wada and Snell, 1961). Other reports that transamination between pyridoxal phosphate and pyridoxamine phosphate occurs in micro-organisms (Meister et al., 1951; Cattaneo-Lacombe et al., 1958) may have been a result of non-enzymatic reactions (Wada and Snell, 1961).

The interconversions (indicated in Fig. 1) also appear to take place in isolated duck erythrocytes; pyridoxal phosphate and pyridoxamine phosphate will both stimulate haem synthesis from glycine and succinate in red cells isolated from vitamin B₆-deficient ducks; on the other hand, free pyridoxal and pyridoxamine do not stimulate haem synthesis (Schulman and Richert, 1957). However, this experiment does not rule out inter-conversion at the non-phosphorylated level, with the absence of pyridoxal phosphokinase as the metabolic block.

The extent to which Fig. 1 is applicable to micro-organisms is not yet clear. It has already been stated (p. 161) that pyridoxal phosphokinase is widely distributed in bacteria and fungi, but the

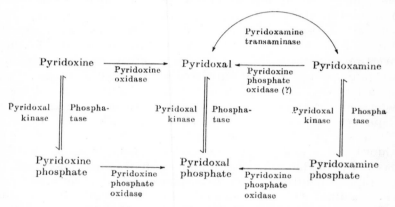

FIG. 1. The metabolic interrelationships of vitamin B₆ in animal tissues (Wada and Snell, 1961).

existence of a microbial pyridoxine oxidase remains to be reported. In *Clostridium* spp. (Boyd *et al.*, 1947) and protozoa (Kidder and Dewey, 1949) and *Lactobacillus casei* (Snell and Rannefeld, 1945), which require vitamin B₆, the affinity of the appropriate enzymes for pyridoxine must be very low, because in all cases pyridoxine has only very slight biological activity. The low affinity has now been demonstrated in *Lact. casei* (Table 2). However, it is still possible that cellular permeability may be the limiting factor in controlling the growth-promoting activity of pyridoxine in these organisms.

It appears that the conversion of free pyridoxamine into free pyridoxal occurs in extracts of *Esch. coli* (Gunsalus and Tonzetich 1952) and *Acetobacter rancens* (Hurwitz, 1956).

Pyridoxine oxidase has been purified 67-fold from rabbit liver; it is a flavoprotein which can be separated into its components. The apoenzyme is fully reactivated by FMN, whilst FAD is 1000 times less active. The oxidase has an pH optimum between 9 and 10 and is inhibited by the product of the reaction (pyridoxal phosphate), Cu^{2+} and Hg^{2+} (1mM), p-chloromercuribenzoate and some phosphorylated analogues (for example, pyridoxal phosphate oxine and 4-deoxypyridoxine phosphate). Some of the last named compounds are very potent inhibitors with enzyme affinities of the same order as the true substrates. The inhibition by the product of the reaction is decreased by Tris buffer, cysteine and other compounds which can form Schiff's bases or thiazolidine derivatives of pyridoxal phosphate.

REFERENCES

Beechey, R. B., and Happold, F. C. (1957). *Biochem, J.* **66**, 520.

Bellamy, W. D., Umbreit, W. W., and Gunsalus, I. C. (1945). *J. biol. Chem.* **160**, 461.

Binkley, F., and Christensen, G. M. (1951). *J. Amer. chem. Soc.* **73**, 3535.

Bonner, J. (1943). *Bull. Torrey bot. Club*, **70**, 184.

Bonner, J., and Dorland, R. (1943). *Arch. Biochem.* **2**, 451.

Bonner, J., and Bonner, H. (1948). *Vitam. & Horm.* **6**, 225.

Boyd, M. J., Logan, M. A., and Lytell, A. A. (1947). *J. biol. Chem.* **174**, 1013.

Braunstein, A. E., and Bukin, Y. V. (1956). *Proc. Acad. Sci. Armen. S.S.R.* **106**, 95.

Burkholder, P. R. (1943). *Science* **97**, 562.

Burkholder, P. R., and McVeigh, I. (1945). *Plant Physiol.* **20**, 76, 301.

Cattaneo-Lacombe, J., Senez, J. C., and Beaumont, P. (1958). *Biochim. biophys. Acta* **30**, 458.

Cheldelin, V. H., and Lane, R. L. (1943). *Proc. Soc. exp. Biol., N.Y.* **54**, 53.

Chick, H., El Sadr, M. M., and Worden, A. N. (1940a). *Biochem. J.* **34**, 595.

Chick, H., Macrae, T. F., and Worden, A. N. (1940b). *Biochem. J.* **34**, 580.

Gunsalus, C. F., and Tonzetich, J. (1952). *Nature, Lond.* **170**, 162.

György, P. (1938). *J. Amer. chem. Soc.* **60**, 983.

Holden, J. T., and Snell, E. E. (1951). *J. biol. Chem.* **190**, 403.

Holden, J. T., Furman, C., and Snell, E. E. (1949). *J. biol. Chem.* **178**, 789.

Hurwitz, J. (1953). *J. biol. Chem.* **205**, 935.

Hurwitz, J. (1955). *J. biol. Chem.* **212**, 757; **217**, 513.

Hurwitz, J. (1956). *In* "National Vitamin Foundation Nutrition Symposium Series" No. 13, 49.

Kidder, G. W., and Dewey, V. C. (1949). *Arch. Biochem.* **20**, 433; **21**, 58.

Keresztesy, J. C., and Stevens, J. R. (1938). *J. Amer. chem. Soc.* **60**, 1267.

Kuhn, R., and Wendt, G. (1938). *Ber. dtsch. chem. Ges.* **71**, 780, 1118.

Kuhn, R., Andersag, H., Westphal, K., and Wendt, G. (1939a). *Ber. dtsch. chem. Ges.* **72**, 309.

Kuhn, R., Wendt, G., and Westphal, K. (1939b). *Ber. dtsch. chem. Ges.* **72**, 310.

Luckey, T. D., Briggs, G. M., Elvehjem, C. A., and Hart, E. B. (1945). *Proc. Soc. Exp. Biol. Med., N.Y.* **58**, 340.

McCormick, D. B., and Snell, E. E. (1959). *Proc. Nat. Acad. Sci., Wash.* **45**, 1371.

McCormick, D. B., and Snell, E. E. (1960). *Fed. Proc.* **19**, 413.

McCormick, D. B., and Snell, E. E. (1961). *J. biol. Chem.* **236**, 2085.

McCormick, D. B., Gregory, M. E., and Snell, E. E. (1961). *J. biol. Chem.* **236**, 2076.

Meister, A., Sober, H. A., and Tico, S. V. (1951). *J. biol. Chem.* **189,** 577.
Melnick, D., Hockberg, M., Himes, H. W., and Oser, B. L. (1945). *J. biol. Chem.* **160,** 1.
Nurmikko, V., and Raunio, R. (1961). *Acta chem. scand.* **15,** 856.
Pogell, B. M. (1957). *Abst. Fall Meeting Amer. Chem. Soc.* 85C.
Rabinowitz, J. C., and Snell, E. E. (1947). *J. biol. Chem.* **169,** 631, 643.
Robbins, W. J. (1942). *Amer. J. Bot.* **29,** 241.
Robbins, W. J., and Schmidt, M. B. (1939). *Amer. J. Bot.* **29,** 149.
Roberts, E., and Frankel, S. (1957). *J. biol. Chem.* **190,** 505.
Robinson, F. A. (1951). "The Vitamin B. Complex". Chapman and Hall, London.
Schulman, M. P., and Richert, D. A. (1957). *J. biol. Chem.* **226,** 181.
Snell, E. E. (1960). *In* "Proceedings of the 4th International Congress of Biochemistry, Vienna", XI p. 250. Pergamon Press, London.
Snell, E. E., and Guirard, B. M. (1943). *Proc. nat. Acad. Sci., Wash.* **29,** 66.
Snell, E. E., and Rannefeld, A. N. (1945). *J. biol. Chem.* **157,** 475.
Snell, E. E., and Guirard, B. M., and Williams, R. J. (1942). *J. biol. Chem.* **143,** 519.
Stiller, E. T., Keresztesy, J. C., and Stevens, J. R. (1939). *J. Amer. chem. Soc.* **61,** 1237.
Strauss, B. S. (1951). *Arch. Biochem.* **30,** 292.
Trufanov, A. V., and Kirsanova, J. A. (1946). *Bull. Biol. Med. exp. URSS,* **22,** No. 6.
Turner, J. M., and Happold, F. C. (1961). *Biochem. J.* **78,** 364.
Wada, H., and Snell, E. E. (1961). *J. biol. Chem.* **236,** 2089.
Wada, H., Morisue, T., Nishimura, Y., Morino, Y., Sakamoto, Y. and Ichihara, K. (1959). *Proc. imp. Acad. Japan,* **35,** 299.
White, P. R. (1939). *Plant. Physiol.* **14,** 527.
White, P. R. (1943). *Amer. J. Bot.* **30,** 33.

CHAPTER 8

VITAMIN B$_{12}$ AND RELATED COMPOUNDS (COBAMIDES)

I. INTRODUCTION

Vitamin B$_{12}$, the antipernicious anaemia factor, was first obtained crystalline from liver almost simultaneously by Smith (1948) in England and by Folkers and his colleagues (Rickes et al., 1948) in the United States. Rickes et al. (1948) also indicated that vitamin B$_{12}$ was a microbial fermentation product, a conclusion arrived at a few months previously by Stokstad et al. (1948). It soon became clear that many bacteria produced materials with vitamin B$_{12}$ activity (see Darken, 1953; Perlman, 1959), but that in general it was species of the genus *Streptomyces* which produced significant amounts. The vitamin B$_{12}$ remains intracellular and is not excreted into the culture medium to any significant extent (Ford and Hutner, 1955; Brown et al., 1956; Provasoli, 1958; Perlman, 1959). Various moulds (e.g. *Ustilago zeae*, *Aspergillus niger*, *Eremothecium* sp., *Neurospora* sp.) show vitamin B$_{12}$ activity (see Perlman, 1959), but the activity reported in some algae in early work (Ericson and Lewis, 1953) may, in part, be the result of bacterial contamination of the algae examined. For example, Scott and Ericson (1955) in following the metabolism of ^{60}Co in the red alga *Rhodymenia palmata*, found that the vitamin B$_{12}$ present was not labelled; they concluded that this and possibly other marine algae did not synthesize the vitamin but obtained it by absorbing vitamin B$_{12}$-synthesizing bacteria. It should be emphasized here that, unlike other known vitamins, it is usually considered that the vitamins B$_{12}$ are not synthesized by higher plants, although recently Fries (1962) has cultured peas aseptically and found that extracts show vitamin B$_{12}$ activity in *Esch. coli*, *Euglena gracilis* and a vitamin B$_{12}$-heterotrophic red alga *Goniotrichum*. The photosynthetic bacteria apparently do synthesize these compounds (Kondrat'eva and Uspenskja, 1961).

The micro-organisms most frequently used in the industrial synthesis of vitamin B$_{12}$ are listed in Table 1. Frequently the vitamin is a by-product of a fermentation carried out primarily for

TABLE 1. Organisms Used for Industrial Production of Vitamin B_{12}

Organism	Reference
Bacillus megaterium	Lewis *et al*. (1949)
Propionibacterium freudenreichii	Sudarsky and Fischer (1957)
Streptomyces olivaceus	Hester and Ward (1954)
Streptomyces sp. (ATCC 11072)	Pagano and Greenspan (1954)

the production of an antibiotic. Mixed fermentations have also been investigated. In one such fermentation a lactose-containing medium was fermented with lactobacilli until maximum lactic acid production was achieved, then the appropriate propionibacteria were added (Leviton, 1956). Hodge *et al*., (1952) used a mixture of *Pseudomonas* sp., *Streptococcus bovis*, *Proteus vulgaris* and *Clostridium putrificum* to ferment a medium based on soya bean oil meal; the vitamin B_{12} yields were higher then when any of the organisms was used singly.

The media proposed in the literature for the growth of the vitamin B_{12}-synthesizing organisms are legion (see Darken, 1953; Perlman, 1959; Goodwin, 1963).

II. CHEMISTRY AND NOMENCLATURE

A. *Vitamin B_{12} and its Analogues*

As investigations into the compounds exhibiting vitamin B_{12}-like activity progressed it became clear that numerous closely related compounds (vitamin B_{12} analogues) existed. The elucidation of the structure of vitamin B_{12} (cyanocobalamin) (I) as a result of the brilliant co-ordination of classical organic chemistry and X-ray crystallography (Hodgkin *et al*., 1955) [see Johnson and Todd (1957) for a full discussion] made it possible to define the structures of the various naturally occurring analogues and to rationalize the nomenclature of these compounds (Smith, 1960). The basic tetra-pyrrole residue, which differs from a porphyrin macro-ring in that it lacks a methine bridge between pyrrole rings D and A, and which has frequently been referred to as a pseudoporphyrin ring system, has now been termed the *corrin* ring; the numbering of the constituent atoms is indicated in (II).

Cobrynic acid has structure (III) and it should be noted that the terminal carboxyl groups or modified carboxyl groups are designated by the letters *a* to *g*. The amidated cobrinic acid to

which D_g-1-amino-2-propanol is attached at C-f is named cobinamide (IV); cobinamide to which 3-phosphoribose is attached at the

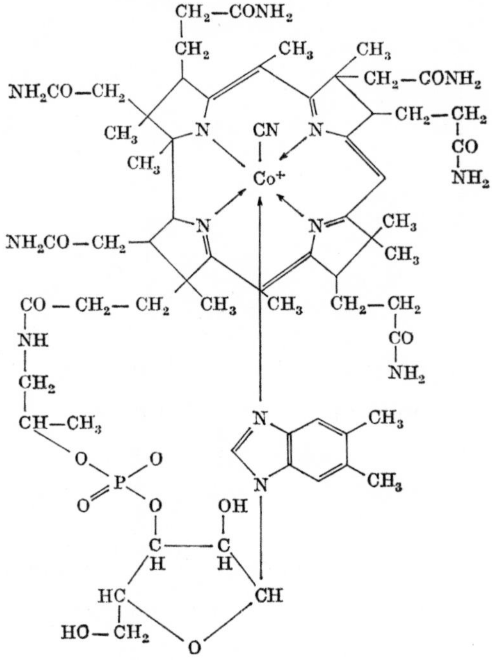

(I)

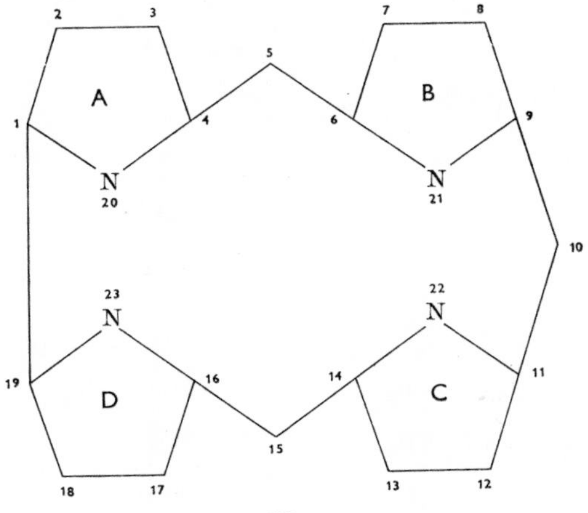

(II)

hydroxyl group of the aminopropanol residue is termed cobamide
(V). The names now proposed for the various vitamin B_{12} analogues

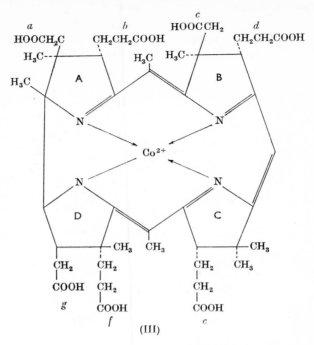

(III)

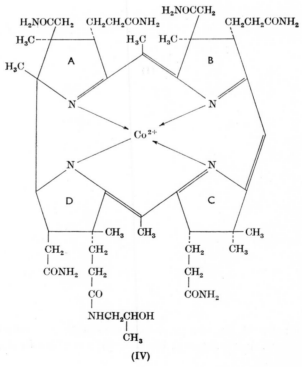

(IV)

which have well authenticated structures are summarized in Table 2. These compounds thus differ from vitamin B$_{12}$ either by containing no nucleotide (Factor B, cobinamide, IV) or a nucleotide different from that in vitamin B$_{12}$. Factor B was first isolated from calf rumen contents (Ford *et al.*, 1951). Cobamide (V) has been obtained

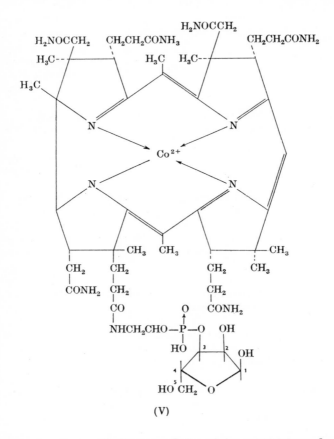

(V)

from the same source (Dellweg and Bernhauer, 1957), and cobinam-de phosphate occurs in cultures of *Nocardia rugosa* (di Marco *et al.*, 1957); of special importance is cobinamide-guanosine disphosphate, which has been obtained from *P. shermanii* (Pawelkiewitz *et al.*, 1959) and *N. rugosa* (Barchielli *et al.*, 1960). It is the guanosine 5'-pyrophosphate derivative of cobinamide in which the ribose is linked to N-9 of guanine; in the other known guanine derivative (Factor C, Table 2) the ribose is linked to N-7 (Friedrich and Bernhauer, 1959) as it is the other purine analogues of vitamin B$_{12}$ e.g. α-adenylcobamide (pseudovitamin B$_{12}$) (Hodgkin *et al.*, 1955).

TABLE 2. Some Naturally Occurring Nucleotide Analogues of Vitamin B_{12}*

Trivial Name	Systematic name	Base of nucleotide	Occurrence
Pseudovitamin B_{12}	α-Adenylcobamide cyanide	Adenine	Sewage sludge; unidentified rumen organism, marine algae, *Corynebact. diphtheriae*, *Prop. shermanii*, *P. arabinosum* *P. pentosaccum*
Factor A (vitamin B_{12m}; pseudovitamin)	2-Methyl-α-adenylcobamide cyanide	2-Methyladenine	Calf gut contents; calf and pig faeces; sewage sludge; marine algae, *Corynebact. diphtheriae*
Factor C (Nocardia factor 1)	Guanylcobamide cyanide	Guanine	Calf faeces; *Nocardia rugosa*
Factor F	2-Methylthio-α-adenylcobamide cyanide	2-Methylthio-adenine	Chicken faeces; sewage sludge
Factor G	α-Hypoxanthyl-cobamide cyanide	Hypoxanthine	Pig faeces
Factor H	2-Methyl-α-hypoxanthylcobamide cyanide	2-Methylhypoxanthine	Pig and calf faeces
Factor I (vitamin B_{12III})	5-Hydroxy-α-benzimidazolycobamide cyanide	5-Hydroxy-benzimidazole	Pig faeces; sewage sludge

It has been suggested that various mono- and dicarboxylic acid derivatives of vitamin B_{12} exist in sewage sludge (Friedrich and Bernhauer, 1953) and in *Propionibact. shermanii* (Kelemen and Csanyi, 1961); one of these, Factor VIa, has been isolated and shown to be cobrynic acid *abcdeg* hexamide (Bernhauer *et al.*, 1960a,b); however, Dellweg *et al.* (1956) and Pawelkiewicz and

* These compounds almost certainly exist as cobamide coenzymes (see p. 173).

Zodrow (1957) from their investigations with *Esch. coli* and *Cory-nebact. diphtheriae* respectively, consider that these compounds are breakdown products because they only appear late in the fermentations; however, this view appears to be ruled out by the observation that an adenine derivative of Factor VIa accumulates in a vitamin B_{12} auxotroph of *Nocardia rugosa* (Migliacci and Rusconi, 1961).

Various other "incomplete" factors, which have not yet been unequivocally characterized are discussed by Coates and Kon (1957) and Kon and Pawelkiewicz (1960).

It is becoming increasingly clear that the main naturally occurring forms of vitamin B_{12} are the "cobamide coenzymes" which are discussed in the following paragraphs and that the "free" vitamins B_{12} which are found naturally are mainly aquocobamides and not cyanocobamides. The aquocobamides, which were first isolated from *Strept. aureofaciens* (Pierce *et al.*, 1950) have OH^- instead of CN^- in co-ordinate linkage with cobalt. The isolation procedures normally used split adenosine from the cobamide coenzymes and replace it by CN^-, which probably originates from the charcoal used during the isolation of the vitamin (Toohey and Barker, 1961).

B. *Cobamide Coenzymes*

Barker and his colleagues (see Barker, 1961) were first to note that derivatives of vitamin B_{12} were coenzymes in certain enzymatic reactions, in particular *glutamate isomerase* (the isomerization of L-glutamate to β-methylaspartate), in micro-organisms. These cobamide coenzymes were found to contain adenosine* attached at C-5 to divalent cobalt in the cobamide residue (Barker *et al.*, 1960; Weissbach *et al.*, 1960; Ladd *et al.*, 1960; Lenhert and Hodgkin, 1961). The conclusion that the cobalt in Coenzyme B_{12} is divalent is based on the report that cyanocobalamin is diamagnetic whilst Coenzyme B_{12} is paramagnetic; there is also a similarity between the absorption spectrum of the reduced cobalamin and Coenzyme B_{12}(Bernhauer *et al.*, 1961a). Crystallographic evidence is not so clear-cut (Lenhert and Hodgkin, 1961). The adenosine derivative of α-adenylcobamide (VI) is the coenzyme for glutamate isomerase (Barker *et al.*, 1958), but coenzymes containing other bases have been obtained (Barker, 1961). Other reactions in with cobamide coenzymes have been implicated include the isomerization of methyl-malonyl-CoA to succinyl-CoA, the formation of methionine (see Chapter 9) and thymidine, and the incorporation of amino acids into proteins (see Barker, 1961; Plaut, 1961).

* Now known to be deoxyadenosine.

Frequently over 80% of the vitamin B_{12} found in micro-organisms is in the coenzyme form (Volcani *et al.*, 1961; Perlman *et al.*, 1960)

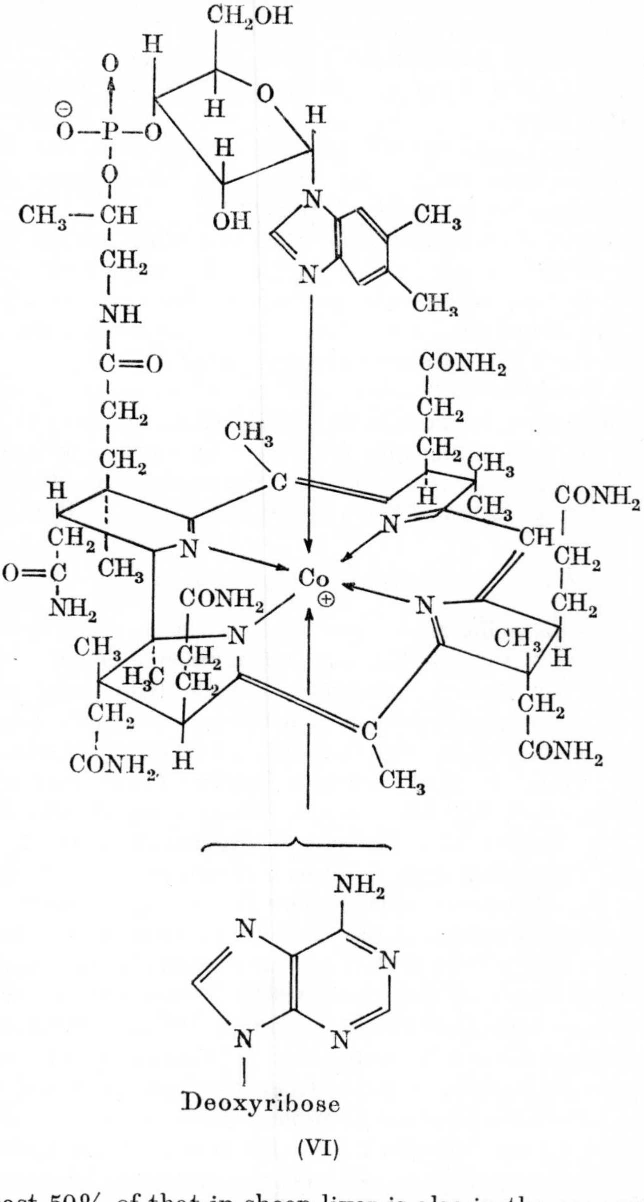

Deoxyribose

(VI)

and at least 50% of that in sheep liver is also in the coenzyme form (Toohey and Barker, 1961; Barker, 1961).

C. *Cobamide Peptides*

Cobamide peptides have been isolated from *Streptomyces griseus* by, for example, Hausmann *et al.* (1953). The purest preparation so far obtained from micro-organisms contained about 23% of cobamide (Mulli and Schmid, 1956). The function of these peptides is unkown, and their relationship to the cobamide-coenzymes has not yet been clarified. It is possible that they are artefacts. A peptide which contains cobalamine has also been isolated from ox liver (Hedbom, 1961).

III. THE BIOSYNTHESIS OF VITAMIN B$_{12}$

A. *General*

It is not intended here to discuss the considerable body of work which has been carried out on the control of the microbiological synthesis of vitamin B$_{12}$ by alterations in various complex consti-tuents of the culture medium and which have been specifically aimed at developing industrial processes. These have been fully discussed by, *inter alia*, Darken (1953), Tanaka, (1957) and Perlman, (1959). However, a few typical examples of the media used and the yields obtained are given in Table 3.

The problem of the effect of the cobalt content of the medium on vitamin B$_{12}$ synthesis is, however, important in the present context. If the cobalt concentration is below a certain critical concentration in a particular fermentation, then its addition to the medium will stimulate vitamin B$_{12}$ synthesis. This has been demonstrated with *Mycobact.* spp. (Kocher and Sorkin 1952) and with *S. griseus* (Hend-lin and Ruger, 1950) and in bacteria isolated from maize and potato rhizospheres (Bershova and Kozlova, 1962) and in a *Candida* sp. (Shadkhan *et al.*, 1962). If the cobalt content of the medium is not limiting, then no stimulation of vitamin B$_{12}$ synthesis can be expect-ed on further addition of the element; indeed cobalt levels above 50 p.p.m. inhibit synthesis (Principe and Thornberry, 1952). With limiting concentrations of cobalt (1 p.p.m. or less), as much as 75% of the added element can be incorporated into the vitamin, although the degree of incorporation falls rapidly with increasing concentra-tions of cobalt (Perlman and O'Brien, 1954; Smith *et al.*, 1952). Vitamin B$_{12}$ labelled with ^{60}Co is obtained with a high specific acti-vity (0·8 mc/mg) if a *S. griseus* fermentation is carried out in a medium containing sub-optimal levels of cobalt (Smith, 1955). Much higher activities (12 mc/mg) can be obtained if carrier-free ^{56}Co or

TABLE 3. Media Used for Industrial Fermentation of Vitamin B_{12}

Organism	Medium	Yield B_{12} (mg/l)	Reference
Bacillus megaterium	Beet molasses; ammonium phosphate, cobalt salts, inorganic salts	0·45	Lewis *et al.* (1949)
Propionibacterium freudenreichii	Glucose, casein hydrolysate; yeast extract; cobalt salts. lactic acid	3·0	Leviton and Hargrove (1952)
Streptomyces griseus	Glucose: soyabean meal; cobalt salts	0·3	Wood and Hendlin (1952)
S. fradiae	Glucose, brewers' yeast; soyabean meal; cobalt salts: inorganic salts	0·7	Nelson *et al.* (1950)
S. olivaceus	Glucose: soyabean meal; distillers' solubles; cobalt salts; inorganic salts.	3·3	Hall *et al.* (1953)
Streptomyces sp.	Soyabean meal; glucose; K_2HPO_4; $CoCl_2$	5·7	Pagano and Greenspan (1954)

[57]Co are used (Mollin and Smith, 1956; Smith, 1957). The feeding to sheep of a "cobalt bullet", which remains in the rumen, increased the vitamin B_{12} content of ewes' milk by up to ten times (O'Halloran and Skerman, 1961).

The mechanism of incorporation of cobalt into vitamin B_{12} is not known, but Perlman and O'Brien (1954) found that organically bound cobalt, produced by growing yeast in a cobalt-containing medium, was more effectively utilized by *S. griseus* than was Co^{2+}. Fluoride inhibits the incorporation of Co^{2+} into vitamin B_{12} by *S. griseus* (Iwamoto, 1952).

Maitra and Roy (1960) have examined the effect of trace elements on vitamin B_{12} production by *Streptomyces olivaceus* when growing on a basal glucose/inorganic salt medium freed from trace elements. They found that iron and zinc (1·0 p.p.m.) are essential for vitamin B_{12} synthesis; and that copper, up to 10 p.p.m. favours both growth and vitamin synthesis. On the other hand molybdenum, chromium and manganese, up to 5,2 and 100 p.p.m., respectively, favour growth but have no significant effect on vitamin production. Nickel (0·2 p.p.m.) inhibits both growth and vitamin synthesis, whilst boron inhibits only growth.

B. *Formation of the Corrin Ring*

A considerable amount of work on "guided biosynthesis" in the vitamin B$_{12}$ field (see p. 182) indicates that cobinamide (Factor B) is first synthesized and then coupled to the appropriate nucleotide. It is now also clear that the pyrrole residues of the corrin ring system are synthesized in the same way as the pyrrole residues of the porphyrins. The elegant investigations of Shemin, Neuberger and Rimington and their colleagues (see Goodwin, 1960) have shown that the pyrrole ring arises as porphobilinogen from succinate and glycine via δ-aminolaevulic acid (ALA) (reaction 1). Similarly Neuberger *et al.* (see Smith, 1960), Shemin *et al.* (1956) and Schwartz *et al.* (1858) have demonstrated that in vitamin B$_{12}$-synthesizing Actinomycetes [1,4-^{14}C]-δ-aminolaevulic acid and [^{14}C]porphobilinogen were rapidly incorporated into cobinamide. Furthermore, if the pathway of incorporation of [1,4-^{14}C]-δ-aminolaevulic acid is the same as into the porphyrin ring then the atoms starred in (VII) should be labelled. That is, 6 of the 15 labelled atoms (40% of the total activity) should reside in the carboxyl carbons of the side chains. Corcoran and Shemin (1957) found experimentally a value of 30% and concluded that δ-aminolaevulic acid is a true intermediate in the synthesis of the corrin ring and that it is incorporated in the same way as into porphyrins.

$$\text{Succinyl} - \text{CoA} + \text{glycine} \rightarrow \text{ALA} \rightarrow \text{porphobilinogen} \qquad (1)$$

A further characteristic of the cobinamide residue of vitamin B$_{12}$ compared with the porphyrins is the existence of supernumerary methyl groups. According to Bray and Shemin (1959) the six methyl groups marked with dots in (VII) arise from the methyl group of methionine. [^{14}C-Methyl]choline and [^{14}C-methyl]betaine are not incorporated. The transfer reaction probably involves S-adenosyl methionine (see Chapter 9). There is at present no direct information as to when the methyl groups are incorporated; Bukin and Mantrova (1961a,b), Mantrova *et al.* (1961) and Pronyakova (1960) consider that the macro-ring is not formed from δ-aminolaevulic acid but possibly from methylated ALA. Their conclusion is based on the following observations on *Propionibact. shermanii*: (a) toxopyrimidine (VIII) does not inhibit vitamin B$_{12}$ formation but does inhibit the synthesis of porphyrins, presumably by inhibiting the pyridoxine-dependent ALA-synthetase; (b) addition of ALA stimulated porphyrin production but not vitamin B$_{12}$ synthesis; (c) iron

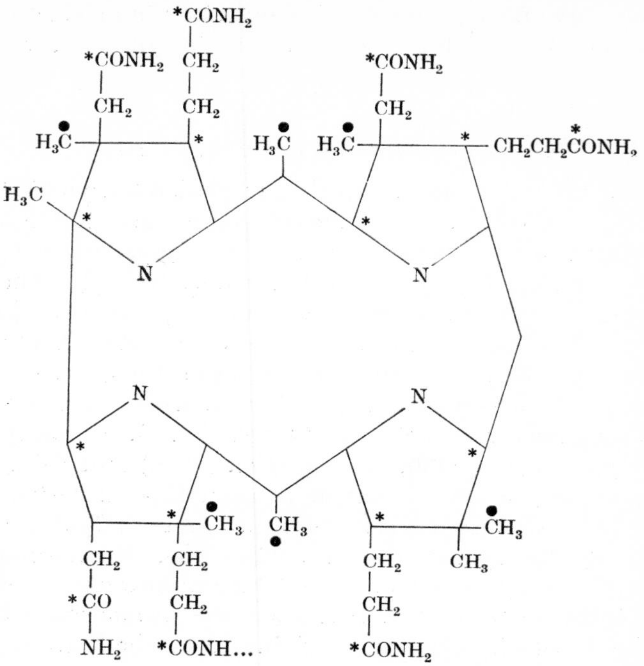

(VII)

salts inhibited porphyrin synthesis but had no effect on vitamin B_{12} synthesis; and (d) aminopterin suppressed vitamin B_{12} synthesis without affecting porphyrin synthesis.

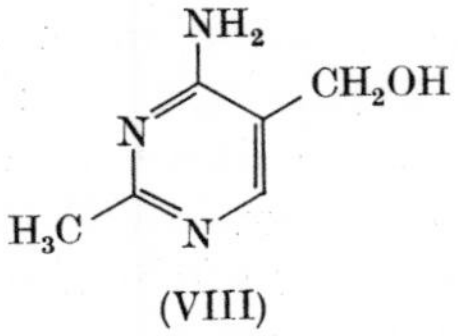

(VIII)

D_g-1-Amino-2-propanol, which represents the link between the cobinamide and the nucleotide portions of vitamin B_{12} (I), probably arises from threonine, because in the presence of L-[^{15}N]threonine, *Streptomyces griseus* concentrates ^{15}N into the aminopropanol residue of vitamin B_{12} (Krasna *et al.*, 1957); the decarboxylation of threonine probably occurs before acylation with the corrin derivative. Bernhauer and Wagner (1962) found that *P. shermanii* and *Esch. coli* 113–3 would not utilize the threonine derivative of cobrynic acid *abcdeg* hexamide (cobrinyl *abcdeg* hexamide-*f*-N-L-threonine), whereas the aminoethanol derivative and its monophosphate were actively utilized. The monophosphate may be the true precursor because it is more effectively converted than is the free aminoethanol derivative.

The exact mechanism of the incorporation of the constituent pyrrole units into the corrin ring system is not known. It will be recalled that the first macro-ring formed in porphyrin synthesis is the octacarboxylated compound uroporphyrinogen (see Goodwin, 1960). By analogy with this, it would be reasonable to assume that the first macro-ring formed during vitamin B_{12} biosynthesis would be the corresponding octacarboxylated hydrogenated corrin which could be converted by dehydrogenation, methylation, decarboxylation and co-ordination with cobalt into cobrynic acid (III); this in turn would be amidated, stepwise to cobrynic acid *abcdeg* hexamide which on attachment of aminopropanol would yield cobinamide (IV) (reaction 2). Support for this view comes from the observations, mentioned previously, that cobrynic acid *abcdeg* hexamide accumulates in a vi-

Octacarboxy-corrin → cobrynic acid → cobrynic acid *abcdeg* hexamide →
cobinamide   (2)

tamin B_{12} deficient mutant of *Nocardia rugosa*, and that it is utilized for vitamin B_{12} synthesis by another mutant strain (635) of, the same organism (Migliacci and Rusconi, 1961) and also by *P. shermanii* (Bernhauer *et al.*, 1960). However, it should be borne in mind that these reactions may take place at the "coenzyme" level, because the hexamide exists *in vivo* with an adenyl derivative attached to the cobalt atom (see p. 184).

C. *Incorporation of the Nucleotide Residue*

Kon and his colleagues (Kon, 1955) using a vitamin B_{12}-requiring mutant of *Esch. coli* (113–3) have biosynthesized vitamin B_{12} from cobinamide and 5,6-dimethylbenzimidazole (Ford and Holdsworth, 1952; Ford *et al.*, 1954, 1955a). When ^{60}Co cobinamide is used, there is very little dilution out of radioactivity in the resulting vitamin B_{12}. Similar results were obtained with wild strains of *Esch. coli* (Bernhauer and Friedrich, 1954), *Propionibacterium shermanii* (Janicki and Pawelkiewicz, 1954) and *Streptomyces griseus* (Fantes and O'Callaghan, 1955). *Euglena* spp., which require vitamin B_{12}, can also condense cobinamide with 5,6-dimethylbenzimidazole (Provasoli, 1958), whilst *Ochromonas malhamensis* cannot (Ford *et al.*, 1954). In this respect *O. malhamensis* resembles humans and chicks, which also require the intact vitamin B_{12} molecule (Coates and Ford, 1955).

Most of the other naturally occurring vitamins B_{12} can be similarly synthesized by *Esch. coli* (113–5) in the presence of cobinamide and the appropriate base, but Factors G and H (Table 2) cannot be synthesized. The reason for this is unknown, and it is all the more inexplicable when it is realized that a great number of "unnatural" analogues can be synthesized by this organism (see p. 182).

The α-D-nucleoside of 5,6 dimethylbenzimidazole (α-ribasole) and α-ribasole phosphate are much less efficient than the free base in the conversion of cobinamide into vitamin B_{12} by *Esch. coli* (Dellweg *et al.*, 1956). This could be ascribed to differences in permeability of the cell membrane to the various compounds, but an alternative explanation is that the "activated" base which is attached to the cobinamide residue, is not an α-riboside or ribotide. However, according to the work of Boretti *et al.* (1960) discussed below, dimethyl benzimidazole α-D-riboside is an intermediate in *Nocardia rugosa* and Friedman and Harris (1962) have reached the same conclusion with *Propionibact. shermanni*. On the other hand, this suggested explanation is particulary attractive in the case of the purine-containing vitamins B_{12}, because, as indicated earlier in the chapter the constitutent nucleoside is the 7-α-nucleoside (IX) whilst the purine nucleotides found in nucleic acids, ATP and similar compounds, always have the 9-β-nucleoside structure (X). Furthermore

(IX)   (X)

none of the 9-β-purine nucleosides investigated by Ford *et al.* (1955a, b) was incorporated into vitamin B_{12} analogues.

It has been suggested that GDP-cobinamide (p. 171) is an important intermediate in vitamin B_{12} biosynthesis in *Nocardia rugosa* (Barchielli *et al.*, 1960; Boretti *et al.*, 1960; di Marco *et al.*, 1961; Barbieri *et al.*, 1962). Reactions (3), (4), and (5) represent the proposed pathway. Evidence for this pathway includes the following: (a) cobinamide phosphate and cobinamide-GDP appear during initial stages of a *Nocardia rugosa* fermentation; (b) these two compounds accumulate in a mutant of *N. rugosa* in which vitamin B_{12} biosynthesis is blocked; (c) a mutant of *N. rugosa* blocked before cobinamide phosphate will convert this compound and cobinamide-GDP into vitamin B_{12}; (d) in the presence of $^{32}P_i$ the vitamin is unlabelled when cobinamide-GDP is the substrate, and is only

$$\text{Cobinamide} \xrightarrow{\quad \overset{\text{ATP} \quad \text{ADP}}{\smile} \quad} \text{cobinamide}-P \qquad (3)$$

$$\text{Cobinamide}-P \xrightarrow{\quad \overset{\text{GTP} \quad \text{P-P}}{\smile} \quad} \text{cobinamide}-\text{GDP} \qquad (4)$$

$$\text{Cobinamide}-\text{GDP} \xrightarrow{\quad \underset{\substack{\text{Dimethyl} \quad \text{GMP} \\ \text{benzimidazole} \\ \alpha\text{-riboside}}}{\frown} \quad} \text{vitamin } B_{12} \qquad (5)$$

very slightly labelled when cobinamide phosphate is the substrate; and (e) 5,6-dimethylbenzimidazole α-riboside is incorporated as a unit.

D. *Formation of 5,6-Dimethylbenzimidazole-α-D-Riboside*

Ford *et al.* (1955a, b) showed that *Esch. coli* 113–3 would synthesize vitamin B_{12} from cobinamide in the presence of 1,2-dimethyl-4,5-diaminobenzene. This indicates that the organism can attach a 1-C unit to the *o*-phenylenediamine derivative and cyclize this derivative to dimethylbenzimidazole. These observations do not prove conclusively that the benzimidazole derivative is normally derived from *o*-phenylenediamine. The effectiveness of *o*-phenylenediamine in vitamin B_{12} biosynthesis should be contrasted with the inability of this and related compounds to be incorporated into ring A of riboflavin (p. 57).

There is no information available on whether the dimethylbenzimidazole is synthesized at the α-D-riboside or ribotide level or as the free base. Furthermore the mechanism of the formation of the α-D-riboside linkage is unknown.

E. *Formation of Purine Residues in Vitamins B_{12}*

The pathway of biosynthesis of the common naturally occurring purines is now well established (see e.g. Goodwin, 1960) and need not be discussed here; the general pathway involved has already been summarized in Chapter 2 (p. 48). However, new and important problems arise when the purine-containing vitamins B_{12} are considered. Firstly, it will be remembered that the purines are synthesized at the nucleoside 5'-phosphate level and that the sugar is attached at N-9-in a β-glycosidic linkage. In the vitamins B_{12} the sugar is attached to N-7 in an α-glycosidic linkage. If a reaction analogous to reaction (5) (p. 181) applies to the incorporation of purines into the cobinamide residue, then enzymes must exist which convert 9-β-nucleotides into 7-α-nucleosides. Investigations on this problem have not yet been reported, but whilst a mechanism of this type may exist in *Propionibact. shermanii*, it is probably absent from *Nocardia rugosa* which cannot synthesize purine analogues of vitamin B_{12} (Barbieri *et al.*, 1961).

Secondly methyl groups appear at C-2 of the purine residues in Factors A and H (Table 2). Such methylated purines are rare outside the vitamin B_{12} field and the question which arises is "at what point on the biosynthetic pathway is the methyl group inserted?". No direct evidence is available, but experiments on guided biosynthesis (p. 183) would suggest that it occurs before the condensation of the base with cobinamide. Finally, the appearance of a sulphur derivative, 2-methylthioadenine, in Factor F, raises similar problems because this purine has not been found naturally elsewhere.

F. *Guided Biosynthesis — Synthesis of Vitamin B_{12} Analogues*

The original observation of Sahashi *et al.* (1950) that addition of 5,6-dimethylbenzimidazole to a *Streptomyces* sp. increased the yield of vitamin B_{12}, has been confirmed many times and extended to a number of other organisms. Janicki and Pawelkiewicz (1954) pursued this report and demonstrated that another benzimidazole, the 5-methyl derivative, was utilized by *Propionibacterium shermanii* to synthesize a vitamin B_{12} analogue which, on hydrolysis, yielded 5-methylbenzimidazole. This stimulated a vast amount of painstaking research on the synthesis of other analogues, which has been fully outlined by Kon and Pawelkiewicz (1960). Three main approaches have been developed; (a) cobinamide and an appropriate base are added to growing cells of a vitamin B_{12}-requiring bacterium (*Esch. coli* mutant 113–3) (Kon, 1955); (b) cobinamide and the appropriate base are added to resting cells of an organism which can synthesize "metabolic" amounts of vitamin B_{12} (native strains of *Esch. coli*) (Bernhauer and Friedrich, 1954); (c) the appropriate base only is added to organisms such as *Streptomyces* spp. (Fantes and O'Callaghan, 1954) *Propionibact. arabinosum* and *Propionibact. pentosaceum* (Perlman and Barrett, 1959) which produce relatively large amounts of vitamin B_{12}.

Only small amounts of analogues are synthesized by system (a), but it is the most versatile system in that it will form analogues with various substituted benzimidazoles, purines (including azapurines) and benztriazoles (Kon and Pawelkiewicz, 1960). System (b) will give improved yields but only of benzimidazole derivatives. System (c) gives the best yields, and a further advantage is that cobinamide does not need to be added to the fermentation. However, only the benzimidazole bases can be incorporated and, furthermore, a high level of the analogue base has to be present in the medium, presumably in order to compete with the synthesis of the natural vitamin, which under these conditions is greatly suppressed but not entirely eliminated.

Most bases which can be converted into analogues are incorporated unchanged, but substituents on position 2 of the benzimidazole ring appear to be eliminated; for example, 2-carboxybenzimidazole yields the analogue containing the unsubstituted base (Dellweg et al., 1956). Furthermore, nitro derivatives are often reduced to amino derivatives (Smith, 1960).

Although the base present in the cobamide coenzyme of Cl. tetanomorphum is adenine, benzimidazole cobamide coenzyme and 5,6-dimethylbenzimidazole coenzyme have been obtained by growing Cl. tetanomorphum in the presence of these bases (Weissbach et al., 1961; Ladd et al., 1961). Similar results have been obtained with other bacteria (Toohey and Barker, 1960; Barker et al., 1960; Mattern, 1960). In particular, analogues containing 2,6-diaminopurine, 5-methylbenzimidazole, 5-trifluorobenzimidazole, 5-aminobenzimidazole or 5-nitrobenzimidazole have been isolated from Propionibacterium arabinosum (Toohey et al., 1961). In all cases an adenine nucleoside was linked to reduced cobalt. Similar results have been observed with P. shermanii and P. petersonii as well as with P. arabinosum (Bernhauer et al., 1961b).

It is important to note that pyrimidines will not yield vitamin B_{12} analogues.

G. Biosynthesis of Coenzymes B_{12}

The addition of the adenosine nucleoside to vitamin B_{12} and the reduction of the valency of the cobalt from three to two resulting in the production of coenzyme B_{12} has been reported to occur in cell-free extracts of Propionibacterium shermanii (Brady and Barker, 1961; Brady et al., 1962) and Clostridium tetanomorphum (Pawelkiewicz et al., 1961b; Bernhauer et al., 1961a; Weissbach et al., 1961, Peterkofsky and Weissbach, 1962). The cofactors required for this synthesis are glutathione NADH, $FADH_2$, $MnCl_2$ and ATP. Peterkovsky et al. (1961), by use of [U-^{14}C]-ATP, have shown that ATP contributes both the adenine and the sugar residues to the coenzyme B_{12}.

On the assumption that the valency is changed Brady *et al.* (1962) propose the following mechanism:

$$\text{Hydroxobenzimidazoylcobamide} + \text{ATP} + \text{FADH}_2 + e \xrightarrow{\text{Mn}^{2+}} \text{benzimidazoylcobamide coenzyme} + \text{P} - \text{P} + \text{P}_i + \text{FAD}$$

and this is not inconsistent with the recent observations of Weissbach *et al.* (1962) that reduced benzimidazoylcobamide is not an obligatory intermediate in the reaction.

Under normal fermentation conditions adenosine may be bound to the ring system of vitamin B_{12} before completion of the molecule. Migliacci and Rusconi (1961) found that cobrynic acid *abcdeg* hexamide which accumulated in a mutant strain of *Nocardia rugosa* was linked via cobalt to an adenine derivative.

REFERENCES

Barbieri, P., Boretti, G., di Marco, A., Migliacci, A., and Spalla, C. (1961). *In* "Procedings of the 5th International Congress of Biochemistry, Moscow," p. 274. Pergamon Press, London.

Barbieri, P., Boretti, G., di Marco, A., Migliacci, A., and Spalla, C. (1962). *Biochim. biophys. Acta* **57,** 599.

Barchielli, R., Boretti, G., di Marco, A., Julita, P., Migliacci, A., Minghetti, A., and Spalla, C. (1960). *Biochem. J.* **74,** 382.

Barker, H. A. (1961). *Fed. Proc.* **20,** 956.

Barker, H. A., Weissbach, H., and Smyth, R. D. (1958). *Proc. nat. Acad. Sci., Wash.* **44,** 1093.

Barker, H. A., Smyth, R. D., Weissbach, H., Toohey, J. I., Ladd, J. N., and Volcani, B. E. (1960). *J. biol. Chem.* **235,** 480.

Bernhauer, K., and Friedrich, W. (1954). *Angew. Chem.* **66,** 776.

Bernhauer, K., Dellweg, H. W., Friedrich, W., Gross, G., Wagner, F., and Zeller, P. (1960a). *Helv. chim. Acta* **43,** 693.

Bernhauer, K., Wagner, F., and Zeller, P. (1960b). *Helv. chim. Acta* **43,** 696.

Bernhauer, K., and Wagner, F. (1962). *Biochem. Z.* **335,** 325.

Bernhauer, K., Becher, E., Gross, G., and Wilharm, G. (1960). *Biochem. Z.* **332,** 562.

Bernhauer, K., Gaiser, P., Müller, O., Muller, E., and Gunter, F. (1961a). *Biochem. Z.* **333,** 560.

Bernhauer, K., Müller, O., and Müller, G. (1961b). *Biochem. Z.* **335,** 37.

Bershova, I. O. I., and Koslova, I. A. (1962). *Mikrobiol. Zh. Akad. Nauk. S. S. R.* **24,** 30.

Boretti, G., di Marco, A., Fuoco, L., Marnati, M. P., Migliacci, A., and Spalla, C., (1960). *Biochim. biophys. Acta* **37,** 379.

Brady, R. O., and Barker, H. A. (1961). *Biochim. biophys. Res. Comm.* **4,** 464.

Brady, R. O. Castanera, E. G., and Barker, H.A. (1962). *J. biol. Chem.* **237,** 2325.

Bray, R., and Shemin, D. (1959). *Biochim. biophys. Acta* **30,** 647.

Brown, F., Cuthbertson, W. F. J., and Fogg, G. E. (1956). *Nature, Lond.* **177**, 188.

Bukin, V. N., and Mantrova, G. V. (1961a). *C.R. Acad. Sci. U.R.S.S.* **137**, 713.

Bukin, V. N. and Mantrova, G. V. (1961b). *Vitamin Resussy Akad. Nauk. S. S. R. Inst. Biochem.* p. 32.

Coates, M. E., and Ford, J. E. (1955). *Biochem. Soc. Symp.* **13**, 361.

Coates, M. E., and Kon, S. K. (1957). *In* "Vitamin B$_{12}$ and Intrinsic Factor". p. 72, F. Enke. Stuttgart.

Corcoran, J. W., and Shemin, D. (1957). *Biochim. biophys. Acta* **25**, 661.

Darken, M. A. (1953). *Bot. Rev.* **19**, 99.

Dellweg, H., and Bernhauer, K. (1957). *Arch. Biochem. Biophys.* **69**, 74.

Dellweg, H., Becher, E., and Bernhauer, K. (1956). *Biochem. Z.* **327**, 422; **328**, 81, 88, 96.

Di Marco, A., Boretti, G., Migliacci, A., Julita, P., and Minghetti, A. (1957). *Boll. Soc. ital. Biol. sper.* **33**, 1513.

di Marco, A., Boretti, G., and Spalla, C. (1961). *Sci. Rept. Inst. Sup. Sanita*, 1, 355.

Ericson, L. E., and Lewis, L. (1953). *Ark. Kemi.* **6**, 427.

Fantes, K. H., and O'Callaghan, C. H. (1954). *Biochem. J.* **58**, xxi.

Fantes, K. H., and O'Callaghan, C. H. (1955). *Biochem. J.* **59**, 79.

Ford, J. E., Kon, S. K., and Porter, J. W. G. (1951). *Biochem. J.*, **50**, ix

Ford, J. E., and Holdsworth, E. S. (1952). *Biochem. J.* **53**, xxii.

Ford, J. E., and Hutner, S. H. (1955). *Vitam. & Horm.* **13**, 101.

Ford, J. E., Holdsworth, E. S., and Kon, S. K. (1954). *Biochem. J.* **58**, xxi.

Ford, J. E., Gregory, M. E., and Holdsworth, E. S. (1955a). *Biochem. J.* **61**, xxiii.

Ford, J. E., Holdsworth, E. S., and Kon, S. K. (1955b). *Biochem. J.* **59**, 86.

Friedmann, H. C., and Harris, D. L. (1962). *Biochem. biophys. Res. Comm.* 8, 164.

Friedrich, W., and Bernhauer, K. (1953). *Angew. Chem.* **65**, 627.

Friedrich, W., and Bernhauer, K. (1959). *Med. Grundlagenforsch.* **2**, 661; *Hoppe-Seyl. Z.* **317**, 166.

Fries, L. (1962). *Physiol. Plant.* **15**, 566.

Goodwin, T. W. (1960). "Recent Advances in Biochemistry". Churchill London.

Goodwin, T. W. (1963). *In* "Biochemistry of Industrial Micro-organisms" (A. H. Rose and C. Rainbow, ed.). Academic Press, London.

Hall, H. H., Benedict, R. G., Wiesen, C. F., Smith, C. E., and Jackson, R. W. (1953). *Appl. Microbiol.* 1, 124.

Hausmann, K., Ludwig, L., and Mulli, K. (1953). *Acta Haematol.* **10**, 282.

Hedbom, A. (1961). *Arkiv. Kemi* **17**, 551.

Hendlin, D., and Ruger, M. L. (1950). *Science*, **111**, 541.

Hester, A. S., and Ward, G. E. (1954). *Industr. Engng. Chem.* **46**, 238.

Hodge, H. M., Hanson, C. T., and Allgeier, R. J. (1952). *Industr. Engng. Chem.* **44**, 132.

Hodgkin, D. C., Pichworth, J., Robertson, J. H., Trueblood, K. N., Prosen, R. J., White, J. G., Bonnet, R., Cannon, J. R., Johnson, A. W., Sutherland, I., Todd, A. R., and Smith, E. L. (1955). *Nature, Lond.* **176**, 325.

Iwamoto, K., (1952). *Nippon Nogei-Kagaku Kaishi* **26**, 553.

Janicki, J., and Pawelkiewicz, J. (1954). *Acta Biochem. Polon.* 1, 307.

Johnson, A. W., and Todd, A. R. (1957) *Vitam. and Horm.* 15, 1.

Kelemen, A. M., and Csanyi, E. (1961). *In* "Proceedings of the 5th International Congress of Biochemistry, Moscow", p. 232. Pergamon Press, London.

Kocher, V., and Sorkin, E. (1952). *Helv. chim. Acta* **35**, 1741.

Kon, S. K. (1955). *Biochem. Soc. Symp.* **13,** 17.

Kon, S. K., and Pawelkiewicz, J. (1960). *In* "Proceedings of the 4th International Congress of Biochemistry, Vienna", XI, p. 115. Pergamon Press, London.

Kondrat'eva, E. N., and Uspenskja, V. E. (1961). *C. R. Acad. Sci. U.R.S.S.* **136,** 718.

Krasna, A. I., Rosenblum, C., and Sprinson, D. B. (1957). *J. biol. Chem.* **225,** 745.

Ladd, J. N., Hogenkamp, H. P. C., and Barker, H. A. (1960). *Biochem. biophys. Res. Comm.* **2,** 143.

Ladd, J. N., Hogenkamp, H. P. C., and Barker, H. A. (1961). *J. biol. Chem.* **236,** 2114.

Lenhert, P. G., and Hodgkin, D. C. (1961). *Nature, Lond.* **192,** 937.

Leviton, A. (1956). *U.S. Pat. Syst. Leafl.* 2, 753, 289; 2, 764, 52.

Leviton, A., and Hargrove, R. E. (1952). *Industr. Engng. Chem* **44,** 2651.

Lewis, J. C., Ijichi, K., Snell, N. S., and Garibaldi, J. A. (1949). *U.S. Dept. Agric. Bull. AIC,* **254.**

Mattern, C. F. T. (1960). *J. biol. Chem.* **235,** 489.

Mollin, D. L., and Smith, E. L. (1956). *Proceedings of the International Conference on Peaceful Uses of Atomic Energy,* **10,** 475.

Migliacci, A., and Rusconi, A. (1961). *Biochim. biophys. Acta* **50,** 370.

Mulli K., and Schmid, O. J. (1956). *Z. Vitamin-, Hormon-, u. Fermentforsch.* **8,** 225.

Nelson, H. A., Calhoun, K. M., and Colingsworth, D. R. (1950). *Abst. 118th Meeting Amer. chem. Soc.* p. 16A.

O'Halloran, M. W., and Skerman, K. D. (1961). *Brit. J. Nutr.* **15,** 99.

Pagano, J. F., and Greenspan, G. (1954). *U.S. Pat. Syst. Leafl.* 2, 695, 864.

Pawelkiewicz, J., and Zodrow, K. (1957). *Acta Biochim. Polon.,* 4, 203.

Pawelkiewicz, J., Bartosinski, B., and Walerych, W. (1960). *Bull. acad. polon. Sci. Classe II,* 8, 123.

Pawelkiewicz, J., Bartosinski, B., and Walerych, W. (1961). *Acta Biochim. Polon.* 8, 131

Pawelkiewicz, J., Walerych, W. and Bartosinski, B. (1959). *Acta Biochim. Polon.* 6, 431

Perlman, D. (1959) *In* "Advances in Applied Microbiology" 1, 87. Academic Press, New York and London.

Perlman, D., and O'Brien, E. (1954). *J. Bact.* **68,** 167.

Perlman, D., and Barrett, J. M. (1959). *J. Bact.* **78,** 171.

Perlman, D., Semar, J. B., and Frazier, W. B. (1960). *Abst. 138th Meeting Amer. chem. Soc.,* p. 10A.

Peterkofsky, A., and Weissbach, H. (1962). *Fed. Proc.* **21,** 470.

Peterkofsky, A., Redfield, B., and Weissbach, H. (1961). *Biochem. biophys. Res. Comm.* **5,** 213.

Pierce, J. V., Page, A. C. Jr., Stokstad, E. L. R., and Jukes, T. H. (1950). *J. Amer. chem. Soc.* **72,** 2615.

Plaut, G. W. E. (1961). *Annu. Rev. Biochem.* **30,** 409.

Principe, P. A., and Thornberry, H. H. (1952). *Phytopathology,* **42,** 123.

Pronyakova, G. V. (1960). *Biokhymia* **25,** 296.

Provasoli, L. (1958). *Annu. Rev. Microbiol* **12,** 279.

Rickes, E. L., Brink, N. G., Koniuszky, F. R., Wood, T. R., and Folkers, K. (1948). *Science* **107,** 396.

Sahashi, Y., Mitaka, M., and Skai, H. (1950). *Bull. chem. Soc. Japan* **23,** 247.

Schwartz, S., Ikeda, K., Miller, I. A., and Watson, C. J. (1958). *Science* **129,** 40.

Scott, R., and Ericson, L. E. (1955). *J. exp. Bot.* **6**, 348.
Shadkhan, K. B., Cirite, L. and Kokileva, L. (1962). *Latvijas PSR Zinaļna Akad. Vestis*, p. 89
Shemin, D., Corcoran, J. W., Rosenblum, C., and Miller, I. M. (1956). *Science* **124**, 272.
Smith, E. L. (1948). *Nature, Lond.* **162**, 144.
Smith, E. L. (1955). *Biochem. Soc. Symp.* **13**, 3.
Smith, E. L. (1957). *In* "Vitamin B$_{12}$ and Intrinsic Factor", p. 1. (H. C. Heinrich, ed.). Enke, Stuttgart.
Smith, E. L. (1960). "Vitamin B$_{12}$". Methuen, London.
Smith, E. L., Fantes, K. H., Ball, S., Waller, J. G., Emery, W. B., Anslow, W. K., and Walker, A. D. (1952). *Biochem. J.* **52**, 389.
Stokstad, E. L. R., Page, A. C. Jr., Pierce, J., Franklin, A. L., Jukes, T. H., Heinle, R. W., Epstein, M., and Welch, A. D. (1948). *J. Lab. clin. Med.* **33**, 860.
Sudarsky, J. M., and Fisher, R. A. (1957). *U.S. Pat. Syst. Leafl.* **2**, 816, 856.
Takata, R. (1957). *Vitamins (Kyoto)*, **12**, 1.
Toohey, J. I., and Barker, H. A. (1960). *Fed. Proc.* **19**, 417.
Toohey, J. I., and Barker, H. A. (1961). *J. biol. Chem.* **236**, 560.
Toohey, J. I., Perlman, D., and Barker, H. A. (1961). *J. biol. Chem.* **236**, 2119.
Volcani, B. E., Toohey, J. I., and Barker, H. A. (1961). *Arch. Biochem. Biophys.* **92**, 381.
Weissbach, H., Ladd, J. N., Volcani, B. E., Smyth, R. D., and Barker, H. A. (1960). *J. biol. Chem.* **235**, 1462.
Weissbach, H., Redfield, B., and Peterkofsky, A. (1961). *J. biol. Chem.* **236**, PC40.
Weissbach, H., Redfield, B. G., and Peterkofsky, A. (1962). *J. Biol. Chem.* **237**, 3217.
Wood, T. R., and Hendlin, D. (1952). *U.S. Pat. Syst. Leafl.* 2, 595, 499.

CHAPTER 9

CHOLINE AND RELATED COMPOUNDS

I. INTRODUCTION

It could be thought that choline (I), rather like inositol (Chapter 10), has crept into the pages of this book under false pretences. It is now clear that animals have the ability to synthesize large amounts of choline, provided that a sufficient supply of "labile methyl groups" is available. The diet of most animals usually provides all the labile methyl groups required for choline synthesis in the form of the essential amino acid methionine (II). If labile methyl groups (i.e. methi-

$$(CH_3)_3\overset{+}{N}CH_2CH_2OH$$

(I)

$$S—CH_3$$
$$|$$
$$CH_2$$
$$|$$
$$CH_2$$
$$|$$
$$CHNH_2$$
$$|$$
$$COOH$$

(II)

onine) are in short supply, pathological manifestations of a nutritional deficiency disease appear. The best known characteristic of such a condition is a fatty degeneration of the liver, although this can also occur in other deficiencies, such as in the absence of the essential unsaturated fatty acids (see Chapter 12).

Choline has never been reported as a growth factor for micro-organisms although it is present in numerous fungi (Stoll, 1952). As a component of phospholipids it is also widely distributed in nature.

This chapter will be concerned with (a) the biosynthesis of methionine in micro-organisms, animals and plants, (b) the biosynthesis of choline as such and in phospholipids, (c) the biosynthesis of phospholipids which contain choline.

II. Biosynthesis of Methionine

A. *Formation of Methyl Groups and Their Transfer to Homocysteine*

(i) *In Bacteria.*

Nutrition experiments with micro-organisms indicated that the vitamin B_{12} requirements of some bacteria could be spared by either thymine or methionine (Lascelles and Cross, 1955). The first *in vitro* demonstration of the effect of vitamin B_{12} on methionine biosynthesis was reported by Woods and his colleagues who worked with an *Escherichia coli* mutant (strain 121/176) which requires either methionine or vitamin B_{12} for growth. Cell-free preparations require vitamin B_{12} for the synthesis of methionine from homocysteine and serine in the presence of FAH_4 (Helleiner and Woods, 1956; Helleiner *et al.*, 1957; Kisliuk and Woods, 1957; Guest *et al.*, 1960). It was later shown that a vitamin B_{12}-containing protein was an integral part of the system (Kisliuk and Woods, 1959). A similar situation was found to exist in *Esch. coli* strain PA15, a serine or glycine-requiring auxotroph (Cross and Woods, 1954; Gibson and Woods, 1960; Szulmajster and Woods, 1960; Guest *et al.*, 1960) and the vitamin B_{12}-containing factor has been purified 150 times from this source (Foster *et al.*, 1961); it has all the properties of an enzyme. Kisliuk (1960) has also reported briefly on the purification of this enzyme.

Hatch *et al.* (1959) and Larrabee and Buchanan (1961) in similar investigations have found that two enzymes are concerned with the synthesis of methionine from $N^{5,10}$-methylene FAH_4 [the active C_1 unit derived from serine (see p. 119)] and homocysteine in *Esch. coli* strain 113–3. The first enzyme, when incubated with NADH and $N^{5,10}$-methylene FAH_4, produces a compound now identified as 5-methyl-FAH_4 (see p. 122) (reaction 1). The second enzyme, which contains vitamin B_{12}, will transfer the methyl group from 5-methyl-FAH_4 to homocysteine in the presence of NADH, FAD, ATP and Mg^{2+} (reaction 2). Grossowicz and Aronovitch (1961) also report the involvement of vitamin B_{12} in methionine biosynthesis in *Arthrobacter* spp., and a similar effect with vitamin B_{12} was found in studies on the formation of the methyl group of thymine from formate (Dinning *et al.*, 1958).

$$N^{5,10}\text{-Methylene FAH}_4 \xrightarrow[\text{NAD}]{\text{NADH}_2} N^5\text{-Methyl FAH}_4 \qquad (1)$$

$$N^5\text{-Methyl-FAH}_4 + \text{``homocysteine''} \xrightarrow[\text{ATP, Mg}^{2+}]{\text{NADH FAD}} \text{Methionine} + \text{FAH}_4 \qquad (2)$$

The details of reaction (2) have not yet been elucidated but almost certainly S-adenosylhomocysteine (III) is first formed and this is methylated to S-adenosylmethionine (IV) (Duerre and Schlenk, 1962). Furthermore, Shapiro (1961) has shown with the aid of bacterial mutants that S-adenosylmethionine is probably the immediate source of methionine in his organisms.

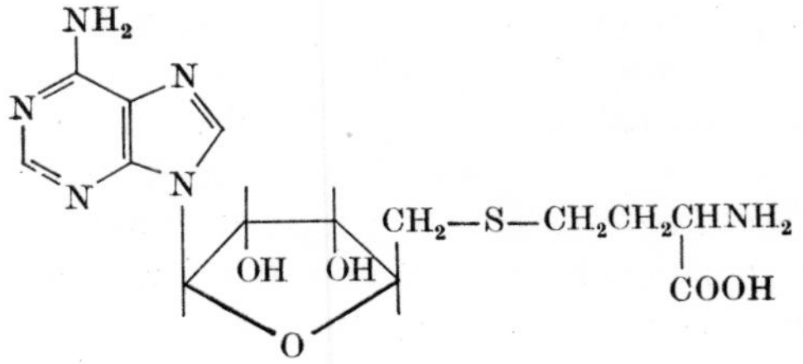

(III)

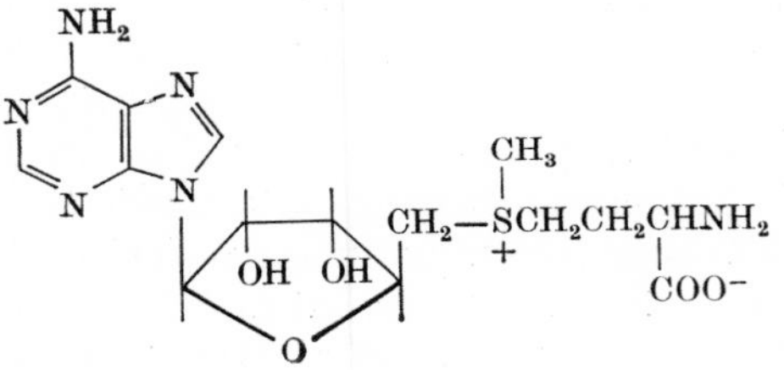

(IV)

(ii) *In Fungi*

In bakers' yeast the final reaction in the biosynthetic sequence is the direct methylation of homocysteine (Pigg *et al.*, 1962).

(iii) *In Animals*

Jaenicke (1961) has purified an enzyme system from pig liver which converts $N^{5,10}$-methylene-FAH$_4$ into N^5-methyl-FAH$_4$ which, in turn, transfers the methyl group to S-adenosylhomocysteine to form S-adenosylmethionine. This suggests that the formation of a 1-C unit at the oxidation level of "methyl" can take place in animals and probably occurs in a very similar fashion to that in bacteria. Vitamin B$_{12}$ has not yet been involved in these reactions in animals, but it has long been apparent from nutrition experiments with intact animals that vitamin B$_{12}$-deficient animals have an impaired ability to synthesize methyl groups (see e.g. Arnstein, 1955).

It is possible, however, that the vitamin B$_{12}$ may not be functioning at exactly the same site as in the bacterial system. Dinning and Young (1959) found that the incorporation of label from [^{14}C] formaldehyde or [3-^{14}C]serine into the methyl group of thymine in bone marrow preparations was not stimulated by the addition of vitamin B_{12}, and suggested that the vitamin B_{12}-dependent enzyme in this system was N^5-hydroxymethyl-FAH_4 dehydrogenase which produced N^5,^{10}-methylene-FAH_4 from N^5-hydroxymethyl-FAH_4. In support of this view Dinning and Hogan (1960) found that the activities of this enzyme in the bone marrow and liver of vitamin B_{12}-deficient chicks were lower than normal; addition of vitamin B_{12} to bone marrow preparation from deficient chicks stimulated the activity of the dehydrogenase but with the partly purified liver extracts results were erratic. It is interesting that vitamin B_{12} was more effective than vitamin B_{12}-coenzyme in the bone marrow system (Dinning, 1960) (see also p. 123).

It should be pointed out at this stage that Woolley and Koehelik (1961) claim that in *Esch. coli* a FAH_4-independent but vitamin B_{12}-coenzyme-dependent synthesis of thymine does not involve methylation of deoxyuridylic acid but the formation of 3-methylaspartate, which could be a direct intermediate in thymine biosynthesis.

It is clear from this discussion that, fundamentally, methionine is an essential amino acid for animals because they cannot synthesize the homocysteine residue; however, it is also probably true that, quantitatively, the rate of endogenous synthesis of methyl groups is not great enough to fulfil all demands.

(iv) *Plants*

Extracts of barley will synthesize S-adenosylmethionine, which will also act as a methyl donor in the same extracts (Mudd, 1960); these experiments indicate that in higher plants the activation of the methyl group and its transfer are analogous to the reactions which occur in animals and micro-organisms. Cell-free extracts of a number of plants will transfer methyl groups from either S-methylmethione or S-adenosylmethionine to homocysteine to form methionine, the former being more effective (Turner and Shapiro 1961). The activity of the plant extracts was much lower than that of similar extracts from yeast.

B. *Formation of Homocysteine*

The steps involved in the biosythesis of homocysteine are outlined in Fig. 1. The activation of aspartate by its conversion into β-aspartyl phosphate (4-phospho-L-aspartate) (step A, Fig. 1), is carried out by *aspartyl kinase*, which has been purified a hundred fold from brewers' yeast. It is activated by Mg^{2+} (0·03M) and has a very broad pH optimum (5·0–9·0). Aspartyl phosphate, which is a very unstable compound, has not been isolated from the reaction mixture, but the product behaves similarly to authentic aspartyl phosphate on chromatography and yields β-aspartohydroxamic acid on treatment with hydroxylamine (Black and Wright, 1955).

Aspartic β-*semialdehyde* *dehydrogenase* [L-aspartate β-semial-dehyde: NADP oxidoreductase (phosphorylating)] (step B, Fig. 1) has also been purified from brewers' yeast; NADPH is the obligatory

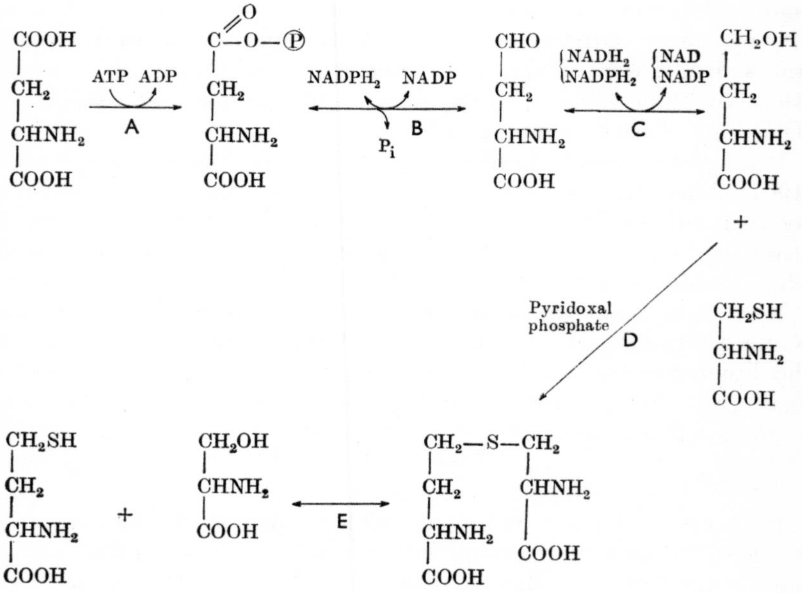

$$
\begin{array}{ccccc}
\text{COOH} & & \overset{\displaystyle O}{\text{C}-\text{O}-\text{P}} & & \text{CHO} & & \text{CH}_2\text{OH} \\
| & & | & & | & & | \\
\text{CH}_2 & \xrightarrow[\text{A}]{\text{ATP}\ \text{ADP}} & \text{CH}_2 & \xrightarrow[\text{P}_i]{\text{NADPH}_2\ \text{NADP}}_{\text{B}} & \text{CH}_2 & \xrightarrow[\text{C}]{\{\text{NADH}_2\ \{\text{NAD} \atop \text{NADPH}_2\ \text{NADP}\}} & \text{CH}_2 \\
| & & | & & | & & | \\
\text{CHNH}_2 & & \text{CHNH}_2 & & \text{CHNH}_2 & & \text{CHNH}_2 \\
| & & | & & | & & | \\
\text{COOH} & & \text{COOH} & & \text{COOH} & & \text{COOH}
\end{array}
$$

Pyridoxal phosphate D

$$
\begin{array}{c}
\text{CH}_2\text{SH} \\
| \\
\text{CHNH}_2 \\
| \\
\text{COOH}
\end{array}
$$

$$
\begin{array}{ccc}
\text{CH}_2\text{SH} & & \text{CH}_2\text{OH} & & \text{CH}_2-\text{S}-\text{CH}_2 \\
| & & | & & |\qquad\quad | \\
\text{CH}_2 & + & \text{CHNH}_2 & \xleftrightarrow{\ \text{E}\ } & \text{CH}_2\qquad \text{CHNH}_2 \\
| & & | & & |\qquad\quad | \\
\text{CHNH}_2 & & \text{COOH} & & \text{CHNH}_2\quad \text{COOH} \\
| & & & & | \\
\text{COOH} & & & & \text{COOH}
\end{array}
$$

FIG. 1. The biosynthesis of homoserine

co-factor and the pH optimum is 8·0 in the forward direction and 9·0 in the reverse direction; the reaction is inhibited by iodoacetate (Black and Wright, 1955). Reaction C (Fig. 1) is catalysed by *homo-serine dehydrogenase* [L-homoserine: NAD oxidoreductase] which, when purified from brewers' yeast, will use both NADH and NADPH as hydrogen donors, although the former is about three times more effective than the latter (Black and Wright, 1955). The incorporation of homoserine into cystathionine (reaction D, Fig. 1) in the presence of cysteine by crystalline *homoserine deaminase* (cystathionase) (Selim and Greenberg, 1955) has been reported by Matsuo and Greenberg (1959); the same enzyme also probably carries out reaction E (Fig. 1). Although no enzyme studies have been reported on higher plants, they can synthesize homoserine (Virtanen *et al.*, 1954).

III. FORMATION OF CHOLINE

A. *In Phospholipids*

It seems clear from recent important investigations that formation of choline occurs in phosphatidyl combination, with phosphatidyl serine as the key precursor (Fig. 2). In 1953 Kennedy demonstrated that the incorporation of $^{32}P_i$ into the phospholipids of rat liver particles was stimulated by the addition of glycerol and that L-α-glycerophosphate was an obligatory intermediate in the process. These observations suggested that phosphorylation of glycerol was the first step in the biosynthesis of phospholipids, and later an enzyme L-α-*glycerophosphate kinase* (A, Fig. 2), the existence of which had been demonstrated in kidney in 1939 by Kalckar, was isolated from liver (Bublitz and Kennedy, 1954) and was later obtained crystalline (Wieland and Suyter, 1957). This enzyme is, however, present only in liver, kidney and heart tissues of mammals so that under normal metabolic conditions L-α-glycerophosphate probably arises from dihydroxyacetone phosphate formed during glycolysis (Buell and Reiser, 1959), and L-α-*glycerophosphate dehydrogenase* [L-glycerol-3-phosphate: NAD oxidoreductase] activity (reaction B, Fig. 2) has been known to occur in brain tissue for some time (von Euler *et al.*, 1937). Step C (Fig. 2) is the conversion of one molecule of L-α-glycerophosphate into an L-phosphatidic acid by condensation with two acyl-CoA molecules in the presence of a phosphoglycerol transacylase system. It is reasonable to assume that Step C takes place in two stages, because in phosphatides such as lecithin, the acyl residues are not randomly distributed between the α and β positions (Tattrie 1959; Hanahan *et al.* 1960). In egg lecithin, for example the β-position is esterified almost exclusively with unsaturated fatty acids, and the α-position with saturated fatty acids. As Kennedy (1961) points out, there is probably one enzyme specifically concerned with acylation at each position. Indications that this is so come from recent experiments by Lands (1961) and Lands and Merkl (1962) who found an enzyme in liver microsomal preparations from rat, pig, chicken and guinea-pig which would acylate monoacylglycerophosphate choline; esterification of the β-position of α'-acylglycerophosphate choline is more effective with unsaturated than with saturated acyl-CoA derivatives. There has been some difficulty in detecting phosphatidic acids as intermediates in the biosynthesis of phospholipids, but Hokin and Hokin (1958) detected them in brain tissue of mice injected with high doses of $^{32}P_i$ (1μc/10g body wt.) one hour before being killed. M. R. Hokin and L. E. Hokin (1959) have also demonstrated phosphatidic acid synthesis in isolated brain microsomes and Hübscher and Clark (1960) have found phosphatidic acids in mammalian liver.

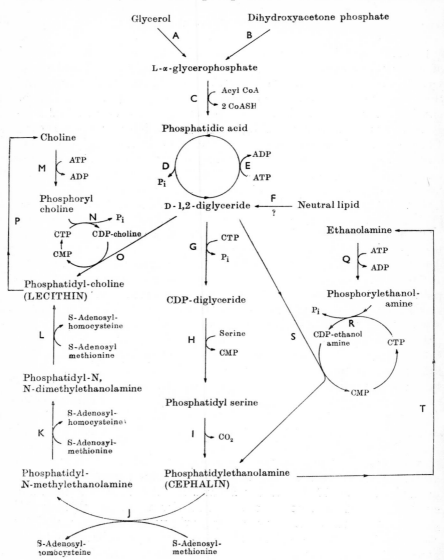

FIG. 2. Biosynthesis of choline

The failure of earlier experiments to reveal the presence of phosphatidic acids was due to the presence of an active *phosphatidic acid phosphatase* [L-α-phosphatidate phosphohydrolase], which cleaves these acids into D-1,2-diglycerides and inorganic phosphate (step D, Fig. 2) (Kennedy 1957; Coleman and Hübscher, 1961), which indeed is the next step in the metabolic sequence. This enzyme, which is strongly inhibited by Mg^{2+}, has been found in liver, brain and other tissues (Smith et al., 1957; Rossiter and Strickland, 1959). M. R. Hokin and L.E. Hokin (1959) have obtained an enzyme from brain tissue, *diglyceride kinase* (step E, Fig. 2) which will convert D-1,2-diglycerides into phosphatidic acids The cyclic dephosphorylation and phosphorylation of phosphatidic acids (Fig. 2) may have important implications in membrane transport (L. E. Hokin and M. R. Hokin, 1959), but it should be emphasized that the diglyceride kinase reaction does not lead to a net synthesis of glycerides. Recently, a third pathway for phosphatidic acid synthesis has been demonstrated in brain tissue. Pieringer and Hokin (1962) have shown that brain preparations will firstly convert an α-or β-monoglyceride into α-lysophosphatidic acid in the presence of ATP and then acylate α-lysophosphate acid with a fatty acyl-CoA to form a phosphatidic acid.

It is also possible that D-1,2-diglycerides can arise in some tissues from food triglycerides by the action of lipases (step F, Fig. 2) (Mattson et al., 1952; Mattson and Beck, 1955; Borgström, 1953, 1954). There is, however, still doubt whether such lipases exhibit stereospecificity; Karnovsky and Wolff (1958) claim that pancreatic lipase, wheat germ lipase and clearing factor lipase (lipoprotein lipase) are not stereospecific.

The D-1,2-diglycerides are then activated by CTP (step G, Fig. 2) and the resulting CDP-diglyceride condenses with serine to give phosphatidyl serine (step H, Fig. 2). It is only recently that this key reaction has been demonstrated in a cell-free extract of *Esch. coli* B (Kanfer and Kennedy, 1962). The reaction remains to be convincingly demonstrated in animal tissues. Experiments have been reported indicating that phosphoserine is incorporated into phosphatidyl serine in brain (Kometiani, 1961), but the mechanism of the reaction was not investigated. However, the recent observation that $^{14}CO_2$ is incorporated into the serine residue of phosphatidyl serine by washed particles from rat kidney, and that this is biotin-dependent, may be of importance in this connection (Fagett and Agranoff, 1962). Phosphatidyl serine is decarboxylated to phosphatidyl ethanolamine (cephalin) by liver microsomes (Wilson et al., 1960) and by extracts from *Esch. coli* B (Kanfer and Kennedy, 1962) (step I, Fig. 2). Experiments by Bremer and Greenberg (1959) first indicated that reaction J, K and L, (Fig. 2) were concerned in the stepwise methylation of cephalin to lecithin; they showed that [^{14}C-methyl]-S-adenosylmethionine injected into rats gave rise to labelled phosphatidyl-N-methylethanolamine and phosphatidyl-N,N-dimethyl-ethanolamine as well as to labelled choline. Later Bremer *et al.* (1960), Bremer and Greenberg (1960), Gibson *et al.* (1961) and Cook-sey and Greenberg (1961) showed that isolated liver microsomes will carry out reactions J and K in the presence of the appropriate sub-strate and S-adenosylmethionine. Phosphatidyl ethanolamine is not readily methylated by this system and it is considered that the inser-tion of the first methyl group is the rate-limiting step in the biosyn-thesis of lecithin and therefore choline. Reaction L (Fig. 2) has been demonstrated in pigeon liver microsomes (Artom and Lofland, 1960; Artom, 1962).

Support for the view that choline is synthesized at the phospho-lipid level is forthcoming from the work of Hall and Nyc (1959); they found that a choline-deficient mutant of *Neurospora crassa* accumulates phosphatidyl mono- and dimethylethanolamine; fur-thermore, the fatty acid composition of lecithin, phosphatidyl mono-methylethanolamine and phosphatidyl dimethylethanolamine in *Neu-rospora* is essentially the same (Hall and Nyc, 1962); this indicates that the precursors contain the same fatty acids during their conver-sion into lecithin.

B. *Formation of "Free" Choline*

The question which naturally arises is whether choline can be synthesized biologically without being attached to phospholipid. As long ago as 1941 Stetten showed that [15N]ethanolamine was incorporated into choline and this was confirmed in experiments with [1,2-14C]ethanolamine by Pilgeram *et al.* (1953), who also later showed that no activity from this substrate appeared in the methyl groups of choline (Pilgeram *et al.*, 1957). These experiments did not preclude the synthesis going on at the phospholipid level, but recently Alexander (1961) obtained a cell-free homogenate from yeast which synthesized labelled choline from ethanolamine and either [14C]formate, [3-14C]serine or [14C-methyl]methionine, and Artom (1962) has reported the conversion of dimethylethanolamine into choline by liver slices. One of the facts which make this pathway of doubtful *in vivo* significance is that no enzyme has yet been reported from any source which will decarboxylate serine or phospho-serine to ethanolamine or phosphoethanolamine, respectively.

In Fig. 2 the important work of Kennedy on the formation of leci-thin from CDP-choline and D-1,2-diglycerides is summarized (reac-tions M, N, O) (see Goodwin, 1960). Its overall *in vivo* significance is now doubtful following the discoveries that choline is synthesized at the phospholipid level, although it should be emphasized that step H (Fig. 2) has not yet been unequivocally demonstrated in animals. It may be an important pathway for reutilizing choline liberated by the breakdown of phospholipids by hydrolytic enzymes (reaction P, Fig. 2); however, *phospholipase D*, [phosphatidylcholine phosphatidohydrolase] which liberates free choline, is present only in higher plants (Kates, 1956). Bremer and Greenberg (1959), for example, found that [^{14}C-methyl]methionine when injected into rats gave rise to activity in CDP-choline as well as in lecithin, but the maximum activity in the former occurred more than one hour after it did in the latter; this suggested that CDP-choline was not the precursor of the bulk of the lecithin which was being synthesized.

The same remarks can probably apply to the significance of the incorporation of ethanolamine into cephalins via CDP-ethanolamine (reactions Q, R, S, Fig. 2).

C. *Plasmalogen Biosynthesis*

Plasmalogens (V) which contain choline [see Gottfried and Rapport (1962) for isolation procedures], can be synthesized in the same

$$
\begin{array}{ll}
\text{O} \ \ \text{CH}_2\text{OCH}{=}\text{CHR} & \text{O} \ \ \text{CH}_2\text{OCH}{=}\text{CHR} \\
\text{RCOCH} \quad\ \ \text{O} & \text{RCOCH} \quad\ \ \text{O} \\
\quad \text{CH}_2\text{O}{-}\overset{\uparrow}{\text{P}}{-}\text{O}{-}\text{CH}_2\text{CH}_2\overset{+}{\text{N}}(\text{CH}_3)_3 & \quad \text{CH}_2{-}\text{O}{-}\overset{\uparrow}{\text{P}}{-}\text{OCH}_2\text{CH}_2\text{NH}_2\text{COOH} \\
\qquad\quad \text{O}^- & \qquad\quad \text{OH} \\
\qquad\quad (\text{V}) & \qquad\quad (\text{VI})
\end{array}
$$

way as lecithins from plasmalogen diglyceride and CDP-choline in the presence of particulate liver preparations (reaction 3) (Kiyasu and Kennedy, 1960).

It remains to be seen whether, in the light of the recent work on lecithin biosynthesis described in the previous sections, the biolo-

$$\text{Plasmalogen diglyceride} + \text{CTP} \rightleftharpoons \text{Choline-plasmalogen} + \text{CMP} \qquad (3)$$

gically significant synthesis of plasmalogen is via a serine derivative such as (VI).

D. *Sphingomyelin Biosynthesis*

The sphingomyelins (VII) represent yet another group of phospholipids which contain choline. A pathway of biosynthesis

$$
\begin{array}{l}
\qquad\qquad\qquad\qquad\qquad \text{O} \\
\qquad\qquad\qquad\qquad\qquad \uparrow \qquad\qquad + \\
\text{CH}_3(\text{CH}_2)_{12}\text{CH}{=}\text{CHCH}{-}\text{CHCH}_2{-}\text{O}{-}\text{P}{-}\text{OCH}_2\text{CH}_2\text{N}(\text{CH}_3)_3 \\
\qquad\qquad\qquad\quad \text{OH} \ \ \text{NH} \qquad \text{O}^- \\
\qquad\qquad\qquad\qquad\qquad \text{C}{=}\text{O} \\
\qquad\qquad\qquad\qquad\qquad \text{R} \\
\qquad\qquad\qquad\qquad (\text{VII})
\end{array}
$$

involving CDP-choline (Fig. 3) has been reported in rat brain homogenates. Palmitic acid is first activated as palmityl-CoA (reaction A, Fig, 3) and free palmityl aldehyde is formed by a NADPH-dependent reduction (step B, Fig. 3) (Brady *et al.* 1958); however, Hoshishima *et al.* (1960) report a NADH-dependent reaction. Brady *et al.* (1958) also demonstrated reactions C and D (Fig. 3) in brain homogenates. The enzymatic formation of ceramide (N-acylsphingosine) has been described by Zabin (1957), by Brady and Koval (1958) and by Sribney (1962), but the exact

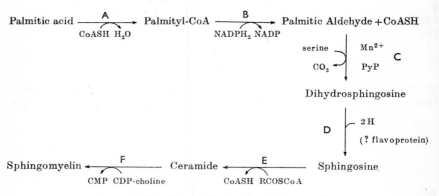

FIG. 3. The biosynthesis of sphingomyelin

point at which acylation occurs is not known; it is assumed for the present to occur at E (Fig. 3). However, it is clear that ceramide is converted into a sphingomyelin because Sribney and Kennedy (1958) have isolated from chicken liver an enzyme, *phosphorylcholineceramide transferase*, which carries out reaction F and produces a marked net synthesis of sphingomyelin. The enzyme is highly specific for both substrates but the stereospecificity of the enzyme towards the ceramide residue was unexpected. The *threo*-configuration of the hydroxyl and amino groups on C-2 and C-3 of the ceramide was very much more reactive than *erythro*-ceramide, although the configuration of the naturally occurring spingomyelins appears to be *erythro* (VII). The reasons for this are not apparent, especially as Fujino and Zabin (1962) have recently synthesized dihydrosphingosine and sphingosine from palmityl-CoA and serine by rat brain homogenates and found that in both cases the configuration of the base was *erythro*.

It is significant that in sphingomyelin biosynthesis as now envisaged serine is the compound from which the ethanolamine residue of dihydrosphingosine is formed (reaction C, Fig. 3) whilst the choline residue is incorporated *in toto* from CDP-choline (reaction F, Fig. 3). It will be important to see whether future investigations will reveal a ceramide-serine condensation, the product of which is then decarboxylated and methylated stepwise to sphingomyelin.

IV. CHOLINE SULPHATE

The sulphate ester, choline sulphate (VIII) was first isolated from *Aspergillus sydowi* by Woolley and Peterson (1937) and later reported in a number of other fungi (de Flines, 1955; Stevens and Vohra, 1955; Ballio *et al.*, 1960; Harada and Spencer, 1960; Takebe, 1960; Itahashi, 1961), in lichens (*Rocella* spp.) (Lindberg, 1955), in the red alga *Gelida cantilaginum* (Lindberg, 1955) and in both roots and green tissues of higher plants (Nissen and Benson, 1961). It has not been reported in bacteria and its distribution in fungi is limited to the higher fungi (Harada and Spencer, 1960).

$$O^- - \overset{\overset{\displaystyle O}{\uparrow}}{\underset{\underset{\displaystyle O}{\downarrow}}{S}} - O - CH_2CH_2N^+(CH_3)_3$$

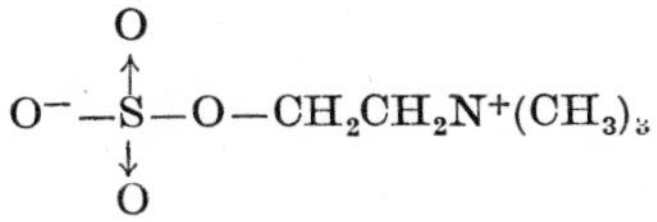

(VIII)

Spencer and Harada (1960) have shown that choline sulphate is synthesized by the transfer of the sulphate radical from adenosine 3'-phosphate 5'-sulphatophosphate ("active sulphate") (IX) to choline in the presence of the enzyme *choline sulphokinase* (reaction 4). Fungi which do not accumulate choline sulphate lack choline

Adenosine 3'-phosphate 5'-sulphatophosphate + choline → choline sulphate + adenosine 3',5'-diphosphate   (4)

sulphokinase.

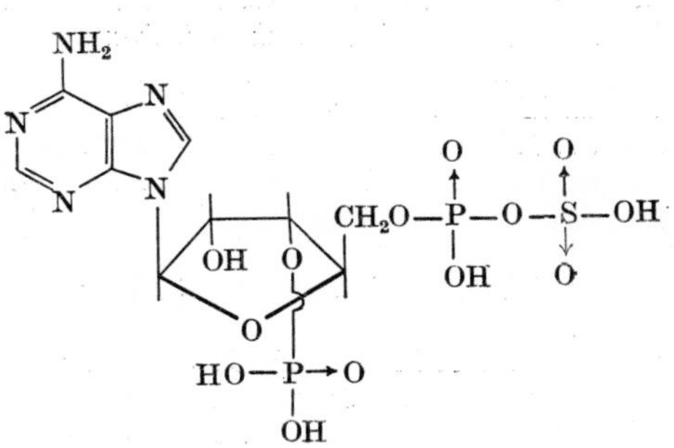

(IX)

The comparatively large amount of choline sulphate (0·2% dry weight in *A. sydowi*) which accumulates in some fungi is thought to be a store of easily assimilable sulphate; the reverse of the last stage of synthesis (reaction 4) would immediately provide "active sulphur" (Spencer and Harada, 1960). Choline sulphate in roots is also considered to be a store of readily available sulphate (Nissen and Benson, 1961).

REFERENCES

Alexander, G. J. (1961). *J. Neurochem.* **6**, 277, 285, 292.
Arnstein, H. R. V. (1955). *Biochem. Soc. Symp.* **13**, 92.
Artom, C. (1962). *Fed. Proc.*, **21**, 297.
Artom, C., and Lofland, H. B. (1960). *Biochem. Biophys. Res. Comm.* **3**, 244.
Ballio, A., Chain, E. B., di Accadia, F. D., Navazio, F., Rossi, C., and Ventura, M. T. (1960). *Selected Scientific Papers from the Istituto Superiore di Sanita*, p. 312.
Black, S., and Wright, N. G. (1955). *J. biol. Chem.* **213**, 27, 39, 51.
Borgström, B. (1953). *Acta chem. scand.* **7**, 557.
Borgström, B. (1954). *Biochim. biophys. Acta* **13**, 491.
Brady, R. O., and Koval, G. J. (1958). *J. biol. Chem.* **233**, 26.
Brady, R. O., Formica, J. V., and Koval, G. J. (1958). *J. biol. Chem.* **233**, 1072.
Bremer, J., and Greenberg, D. M. (1959). *Biochim. biophys. Acta* **35**, 287.
Bremer, J., and Greenberg, D. M. (1960). *Biochim. biophys. Acta* **37**, 173.
Bremer, J., Figard, P. H. and Greenberg, D. M. (1960). *Biochim. biophys. Acta* **43**, 477.
Bublitz, C., and Kennedy, E. P. (1954). *J. biol. Chem.* **211**, 951, 963.
Buell, G. C., and Reiser, R. (1959). *J. biol. Chem.* **234**, 217.
Coleman, R., and Hübscher, G. (1961). *Biochem. J.* **80**, 11P.
Cooksey, K. E., and Greenberg, D. M. (1961). *Biochem. Biophys. Res. Comm.* **6**, 256.
Cross, M. J., and Woods, D. D. (1954). *Biochem. J.* **58**, xvi.
de Flines, J. (1955). *J. Amer. chem. Soc.* **77**, 1676.
Dinning, J. S. (1960). *Proc. Soc. exp. Biol., N.Y.* **104**, 431.
Dinning, J. S., Allen, B. K., Young, R. S., and Day, P. L. (1958). *J. biol. Chem.* **233**, 674.
Dinning, J. S., and Young, R. S. (1959). *J. biol. Chem.* **234**, 1199, 3241.
Dinning, J. S., and Hogan, R. (1960). *Fed. Proc.* **19**, 418.
Duerre, J. A., and Schlenk, F. (1962). *Arch. Biochem. Biophys.* **96**, 575.
Faggett, J. J., and Agranoff, B. W. (1962). *Fed. Proc.* **21**, 296.
Foster, M. A., Jones, K. M., and Woods, D. D. (1961). *Biochem. J.* **80**, 519.
Fujino, Y., and Zabin, I. (1962). *J. biol. Chem.* **237**, 2069.
Gibson, F., and Woods, D. D. (1960). *Biochem. J.* **74**, 160.
Gibson, K. D., Wilson, J. D., and Udenfriend, S. (1961). *J. biol. Chem.* **236**, 673.
Goodwin, T. W. (1960). "Recent Advances in Biochemistry". Churchill, London.
Gottfried, E.L., and Rapport, M.M. (1962). *J. biol. Chem.* **237**, 329.
Grossowicz, N., and Aronovitz, J. (1961). Abstracts of the 5th International Congress of Biochemistry Moscow. p. 30. Pergamon Press. London.
Guest, J. R., Helleiner, C. W., Cross, M. J., and Woods, D. D. (1960). *Biochem. J.* **76**, 396.

Hall, M. O., and Nyc, J. F. (1959). *J. Amer. chem. Soc.* **81**, 2275.
Hall, M. O., and Nyc, J. F. (1962). *Biochim. biophys. Acta* **56**, 370.
Hanahan, D. J., Brokerhoff, H., and Barron, E. J. (1960). *J. biol. Chem.* **235**. 1917.
Harada, T., and Spencer, B. (1960). *J. gen. Microbiol.* **22**, 520.
Hatch, F. T., Takeyama, S., and Buchanan, J. M. (1959). *Fed. Proc.* **18**, 243
Helleiner, C. W., and Woods, D. D. (1956). *Biochem. J.* **63**, 26P.
Helleiner, C. W., Kisliuk, R. L., and Woods, D. D. (1957). *J. gen. Microbiol.* **18**, xv.
Hokin, L. E., and Hokin, M. R. (1958). *J. biol. Chem.* **233**, 800, 818, 822.
Hokin, L. E., and Hokin, M. R. (1959). *J. biol. Chem.* **234**, 1381.
Hoshishima, K., Vignais, P., and Zabin, I. (1960). *Fed. Proc.* **19**, 234.
Hübscher, G., and Clark, B. (1960). *Biochim. biophys. Acta* **41**, 45.
Itahashi, M. (1961). *J. Biochem., Tokyo* **50**, 52.
Jaenicke, L. (1961). "Abstracts of the 5th International Congress of Biochemistry Moscow." p. 32. Pergamon Press, London.
Kanfer, J. N., and Kennedy, E. P. (1962). *J. biol. Chem.* **235**, PC270
Kalckar, H. (1939). *Biochem. J.* **33**, 631.
Karnovsky, M. L., and Wolff, D. (1958). *Comm. 4th Int. Cong. Biochem.* p. 208.
Kates, M. (1956). *Canad. J. Biochem. Physiol.* **34**, 967.
Kennedy, E. P. (1953). *J. biol. Chem.* **201**, 399.
Kennedy, E. P. (1957). *Ann. Rev. Biochem.* **26**, 119.
Kennedy, E. P. (1961). Proceedings of Symposium, 5th International Congress of Biochemistry, Moscow. Pergamon Press, Oxford (In press).
Kisliuk, R. L., and Woods, D. D. (1957). *J. gen. Microbiol.* **18**, xv.
Kisliuk, R. L., and Woods, D. D. (1959). *Fed. Proc.* **18**, 261.
Kisliuk, R. L. (1960). *Fed. Proc.* **19**, 416.
Kiyasu, J., and Kennedy, E. P. (1960). *J. biol. Chem.* **235**, 2590.
Kometiani, P. A. (1961). "Proceedings of Symposium, 5th International Congress of Biochemistry, Moscow." Pergamon Press, Oxford (In press).
Lands, W. E. M. (1961). *Fed. Proc.* **20**, 280.
Lands, W. E. M., and Merkl, I. (1962). *Fed. Proc.* **21**, 295.
Larrabee, A. R., and Buchanan, J. M. (1961). *Fed. Proc.* **20**, 9.
Lascelles, J., and Cross, M. J. (1955). *Biochem. Soc. Symp.* **13**, 109.
Lindberg, B. (1955). *Acta chem. scand.* **9**, 917, 1323.
Matsuo, Y., and Greenberg, D. M. (1959). *J. biol. Chem.* **234**, 507, 516.
Mattson, F. H., Benedict, J. H., Martin, J. B., and Beck, L. W. (1952). *J. Nutrit.* **48**, 335.
Mattson, F. H., and Beck, L. W. (1955). *J. biol. Chem.* **214**, 115.
Mudd, S. H. (1960). *Biochim. biophys. Acta* **37**, 164; **38**, 354.
Nissen, P., and Benson, A. A. (1961). *Science*, **131**, 1959.
Pieringer, R. A., and Hokin, L. E. (1962). *J. biol. Chem.* **234**, 653, 659.
Pigg, C. J., Spence, K. D., and Parks, L. W. (1962). *Arch. Biochem. Biophys.* **97**, 491
Pilgeram, L. O., Gal, E. M., Sassenrath, E. N., and Greenberg, D. M. (1953). *J. biol. Chem.* **204**, 367.
Pilgeram, L. O., Hamilton, R. E., and Greenberg, D. M. (1957). *J. biol. Chem.* **227**, 107.
Rossiter, R. J., and Strickland, K. P. (1959). *Ann. N. Y. Acad. Sci.* **72**, 790.
Selim, A. S. M., and Greenberg, D. M. (1959). *J. biol. Chem.* **234**, 1474.
Shapiro, S. K. (1961). "Abstracts of the 5th International Congress of Biochemistry, Moscow", p. 305. Pergamon Press. Oxford.
Smith, S. W., Weiss, S. B., and Kennedy, E. P. (1957). *J. biol. Chem.* **228**, 915.

Spencer, B., and Harada, T. (1960). *Biochem. J.* **77**, 305.
Sribney, M. (1962). *Fed. Proc.* **21**, 280.
Sribney, M., and Kennedy, E. P. (1958). *J. biol. Chem.* **233**, 1315.
Stevens, C. H., and Vohra, P. (1955). *J. Amer. chem. Soc.* **77**, 4935.
Stetten, D. (1941). *J. biol. Chem.* **140**, 143.
Stoll, A. (1952). *Fortschr. Chem. org. Naturstoffe* **9**, 114.
Szulmajster, J., and Woods, D. D. (1960). *Biochem. J.* **75**, 3.
Takebe, I. (1960). *J. gen. appl. Microbiol.* **6**, 83.
Tattrie, N. H. (1959). *J. Lipid Res.* **1**, 60.
Turner, J. E., and Shapiro, S. K. (1961). *Biochim. biophys. Acta*, **51**, 581.
Virtanen, A. I., Berg, A. M., and Kari, S. (1953). *Acta chem. scand.* **7**, 1423.
Von Euler, H. Adler, E., and Gunther, G. (1937). *Hoppe-Seyl. Z.* **249**, 1.
Wieland, I., and Suyter, M. (1957). *Biochem. Z.* **329**, 320.
Wilson, J. D., Gibson, K. D., and Udenfriend, S. (1960). *J. biol. Chem.* **235**, 3539.
Woolley, D. W., and Koehelik, I. H. (1961). *Fed. Proc.* **20**, 359.
Woolley, D. W., and Peterson, W. H. (1937). *J. biol. Chem.* **122**, 213.
Zabin, I. (1957). *J. Amer. chem. Soc.* **79**, 5834.

CHAPTER 10

INOSITOL

I. INTRODUCTION

The inositols or cyclohexitols are a group of nine isomeric hexa-hydroxycyclohexanes. Only one of the isomers is biologically active, this is *myo*-inositol (I) originally isolated from muscle over one hundred years ago by Scherer (1850). It is also often called *meso*-

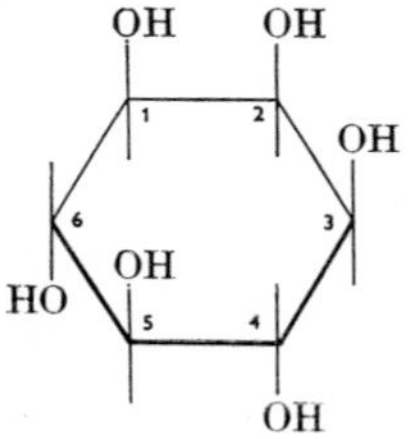

(I) 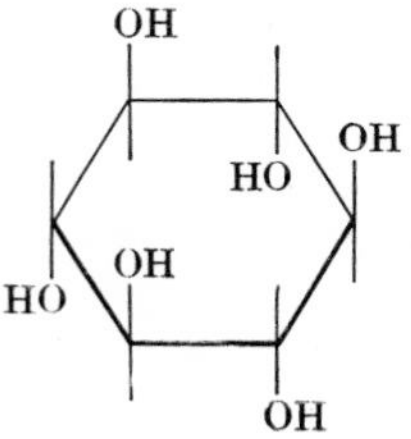 (II)

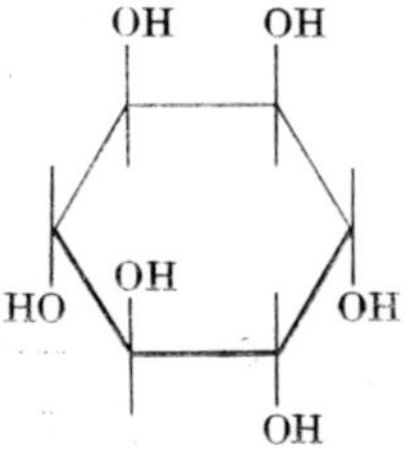

(III) 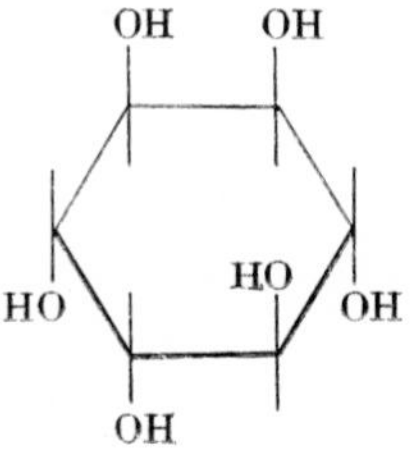 (IV)

inositol and *i*-inositol (*i*-indicates optical inactivity). Other naturally occurring cyclohexitols include scyllitol (II), *d*- and *l*-inositols [(III) (IV)] in the form of monomethylethers, for example, pinitol (*d*-inositol) and quebrachitol (*l*-inositol).

The most widely naturally occuring forms of *myo*-inositol are phytic acid and the inositol-containing phospholipids (phospho-inositides, lipositols, phosphatidyl inositols). Phytic acid, the hexa-phosphoric acid ester of inositol, is widely distributed in higher plants but is present in highest concentrations in seeds and cereal grains, where it can account for up to 86% of the total phosphorus present (Mollgaard *et al.*, 1946).

Phosphatidyl inositols are present in plants, micro-organisms and animals. Typical examples of such compounds are the phytosphingolipid (V) from maize oil (Carter *et al.*, 1958), a phosphatidyl inositol dimannoside (VI) from a virulent strain of the human tubercle bacillus (Vilkas, 1959), and the phosphoinositides from heart and liver (VII) (Hawthorne *et al.*, 1960). The phophoinositide from beef brain is a complex of substances which contains 1-phosphatidyl-L-*myo*-inositol, 1-phosphatidyl-L-*myo*-inositol 4-phosphate and 1-phosphatidyl-L-*myo*-inositol 4-5-diphosphate (Brockenhoff and Ballou, 1961). Free inositol occurs in large quantities in the seminal

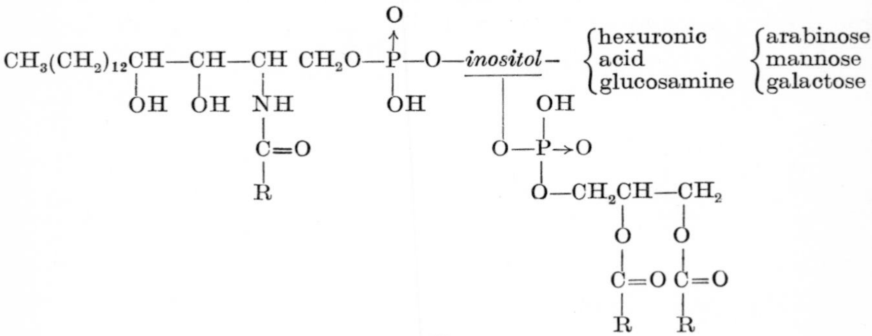

(V)

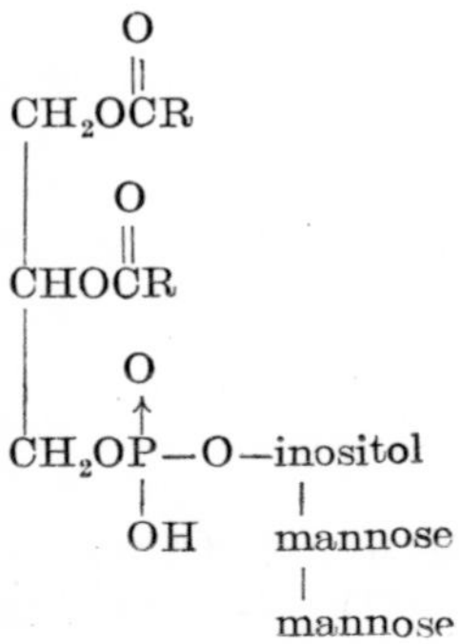

(VI)

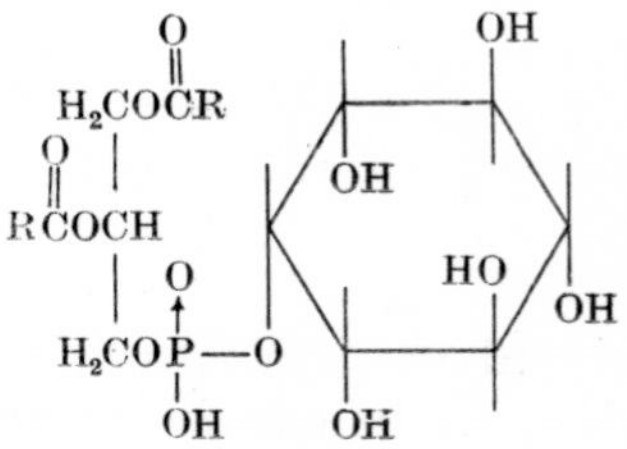

(VII)

fluid of many animals, and in the case of boars can represent 20% of the dry weight (Mann, 1954).

There appears to be little doubt that inositol is a growth factor for a number of strains of yeast (see e.g. Williams *et al.*, 1940) for many other moulds and for some aerobic and anaerobic bacteria (see e.g. Weidlein, 1951). The situation in animals is far more obscure and some authorities feel that in spite of the early work of numerous nutritionists (see Weidlein, 1951) inositol is not a vitamin for most animals, although a need has been demonstrated in a number of species maintained under certain highly specific dietary conditions. Three examples can be quoted of work indicating that inositol is not a vitamin; in the first case rats fed an inositol-free diet over 16 weeks revealed no growth retardation or pathological symptoms; furthermore the urinary and faecal excretion of inositol and the inositol content of the carcass were the same in the control and experimental animals (McCormick *et al.*, 1954); in the second case normal rats injected with [1-^{14}C]glucose synthesized [^{14}C]*myo*-inositol (Halliday and Anderson, 1955) and thirdly germ-free rats and mice synthesize [^{14}C]*myo*-inositol from [1-^{14}C]glucose (Freinkel and Dawson, 1961). In spite of these observations it is clear that inositol is required for growth of all but one of 22 strains of mammalian cells in tissue culture (Eagle *et al.*, 1956, 1957).

II. BIOSYNTHESIS

A. *Inositol*

(i) *Plants.*

Cabbage, maize, mung bean, pea, soya bean and wheat seedlings when germinated in the light show a marked fall in their inositol levels (Richardson and Axelrod, 1957); similar results have been obtained with dark-grown peas and mung beans (Richardson and Axelrod, 1957) as well as oats (Darbre and Norris, 1956) and dwarf beans (Gibbins and Norris, 1963). In the dwarf bean inositol is liberated from its bound form in the cotyledons, probably by the action of phytase, and translocated to the developing embryo; for example, the content of the plumule increases 20 times during two weeks germination (Gibbins and Norris, 1963).

(ii) *Animals.*

The experiments of Halliday and Anderson (1955) quoted in the previous section indicated that the rat can synthesize *myo*-inositol from [1-^{14}C]glucose and this has been confirmed by Daughaday *et al.* (1955) with normal rats and by Freinkel and Dawson (1961) with germ-free rats. Daughaday *et al.* (1955) also showed that labelled inositol was found in chick embryos 64 hr. after [^{14}C]glucose had been injected into the chorioallantoic membrane.

Eagle *et al.* (1960) have shown that the inositol-independent L-929 strain of mouse fibroblast also synthesizes inositol from [^{14}C] glucose. Slight synthesis was also observed in the inositol-dependent HeLa cells and KB cells.

The stereochemical similarity between the C-2 to C-5 segment of glucose and that of inositol had attracted the view that inositol

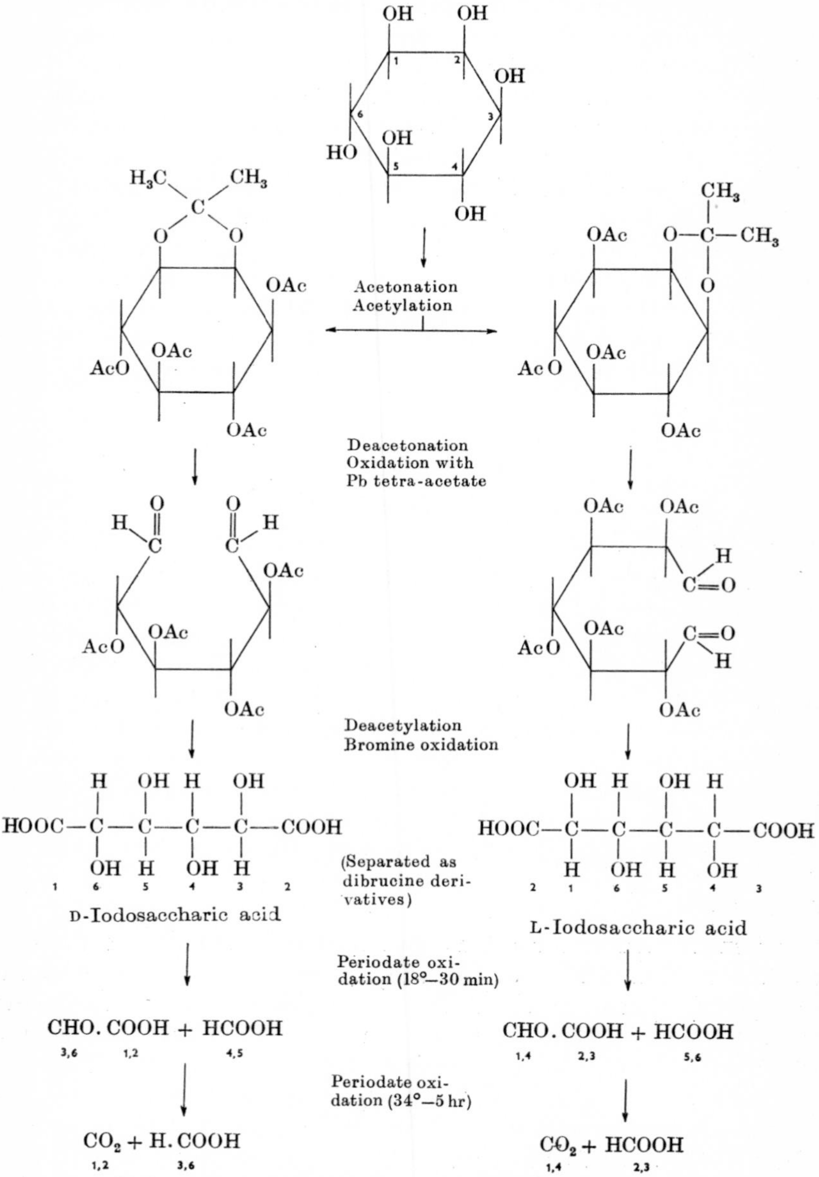

FIG. 1. Degradation of inositol (Charalampous, 1957)

was formed by cyclization of the glucose molecule. The investigations of Charalampous (1957) have ruled out this possibility in yeast. The labelling patterns observed in inositol following addition of [1-^{14}C]-, [2-^{14}C]- and [6-^{14}C] glucose were not consistent with this view. The labelled inositol was degraded as indicated in Fig. 1 and the results obtained are given in Table 1. It is clear the glucose

TABLE 1. Contribution of Glucose Carbon Atoms to Biosynthesis of Inositol (Charalampous, 1957)

[^{14}C]Substrate	Specific activity of inositol (cpm/μmole)	^{14}C Content of carbon atoms (cpm)					
		1	2	3	4	5	6
[1-^{14}C]Glucose	1898	0	0	470	0	752	602
[3-^{14}C]Glucose	1173	154	415	0	629	0	0
[6-^{14}C]Glucose	2418	0	0	1229	0	874	326

is not cyclized to inositol because (a) a mechanism involving cyclization would demand the appearance of C-1 and C-6 of glucose next to each other in the inositol molecule; they clearly occupy the same place and this cannot be explained merely by randomization of C-1 and C-6 of glucose through the triose phosphates of the glycolytic sequence, and (b) the position of the label of C-2 of glucose in inositol is also inconsistent with the cyclization of a 6C molecule.

According to Charalampous (1957) the most likely mechanism to explain the labelling pattern observed would be a condensation of a tetrose, arising from known transaldolase and transketolase reactions, and contributing C-1,2,3,6 of inositol, with a two carbon fragment contributing C-4 and 5. Charalampous noted the similarity between the distribution in inositol and that in shikimic acid. Recent work on the formation of shikimic acid (see Goodwin, 1960) has shown that the synthesis involves erythrose 5-phosphate and phosphoenolpyruvate and dehydroquinic acid (Reaction 1). This is not inconsistent with the data of Charalampous. However, it should be noted that acetate, which is not readily incorporated into shikimic acid, is actively incorporated into inositol. Even more fascinating is the fact that animals can synthesize inositol but not shikimic acid. In higher plants (parsley), glucose appears to be incorporated into inositol by cyclization. For example, the inositol biosynthesized from [1-^{14}C]glucose in parsley leaves was adminis-

tered to detached green strawberries and converted into galac-
turonic acid, which was shown to contain around 80% of the label
in C_1 (Loewus and Kelly, 1962).

B. *Inositol Phosphatides*

A number of investigators demonstrated that in brain, liver and
kidney preparations, the synthesis of phosphoinositides resembled
lecithin biosynthesis (see p. 194) in that a cytidine nucleotide was
involved (see Goodwin, 1960).

Paulus and Kennedy (1960) have recently investigated the details of the synthesis in liver and have demonstrated that inositol
monophosphatide formation proceeds via the steps indicated in
equations 2, 3, 4. Reaction 4 requires Mn^{2+} as a co-factor.

$$\text{L-}\alpha\text{-Glycerophosphate} + 2\text{Acyl-SCoA} \rightarrow \text{phosphatidic acid} + 2\text{CoASH} \qquad (2)$$

$$\text{Phosphatidic acid} + \text{CTP} \rightleftharpoons \text{CDP-diglyceride} + \text{P-P} \qquad (3)$$

$$\text{CDP-Diglyceride} + \text{inositol} \rightleftharpoons \text{inositol monophosphatide} + \text{CMP} \qquad (4)$$

The last reaction was carried out using synthetic CDP-dipalmitin
and CDP-dilaurin. It is now clear from these observations that CTP
is the required co-factor for phosphoinositide synthesis and that it
cannot be replaced by CDP as suggested by Agranoff *et al.* (1958).
This system clearly differs from that which synthesizes lecithins
from choline, in that unlike choline, inositol is incorporated without
prior phosphorylation. However, it resembles the newly observed
pathway for lecithin synthesis in which serine is incorporated into
phosphatidyl serine which is then converted into lecithin. On the
other hand, the pathway may be different in different tissues. In
brain slices, for example, the incorporations of $^{32}P_i$ and [2-^{3}H]
inositol into phosphoinositides were stimulated equally by acetyl-
choline, an observation which suggests the incorporation of inositol as a unit (Hokin and Hokin, 1958).

Reaction (4) is not completely specific for *myo*-inositol, because appreciable activity was also observed with *myo*-inosose-2 and DL-epi-inosose. The same lack of specificity probably exists in the yeast enzyme complex, because Posternak *et al.* (1959) have reported that inositol antagonists are incorporated into yeast phosphatides.

REFERENCES

Agranoff, B. W., Bradley, R. M., and Brady, R. O. (1958). *J. biol. Chem.* **233**, 1077.

Brockenhoff, H., and Ballou, C. E. (1961). *J. biol. Chem.* **236**, 1907.

Carter, H. E., Gigg, R. H., Law, J. H., Nakayama, J., and Weber, E. (1958). *J. biol. Chem.* **233**, 1309.

Charalampous, F. C. (1957). *J. biol. Chem* **225**, 585, 595.

Darbre, A., and Norris, F. W. (1956). *Biochem. J.* **64**, 441

Daughaday, W. H., Larner, J., and Hartnett, C. (1955). *J. biol. Chem.* **212**, 869.

Eagle, H., Oyama, V. I., Levy, M., and Freeman, A. E. (1956). *Science* **123**, 845.

Eagle, H., Oyama, V. I., Levy, M., and Freeman, A. E. (1957). *J. biol. Chem.* **226**, 191.

Eagle, H., Agranoff, B. W., and Snell, E. E. (1960). *J. biol. Chem.* **235**, 1891.

Freinkel, N., and Dawson, R. M. C. (1961). *Biochem. J.* **81**, 250.

Gibbins, L. N., and Norris, F. W. (1963). *Biochem. J.* **86**, 64, 67

Goodwin, T. W. (1960). "Recent Advances in Biochemistry" 3rd Edition. Churchill, London.

Halliday, J. W., and Anderson, L. (1955). *J. biol. Chem.* **217**, 797.

Hawthorne, J. N., Kemp, P., and Ellis, R. B. (1960). *Biochem. J.* **75**, 501.

Hokin, L. E., and Hokin, M. R. (1958). *J. biol. Chem.* **233**, 800, 818, 822.

Loewus, F. A., and Kelly, S. (1962). *Biochem. biophys. Res. Comm.* **7**, 204

Mann, T. (1954). *Proc. Roy. Soc.* B **142**, 21.

McCormick, M. H., Harris, P. N., and Anderson, C. A. (1954). *J. Nutrit.* **52**, 337.

Mollgaard, H., Lorenzen, K., Hansen, I. G., and Christensen, P. E. (1946). *Biochem. J.* **40**, 589.

Paulus, H., and Kennedy, E. P. (1960). *J. biol. Chem.* **235**, 1303.

Posternak, T., Shopfer, W. H., and Deshusses, J. (1959). *Helv. chim. Acta* **42**, 135.

Richardson, K. E., and Axelrod, R. (1957). *Plant Physiol.* **32**, 334

Scherer, J. (1850). *Liebigs Ann.* **73**, 322.

Vilkas, E. (1959). *C. R. Acad. Sci., Paris* **248**, 604.

Weidlein, E. R. (1951). Mellon Institute Bibliographic series. Bull. No. 6.

Williams, R. J., Eakin, R. E., and Snell, E. E. (1940). *J. Amer. chem. Soc.* **62**, 1204.

Chapter 11

ASCORBIC ACID

I. Introduction

Scurvy, the disease which was the scourge of sailors for many generations, is characterized by a tendency to bleeding, especially at the joints, and by pathological changes in gums and teeth. It had been known for some time that fresh vegetables and fruit, especially citrus fruits, were anti-scorbutic, and after the emergence of the concept of accessory food factors it was not long before the active anti-scorbutic principle, vitamin C, was isolated simultaneously by Waugh and King and by Szent-Györgyi. This development was helped enormously by the discovery that in addition to humans, guinea-pigs were also susceptible to scurvy; thus an experimental animal became available for following by bioassay the potency of various vitamin C-active fractions as they were isolated. The structure of ascorbic acid (I) was eventually elucidated mainly by Haworth and Hirst in England and by Reichstein in Switzerland. It will be noted that it has the L-configuration.

The higher plants and animals except primates, guinea-pigs, and the red vented bubul *(Pycnonotus cafer)* and the Indian fruit bat *(Pteropus medius)*, are the main groups of living organisms which synthesize vitamin C. Micro-organisms do not apparently synthesize ascorbic acid or require it for growth. So the organisms which are often the best for studying biosynthetic problems,

(I)   (II)

the protista, are not open to ascorbic acid investigations. Higher plants and animals must be used, but to compensate for the loss of the microbiological approach there is the fascinating problem of the nature of the metabolic lesion which makes the primates and guinea pigs dependent on an exogenous source of vitamin C, whilst most other animals can synthesize sufficient for their needs.

II. FORMATION IN ANIMALS

A. *Biosynthetic Pathway*

Most mammals synthesize their ascorbic acid in the liver, but in birds, reptiles and amphibia, the kidney is the site of synthesis (Grollman and Lehninger, 1957; Roy and Guha, 1958). First experiments on the biosynthesis of ascorbic acid in rats took advantage of the observation that chloretone and other hypnotic drugs greatly stimulate the urinary excretion of L-ascorbic acid and D-glucuronic acid (II) (Longenecker *et al.*, 1940). In these experiments [1-^{14}C]-D-glucose and [6-^{14}C]-D-glucose were administered to rats and the excreted L-ascorbic acid isolated. It was found that with [1-^{14}C]-D-glucose, the resulting L-ascorbic acid was labelled predominantly in C-6 (Horowitz *et al.*, 1952), whilst with [6-^{14}C]-glucose, the label was predominantly in C-1 (Horowitz and King, 1953). Similar results with [1-^{14}C]- and [6-^{14}C]-D-glucose were obtained with rats in which ascorbic acid excretion was not stimulated by chloretone (Burns and Mosbach 1956). These findings indicated that the carbon chain of glucose is converted intact into ascorbic acid by a metabolic pathway which involves inversion, and this was confirmed by observations on rats which indicated that [2-^{14}C]-D-glucose was converted mainly into [5-^{14}C]-L-ascorbic acid (Loewus *et al.*, 1960). It has also been shown that the kidney was not involved because the extent of the conversion of [1-^{14}C]-D-glucose into L-ascorbic acid in nephrectomized animals approximated to that in intact animals (Evans *et al.*, 1959). Glucose in the form of glucose cycloacetoacetate is also converted into ascorbic acid in the rat (Belkhode and Nath, 1962). Two pathways (1,2) have been suggested; in both these schemes C-1 of glucose becomes C-6 of L-ascorbic acid.

Pathway (1) has been ruled out by experiments in which [6-^{14}C] L-sorbose and [U-^{14}C]-2-keto-L-gulonic acid were fed to rats. With the first substrate the isolated L-ascorbic acid was almost equally elablled in C-1 and C-6. This labelling pattern is explicable on the assumption that L-sorbose is converted into triose phosphate which is then incorporated into glucose by the reversal of the well-established Embden-Meyerhof glycolytic sequence (Burns *et al.*, 1955). With the second substrate there was no detectable incorporation of label into L-ascorbic acid (Dayton, 1957).

On the other hand, there is considerable evidence for the existence of pathway (2). Strong circumstantial evidence was obtained by Isherwood *et al.* (1954) when they found that administration of D-glucurono-γ-lactone and L-gulono-γ-lactone to rats stimulated

* In both reaction schemes the numbers in brackets represent the original numbering of the glucose molecule.

the urinary excretion of L-ascorbic acid. Direct evidence was produced with the help of ^{14}C-intermediates. [U-^{14}C]-D-Glucurono-γ-lactone administered to chloretone-treated rats resulted in the excretion of [U-^{14}C]-L-ascorbic acid (Horowitz and King, 1953) and both [6-^{14}C]-D-glucurono-γ-lactone and [6-^{14}C]-L-gulono-γ-lactone yielded [1-^{14}C]ascorbic acid in both normal and chloretone-treated rats (Burns and Evans, 1956). Furthermore, [1-^{14}C]-D-glucose is also converted into [1-^{14}C]-D-glucuronic acid and [6-^{14}C]-L-gulonic acid in chloretone-treated rats (Burns, 1957; Burns et al., 1957).

Investigations into the enzymology of each of the steps indicated in reaction (2) have now been reported. The intermediate reactions in step A are indicated in reaction 3. Glucose-1-phosphate, formed from glycogen by the action of *phosphorylase*, or from glucose via glucose 6-phosphate by the action of *glucokinase* [ATP: D-glucose 6-phosphotransferase] and *phosphoglucomutase* [D-glucose 1,6-diphosphate D-glucose 1-phosphate transferase] respectively, is first converted into uridine diphosphate glucose (UDPG) in a reaction catalysed by *UDPG pyrophosphorylase* [UTP: D-glucose

$$\text{Glucose} \rightarrow \text{G-6-P} \rightarrow \text{G-1-P} \xrightarrow[\text{UTP P-P}]{} \text{UDP-G} \xrightarrow{\overset{2\,\text{NAD}\quad 2\,\text{NADH}_2}{\frown}} \text{UDP-Glucuronic acid} \quad (3)$$

1-phosphate uridylyl transferase]. UDP-Glucuronic acid then arises by the NAD-dependent dehydrogenation of UDPG catalysed by a soluble liver enzyme, *UDPG dehydrogenase* [UDP-glucose:NAD oxidoreductase] (Strominger et al., 1954; Storey and Dutton, 1955). Although two molecules of NAD are utilized for each molecule of glucose oxidized, all attempts to demonstrate the existence of an intermediate at the aldehyde level of oxidation have so far failed. The liberation of glucuronic acid from its UDP-complex has been demonstrated in the microsomal fraction of rat liver (Evans et al., 1959) and also in particulate preparations from rat kidney (Ginsberg et al., 1959). It is assumed that the reaction is a two stage process (reaction 4), the first step involving a reaction similar to UDPG pyrophosphorylase, with the production of glucuronic cid 1-phosphate, the and second involving a phosphatase. Some years ago, however-

$$\text{UDP-Glucuronic acid} + \text{P-P} \rightleftharpoons \text{UTP} + \text{glucuronic acid 1-P}$$
$$\downarrow \text{P}_i \qquad (4)$$
$$\text{glucuronic acid}$$

ever, Smith and Mills (1954) failed to demonstrate the existence of the postulated pyrophosphorylase in liver and yeast, although it is present in mung beans (Feingold *et al.*, 1958); the existence of the phosphatase proposed for the second step also remains doubtful. It has recently been shown that D-galactose is apparently a more direct precursor of L-ascorbic acid than is D-glucose. About 92% of the total activity of [^{14}C]-L-ascorbic acid arising from [1-^{14}C]-D-galactose is located in C-6, whereas the corresponding figure for [1-^{14}C]-D-glucose is 56 (Evans *et al.*, 1959, 1960). These results indicate that D-galactose is converted into L-ascorbic acid without passing through D-glucose; that is, they are consistent with the well-established pathway of conversion of galactose into UDP-glucose via the route outlined in reaction (5) (see e.g. Axelrod, 1960).

$$\text{D-Galactose} \rightarrow \text{D-galactose 1-phosphate} \rightarrow \text{UDP-galactose} \rightleftharpoons \text{UDP-glucose} \qquad (5)$$

The formation of L-gulono-γ-lactone from D-glucuronic acid (step B, reaction 2) can be achieved in two ways. In the first pathway the initial step is the lactonization of D-glucuronic acid in the presence of the enzyme *uronolactonase* [D-glucurono-γ-lactone hydrolase]* which is present in the microsomal fraction of liver cells (Winkelman and Lehninger, 1958; Yamada, 1959). The reduction of the resulting D-glucurono-γ-lactone to L-gulono-γ-lactone is catalysed by the NADP-dependent enzyme, *glucuronolactone reductase* [L-gulono-γ-lactone: NADP oxidoreductase] present in the microsomal fraction of rat liver (Ul Hassan and Lehninger, 1956; Ishikawa and Noguchi, 1957) and goat liver (Kar *et al.*, 1962) homogenates. In an alternative pathway D-glucuronic acid is first reduced to L-gulonic acid by a supernatant enzyme D-glucuronic dehydrogenase; L-gulonic acid is then lactonized by *aldonolactonase* [L-(or D)-gulono-γ-lactone hydrolase], an enzyme also present in the supernatant fraction of rat liver homogenates which reversibly hydrolyses a number of 5-C, 6-C and 7-C aldonolactones as well as L-gulono-γ-lactone, but which will not hydrolyse D-glucurono-γ-lactone (Winkelman and Lehninger, 1958; Mano *et al.*, 1959, Yamada, 1959; Yamada *et al.*, 1959, 1961; Chatterjee *et al.* 1959a; Kawada and Yamada, 1961). The two alternative pathways are indicated in scheme (6). Stubbs and Salomon (1962) consider that the pathway involving aldonolactonase is the preferred pathway and that it is the step involving aldonolactonase which is rate-limiting. The activity of this enzyme, and thus the synthesis of ascorbic acid, is greatly reduced in rats after hypophysectomy.

The final steps in the formation of L-ascorbic acid in rats are carried out in the liver microsomes by L-gulono-oxidase (step C, reaction 2) and is specific for L-gulono-γ-lactone (Burns *et al.*, 1956;

---

* The activity of this enzyme is increased by drugs such as Chloretone which stimulate the secretion of ascorbic acid (Kawada *et al.*, 1961).

Chang and Tung, 1958; Chatterjee, 1959a, b; Yamada *et al.*, 1959; Bublitz and Lehninger, 1959; Kanfer *et al.*, 1959; Isherwood *et al.*, 1960). Some activity is also found in rat liver mitochondria (Isherwood *et al.*, 1960). The intermediate between L-gulono-γ-lac-

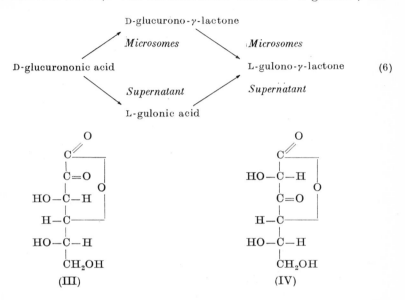

$$D\text{-glucurono-}\gamma\text{-lactone}$$

Microsomes   *Microsomes*

D-glucurononic acid   L-gulono-γ-lactone   (6)

Supernatant   *Supernatant*

L-gulonic acid

(III)   (IV)

tone and L-ascorbic acid is probably 2-oxo-L-gulono-γ-lactone (III), because it is formed during the transformation of L-gulono-γ-lactone into ascorbic acid by a soluble enzyme system from goat liver microsomes (Chatterjee *et al.* 1959b). Bublitz and Lehninger (1959) and Bublitz (1961) have examined the system in detail; L-gulono-γ-lactone dehydrogenase, which uses phenazine methosulphate as electron acceptor, can be obtained in soluble form free from oxidase activity. It would appear that the oxidase is either an autoxidisable dehydrogenase (? flavoprotein) which is altered during fractionation, or an enzyme of similar type to, say succinic oxidase, in which one or more components of the electron transport system have been removed by fractionation. Isherwood and Mapson (1962) have pointed out that this last stage of synthesis differs from that in plants, where no conversion of free aldonic or uronic acids into ascorbic acid has been observed. Nutrition experiments indicate that the impaired conversion of glucose into ascorbic acid in biotin-deficient rats is due to a reduced activity of L-gulono-oxidase. Dakshinamurti and Mistry, 1962).

The earlier suggestion that 3-oxo-L-gulonic acid (IV) was an intermediate (Grollman and Lehninger, 1957) and that the formation of

L-ascorbic acid and L-xylulose from L-gulonic acid passed through a common intermediate has now been withdrawn (Lehninger, 1959); there is not doubt, however, that L-gulonic acid is oxidized to L-xylulose and CO_2 by an NAD-dependent enzyme present in rat and pig kidney (Burns et al., 1959a,b; Ashwell et al., 1959). This is discussed in detail on p. 217.

B. Failure of Primates, the Guinea-pig, the Indian Fruit Bat and the Red Vented Bubul to Synthesize L-Ascorbic Acid

The metabolic lesion which leads to the failure of primates, guinea-pigs, Indian fruit bats and red vented bubuls to synthesis ascorbic acid is the inability of the liver to convert D-glucurono-γ-lactone into L-ascorbic acid owing to the absence of the two microsomal enzymes, D-glucuronoreductase and L-gulono-oxidase; the absence of the latter enzyme was the first deficiency to be detected. Lehninger's group (Ul Hassan and Lehninger, 1956; Grollman and Lehninger, 1957) could demonstrate no net synthesis of L-ascorbic acid from L-gulono-γ-lactone in homogenates prepared from human, monkey and guinea-pig livers whilst homogenates similarly prepared from rat, mouse, rabbit and dog livers carried out an appreciable synthesis. The results obtained by Burns's group (Burns et al., 1956; Burns, 1957), who used [1-^{14}C]-L-gulono-γ-lactone, pointed to the same conclusion. Table 1 shows that human, monkey and guinea pig

TABLE 1. Conversion of [1-^{14}C]-L-Gulono-γ-lactone into L-Ascorbic Acid in Liver Preparations from Various Animals (Burns, 1960)

Species	% Conversion	
	Homogenate	Microsomes
Rat	8·0	10·0
Guinea-pig	0·05	0·05
Monkey	0·07	—
Man	0·07	—

homogenates are less than one hundredth as effective as rat liver homogenates in converting L-gulono-γ-lactone into L-ascorbic acid. Chatterjee et al. (1960a) have also reported the absence of L-gulonooxidase from guinea-pig liver.

The absence of D-glucuronoreductase from guinea-pig liver has recently been reported by Chatterjee *et al.* (1961). The possibility that in guinea-pig liver microsomes the enzyme is present together with an inhibitor was ruled out when it was found that addition of guinea-pig liver microsomes to rat liver microsomes did not inhibit their ability to synthesize vitamin C. Both enzymes are also absent from the livers of the Indian fruit bat and red vented bubul (Kar *et al.*, 1962).

It should be noted, however, that in a recent report, it was claimed that in humans after an oral dose of [6-^{14}C]-D-glucurono-γ-lactone, the urinary ascorbic acid was slightly labelled (Baker *et al.*, 1961).

As it is clear that animals which cannot synthesize L-ascorbic acid can convert glucose into D-glucurono-γ-lactone, the questions arises as to the possible existence of an alternative pathway of metabolism of this compound. It is now clear that D-glucuronic acid can be converted into pentoses and that L-gulonic acid is the branch point. This compound, in addition to being converted into L-gulono-γ-lactone, is also converted into L-xylulose, by L-*gulonic acid dehydrogenase* [L-gulonate:NAD oxidoreductase (decarboxylating)] (scheme 7) which simultaneously decarboxylates the intermediate 3-oxo-L-gulonic acid. The enzyme has been purified from mammalian kidney preparations and is NAD-dependent (Burns *et al.*, 1959a,b; Ashwell *et al.*, 1959). L-Xylulose is converted into its enantiomorph via xylitol (reaction 8). The xylitol dehydrogenase

[xylitol:NADP oxidoreductase (L-xylulose forming)] which converts
xylitol into L-xylulose is highly specific and requires NADP as co-
factor. The dehydrogenase   yielding D-xylulose [xylitol:NAD oxidoreductase (D-xylulose forming)] is, on the other hand, less specific and requires NAD as co-factor. Both enzymes are present in
the insoluble fraction of disrupted mitochondria (Hollman and Touster, 1957). A D-xylulose kinase [ATP:D-xylulose 5-phosphate trans-
ferase] present in mammalian tissues, converts D-xylulose into D-

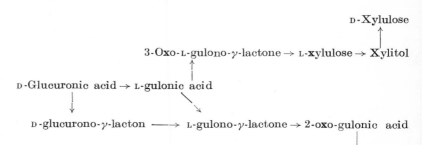

FIG. 1. Relationship between D-glucuronic acid metabolism and synthesis
of L-ascorbic acid and L-xylose.

xylulose 5-phosphate (Hickman and Ashwell, 1956) and thus allows
its entry into the pentose phosphate pathway (see Goodwin, 1960).
This D-xylulose pathway has been demonstrated in all mammalian
tissues examined including those which cannot synthesize vitamin C.
The elucidation of this pathway now yields an explanation for
the excretion of L-xylulose in patients suffering from an essential
pentosuria, an hereditary disease characterized by the presence
of L-xylulose in the urine (Touster et al. 1957). The inter-relation-
ship between the metabolic pathways which have just been discussed is given in Fig. 1.

Key differences between the L-ascorbic acid pathway and the
L-xylulose pathway of glucuronic acid metabolism in mammals
are (i) the L-ascorbic acid system has an absolute requirement for
the lactone ring; (ii) the conversion of L-gulonic acid into L-ascor-
ic acid is not dependent on pyridine nucleotides; (iii) the 2-oxo
derivative of L-gulonic acid is concerned with L-ascorbic acid synthesis and the 3-oxo derivative is concerned with L-xylulose synthesis,
and (iv) L-ascorbic acid synthesis takes place only in the liver whilst
L-xylulose synthesis can also take place in the kidney.

It is interesting to note that bacteria metabolize glucuronic acid
by still other routes, which involve as the first intermediate either
5-keto-L-gulonic acid or D-galacturonic acid (see Rabinowitz, 1959).

C. *Formation in Birds, Reptiles and Amphibia*

Grollman and Lehninger (1957) and Roy and Guha (1958) have demonstrated that, unlike mammals, birds, reptiles and amphibia synthesize vitamin C in the kidney and not in the liver, and this conclusion has been strengthened by the observation that in pigeons the two enzymes D-glucuronolactonase and L-gulonolactonase are found in the kidney and not in the liver, as is the case with mammals (Yamada *et al.*, 1959).

Roy and Guha (1958) have also reported that the red vented bubul cannot synthesize ascorbic acid in either its liver or kidney, and on an ascorbic acid-deficient diet develops a clinical manifestation of scurvy, which can be cured by administering the vitamin. This is the first report of such an occurrence in birds.

D. *General Factors Controlling Biosynthesis in Animals*

(i) *Vitamin A*

A number of early observations indicated that vitamin A deficiency reduced the ascorbic acid levels in the tissues of rats, calves and horses (Sure *et al.*, 1939; Phillips *et al.*, 1941), and that these levels were increased on feeding vitamin A (Phillips *et al.*, 1941). A later re-examination of this problem confirmed these observations in rats but showed that the depressed ascorbic acid levels were due not to vitamin A deficiency *per se* but to the inanition which accompanies the condition; when the food intake of normal animals was reduced to that of the group deprived of vitamin A, then their plasma ascorbic acid levels fell correspondingly (Mapson and Walker 1948).

(ii) *Thiamine and Riboflavin*

There may also be some relationship between ascorbic acid synthesis and the water-soluble vitamins thiamine and riboflavin, for in rats showing signs of thiamine and riboflavin deficiency, the ascorbic acid levels in the blood are low and the chloretone-stimulated excretion of ascorbic acid is not observed (Kennaway and Daff, 1946; Roy *et al.*, 1946). The possibility that inanition was again the cause of these observations was not investigated.

(iii) *Tocopherol*

Caputto *et al.* (1958) and Carpenter *et al.* (1959) found that liver homogenates from tocopherol-deficient rabbits were only 10–30% as effective as liver homogenates from normal rabbits in converting D-glucuronolactone into L-ascorbic acid. Reactivation of the homogenate can be achieved by addition of tocopherol (McCay et al., 1959) or by addition of either Mn^{2+}, Co^{2+}, EDTA or a number of drugs which prevent lipid peroxide formation. However, it should be noted that H_2O_2 stimulates synthesis in soluble preparations obtained from rat microsomes (Feinberg and Caputto, 1960). Recently Kitabchi et al. (1959) and Carpenter et al. (1961) working with rats, have defined the site of tocopherol action more precisely; it controls the conversion of L-gulonolactone into L-ascorbic acid in the liver microsomes. An extract from the liver microsomes of tocopherol-deficient rats inhibits L-gulonolactone oxidase, and this inhibition is overcome by the addition of tocopherol. The nature of the inhibitor, which appears only to have a transient existence, is not known. Vitamin K_1 is also effective and ubiquinone-35 (UQ_7, coenzyme Q_7) partly effective in restoring activity to tocopherol-deficient systems (Chatterjee et al., 1960b).

(iv) Hormones

Hypophysectomy in rats results in decreased ascorbic synthesis from D-glucose; Salmon and Stubbs (1961) have located the metabolic lesion between D-glucuronic acid and ascorbic acid, and this is primarily the result of diminished aldonolactonase activity. The activity of L-gulonolactone oxidase is also affected but to a lesser degree. Touster and Hollman (1961) find that hypophysectomy nullified the increased urinary excretion of ascorbic acid which follows a dose of barbital in normal animals; their conclusion that barbital functions by enhancing UDPG dehydrogenase activity (p. 213) is not contradicted by the observations of Salmon and Stubbs.

E. Effect of Drugs on Ascorbic Acid Synthesis

A variety of drugs, including hypnotics, analgesics, muscular relaxants and antirheumatic agents, as well as carcinogenic hydrocarbons (e.g. 3-methylcholanthrene) stimulate the synthesis of L-ascorbic acid in the rat (Conney and Burns, 1959). The stimulation appears to be the result of an adaptive response to a foreign compound, because not only is the synthesis of D-glucuronic acid, the ascorbic acid precursor, stimulated but the activity of the microsomal enzymes concerned with the metabolism of foreign organic compounds is also increased. In particular, Touster and Hollman (1961) found that barbital and chloretone stimulate UDPG-dehydrogenase (p. 213); however, in vitro experiments indicate that UDP-glucuronic acid pyrophosphatase is inhibited by barbital.

The stimulatory effect of carcinogenic hydrocarbons must be through a different mechanism because they do not stimulate UDPG-dehydrogenase activity (Touster and Hollman, 1961). They also do not stimulate the conversion of L-galacto-γ-lactone into ascorbic acid (Boyland and Grover, 1961).

Lycorine, an alkaloid from *Lycoris radiata*, will produce scurvy in rats but not in guinea-pigs (Mineseta *et al.*, 1959); it was concluded from these observations that lycorine inhibited the biosynthesis of L-ascorbic acid, but the site of action has not yet been determined. Confirmation of this view comes from Yamaguchi (1959) who has demonstrated that lycorine inhibits ascorbic acid synthesis in the developing chick embryo and reduces the stimulatory effect of chlorobutanol.

II. FORMATION IN PLANTS

A. *Biosynthetic Pathways*

(i) *From glucose*

The observation that D-glucurono-γ-lactone and L-gulono-γ-lactone were converted into L-ascorbic acid in cress seedlings, led to the view that L-ascorbic acid was being synthesized in plants in essentially the same way as in animals (Scheme 2), that is by a pathway involving inversion (Isherwood *et al.*, 1954; Mapson *et al.*, 1954; Mapson and Isherwood, 1956). Isotope experiments which indicated the incorporation of [^{14}C]-D-glucorono-γ-lactone into L-ascorbic acid in cress seedlings and ripening strawberry fruit, tended to confirm this view, (Loewus and Jang, 1958; Loewus *et al.* 1958, 1960; Loewus and Kelly, 1961), but a detailed investigation into the location of the label in L-ascorbic acid following introduction into strawberry fruit of [1-^{14}C]-, [2-^{14}C]- or [6-^{14}C]-D-glucose via the stem demonstrated that although the 6-C unit of these compounds was incorporated directly into L-ascorbic acid, there was no inversion of the molecule. For example, [1-^{14}C]-D-glucose yielded L-ascorbic acid with 65–70% of the label in C-1 and only 14–19% in C-6, whilst the values when [6-^{14}C]-D-glucose was the substrate were 18% in C-1 (and C-2) and 71% in C-6 of L-ascorbic acid. Furthermore, D-glucuronate is probably not involved because [6-^{14}C]-D-glucuronate and [6-^{14}C]-D-glucurono-γ-lactone are converted into [1-^{14}C]-L-ascorbic acid under the same conditions (Finkle *et al.*, 1960). These results indicate that two pathways exist in plants, one involving inversion and the other not. A biosynthetic pathway envisaged to account for both routes is that indicated in scheme (9). There is as yet no detailed evidence for the participation of any of these compounds in L-ascorbic acid

(9)

$$\begin{array}{ccccccc}
O= & C- & C-OH & C-OH & C- & HO-C-H & CH_2OH \\
 & & \| & & \| & & \\
 & & & & H-C & & \\
\end{array}$$

CHO—CH—OH—HO—C—H—CH—OH—CH—OH—CH₂OH

synthesis in plants, and the problems still to be solved have been discussed by Isherwood and Mapson (1962) and Loewus (1963).

(ii) *From* D-*galactose*

Mapson and Isherwood, in their investigations on cress seedlings found that L-galactono-γ-lactone very effecively stimulated L-ascorbic acid synthesis, and this has been-confirmed in other plants (Jackson *et al.*, 1961). Mapson and Isherwood also postulated a pathway (scheme 10) analogous to that put forward for the conversion of D-glucose into ascorbic acid and involving L-galactono-γ-lactone. The pathway taken in animals, which involves an initial conversion of D-galactose into D-glucose via UDP-galactose, has already been discussed (p. 214). The UDPG-pathway could also account for the incorporation of D-galactose into ascorbic acid in plants, for Loewus *et al.* (1958) found that strawberries fed [1-^{14}C]-D-galactose produced L-ascorbic acid which was

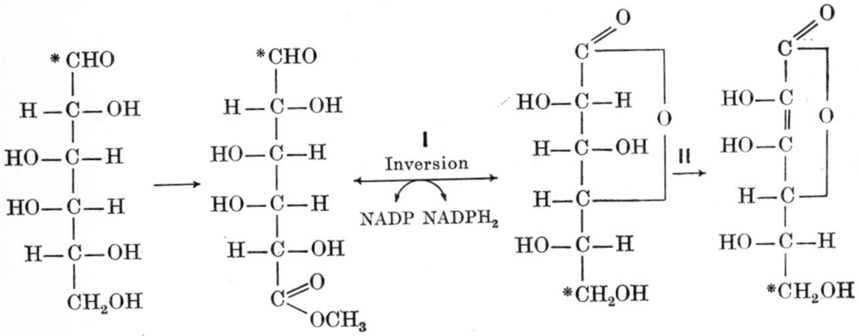

$$
\begin{array}{ccccc}
{}^{*}\text{CHO} & {}^{*}\text{CHO} & & \overset{\displaystyle O}{\underset{\displaystyle |}{\text{C}}} & \overset{\displaystyle O}{\underset{\displaystyle |}{\text{C}}} \\
\text{H}-\text{C}-\text{OH} & \text{H}-\text{C}-\text{OH} & & \text{HO}-\text{C}-\text{H} & \text{HO}-\text{C} \\
\text{HO}-\text{C}-\text{H} & \text{HO}-\text{C}-\text{H} & \xrightarrow[\text{NADP NADPH}_2]{\underset{\text{Inversion}}{\text{I}}} & \text{H}-\text{C}-\text{OH} \quad \overset{\text{II}}{\longrightarrow} & \text{HO}-\text{C} \\
\text{HO}-\text{C}-\text{H} & \text{HO}-\text{C}-\text{H} & & \text{H}-\text{C} & \text{H}-\text{C} \\
\text{H}-\text{C}-\text{OH} & \text{H}-\text{C}-\text{OH} & & \text{HO}-\text{C}-\text{H} & \text{HO}-\text{C}-\text{H} \\
\text{CH}_2\text{OH} & \text{C}\overset{O}{\underset{\text{OCH}_3}{}} & & {}^{*}\text{CH}_2\text{OH} & {}^{*}\text{CH}_2\text{OH}
\end{array}
\tag{10}
$$

predominantly labelled in C-1, indicating that D-galactose is converted into L-ascorbic acid via glucose. In these later experiments Loewus *et al.* (1958) could not confirm the results they previously obtained (Loewus *et al.*, 1956) which suggested that [1-^{14}C]-D-galactose labels L-ascorbic acid equally in C-1 and C-6, and thus must be broken down to a triose before incorporation. Whatever the exact relationship of scheme (10) to L-ascorbic acid biosynthesis, Mapson and his colleagues have purified from plant sources two enzymes concerned with galactose metabolism. The first catalyses a NADPH-specific reduction of esters of D-galacturonic acid to L-galactono-γ-lactone (step I, scheme 10) and is present in the supernatant of cell homogenates of pea seedlings. Free D-galacturonic acid is not reduced whilst the γ-lactones of D-glucuronic acid and D-mannuronic acid are reduced at about 50% the rate of the esters of D-galacturonic acid (Mapson and Isherwood, 1956). The second enzyme, L-galactono-γ-lactone dehydrogenase [L-galactono-γ-lactone: cytochrome *c* oxidoreductase] (step II, scheme 10) is a flavoprotein and has been isolated from the soluble fraction of the mitochondria of cauliflower florets. It shows high specificity towards its substrate, requires SH groups for activity, and cytochrome c and phenazine methosulphate can act as electron acceptors, (Mapson and Breslow, 1958). A mechanism of the overall reaction catalysed by these two enzymes (reactions 11–14) has been proposed by Isherwood and Mapson (1961).

$$\text{L-Galacturonyl-Enz-I} + \text{NADPH} + \text{H}^+ \rightarrow \text{L-Galactonyl-Enz-I} + \text{NADP}^+ \quad (11)$$

$$\text{L-Galactonyl-Enz} + \text{Enz-II} \rightarrow \text{L-Galactonyl-Enz-II} + \text{Enz-I} \quad (12)$$

$$\text{L-Galactonyl-Enz-II} \xrightarrow{\text{O}_2} \text{2-Oxo-L-galactonyl-Enz-II} \quad (13)$$

$$\text{2-Oxo-L-galactonyl-Enz-II} \xrightarrow[\substack{\text{enolization} \\ \text{and ring} \\ \text{formation}}]{\text{Spontaneous}} \text{L-Ascorbic acid} + \text{Enz-II} \quad (14)$$

Mapson *et al.* (1954) demonstrated that intact mitochondria were necessary for the oxidation of L-galactono-γ-lactone to L-ascorbic acid when oxygen is the electron acceptor. The reason for this is probably the need for a functional cytochrome oxidase system. Furthermore, certain components of the tricarboxylic acid cycle, in particlar succinate, inhibit reaction (II) (scheme 10), thus indicating competition for a common electron acceptor. It is possible that this represents a mechanism for control of ascorbic acid synthesis.

B. *General Factors Controlling Ascorbic Acid Synthesis in Plants*

(i) *Light*

Light is not essential for the synthesis of ascorbic acid, which is formed in seedlings germinated in complete darkness (Harris and Roy, 1933). However, it can exert an important controlling influence; there is, for example, a diurnal variation in the ascorbic acid levels of plants grown out of doors, the maximum concentration in potato leaves being observed just before noon (Smith and Gillies, 1940). The transfer of plants from light to darkness, or the shading of a plant results in a drop in ascorbic acid levels (see e.g. Hamner *et al.*, 1945). Indeed, a direct proportionality between ascorbic acid levels and light intensity has been demonstrated in the leaves of turnip and tomato plants (Somers *et al.*, 1948; Åberg, 1953). Similar results have been observed with ripening fruit (McCollum, 1944).

The quality of the illumination is important; red light is most effective (Sugawara, 1939), whilst blue light has very little effect (Åberg, 1953). The unconfirmed claim that red and violet flowers contain less ascorbic acid than white and yellow flowers may be due to the differential effect of light of different wavelengths on ascorbic acid production (Mituda, 1938).

It should be emphasized that most of the observations just described, and others of a similar nature, can be accounted for on the need for photosynthesis to be in progress in order to provide a sufficient supply of hexose from which ascorbic acid is eventually synthesized (see also Isherwood and Mapson, 1962).

(ii) *Oxygen*

Oxygen appears to be obligatory for the synthesis of ascorbic acid in plants (see Mapson, 1955). This would be expected from the pathway of synthesis which has recently been revealed.

(iii) *Temperature*

The effect of temperature on ascorbic biosynthesis in isolated discs of turnip leaves is the same as that observed on photosynthesis (Somers *et al.*, 1948). This again supports the conclusion that ascorbic acid formation is directly dependent on photosynthesized carbohydrate. Harvested potatoes stored at 1° synthesize ascorbic acid, whilst in those stored at higher temperatures, the levels of ascorbic acid eventually fall (Barker and Mapson, 1950, 1952). These observations once more indicate the need for sugars as precursors of ascorbic acid; there is an increased formation of sugar in tubers stored at the lower temperature. Rather similar results have been reported for tomato fruit (Åberg, 1949).

(iv) *pH*

Ascorbic acid synthesis in germinating cress seedlings depends on the pH of the cell sap; increasing the pH above its normal value increased ascorbic acid production, whilst a lowered pH value depressed ascorbic acid synthesis (Mapson *et al.*, 1949).

(v) *Salts*

As might be expected, the general impression gained from the large number of papers published on the effect of salts on ascorbic acid synthesis in plants is of one confusion, probably engendered by

the existence of many uncontrolled variables, such as previous ferti-
lizer treatments (see Isherwood and Mapson, 1962). However, one
clear conclusion which does emerge is that the form in which nitrogen is supplied is important. In cress seedlings, when the cation NH_4^+
is combined with a non-utilizable anion (SO_4^{2-}, Cl^-) synthesis is
inhibited, but when it is combined with a utilizable anion (NO_3^-,
HCO_3^-) synthesis is stimulated (Mapson and Cruickshank, 1947).
The reason for this effect is that certain ammonium salts (in particular $(NH_4)_2SO_4$) depress the synthesis of ascorbic acid from he-
xoses (Mapson et al., 1949; Sastry and Sarma, 1955). The effect must
occur at an early stage in the conversion because the conversion
of D-glucurono-γ-lactone and D-galacturonic acid methyl ester
into L-ascorbic acid by germinating seeds is not inhibited in the
presence of $(NH_4)_2SO_4$ (Sastry and Sarma, 1955; Isherwood and
Mapson, 1962).

(vi) *Trace elements*

(a) *Manganese.* On the basis of the observation that seedlings of
Avena, Triticum, Hordeum, Phaseolus mungo and *Acer auranticum*
contain more ascorbic acid when germinated in the presence of
Mn^{2+}, Rudra (1938, 1939) concluded that manganese plays a role
in the biosynthesis of ascorbic acid. A similar effect reported for
tomatoes (Hester, 1941) was not confirmed (Gunn et al., 1945.)
Mapson (1955) is rightly sceptical about a specific role for manganese
in ascorbic acid biosynthesis; it is well known that it is an activator of many enzymes essential to the metabolic economy of plants.
Furthermore, there is as yet no indication from enzyme studies of
a specific Mn^{2+} requirement in the pathway from glucose to ascorbic acid.

(b) *Molybdenum.* Ascorbic acid levels in molybdenum-deficient plants
are only 25-50% of the normal values. Injection of micro-quanti-
ties of molybdenum into deficient plants immediately stimulates
synthesis so that within 3-5 days the levels become normal (Hewitt et al., 1950). Molybdenum is now known to be part of many dehydrogenase complexes but, as with manganese, the decision as
to whether it plays a specific part in ascorbic acid biosynthesis must
remain unresolved until the enzymology of the biosynthetic pathway is more fully understood. From this point of view it has recently been found that mitochondria from manganese-deficient plants
are as effective as those from normal plants in converting galactur-
onic acid and galactonic acid derivatives into L-ascorbic acid
(Isherwood and Mapson, 1962).

(vii) *Hormones*

Ascorbic acid accumulates in the stems of cucumber plants which had been treated with auxin; at the same time, the ascorbic acid levels in the leaves dropped (Key, 1962).

III. Ascorbigen

Ascorbigen, an indole derivative with the same carbon skeleton as tryptophan, probably (V), was isolated from plant tissues by Proházka *et al.*, (1957). Kutáček *et al.* (1960) further reported that [3-^{14}C]tryptophan is incorporated into ascorbigen by *Brassica oleracea* L. However, it is quite clear from recent investigations (Kutáček *et al.*, 1962) that ascorbigen is an artifact resulting from the action of the enzyme myrosinase, liberated when plant cells are damaged, on the tryptophan derivative glucobrassicin (Gmelin and Virtanen, 1961). No ascorbigen is found if the myrosinase is inacivated before extracting the plant material (Kutáček *et al.*, 1962).

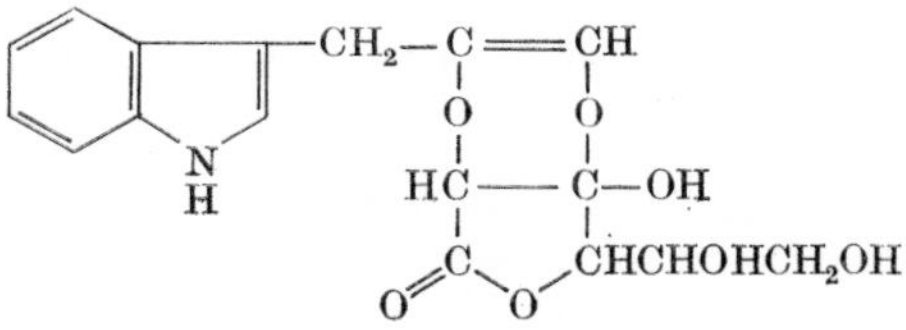

(V)

IV. d-Araboascorbic Acid

According to Takahashi *et al.* (1960, 1961) *Penicillium notatum* 1026 synthesizes d-araboascorbic acid (VI) from d-glucose without rupture or inversion of the carbon chain of the sugar. The mechanism proposed (Takahashi and Mitsumoto, 1961) (reaction 15) is

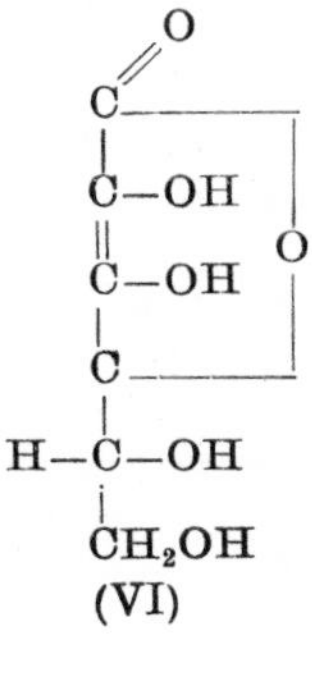

(VI)

carried out by glucose aero-dehydrogenase (step A, reaction 15) and glucono-γ-lactone dehydrogenase (step C, reaction 15). Step B (reaction 15), the conversion of glucono-γ-lactone into glucono-γ-lactone, is said to be a non-enzymatic reaction.

$$
\text{Glucose} \xrightarrow{A}
\begin{array}{c}
\text{C} \!\!\nearrow^{\!\!O} \\
\text{H}-\text{C}-\text{OH} \\
\text{HO}-\text{C}-\text{H} \\
\text{H}-\text{C}-\text{OH} \\
\text{H}-\text{C} \\
\text{CH}_2\text{OH}
\end{array} \; O
\quad \overset{B}{\rightleftarrows} \quad
\begin{array}{c}
\text{C} \!\!\nearrow^{\!\!O} \\
\text{H}-\text{C}-\text{OH} \\
\text{HO}-\text{C}-\text{H} \\
\text{H}-\text{C} \\
\text{H}-\text{C}-\text{OH} \\
\text{CH}_2\text{OH}
\end{array} \; O
\quad \xrightarrow{C} \quad
\begin{array}{c}
\text{C} \!\!\nearrow^{\!\!O} \\
\text{C}-\text{OH} \\
\text{C}-\text{OH} \\
\text{H}-\text{C} \\
\text{H}-\text{C}-\text{OH} \\
\text{CH}_2\text{OH}
\end{array} \; O
\quad (15)
$$

REFERENCES

Åberg, B. (1949). *Physiol. Plantarum.* **2,** 164.

Åberg, B. (1953). *Ann. Roy. Agric. Coll. Sweden* **20,** 125.

Ashwell, G., Kanfer, J., and Burns, J. J. (1959). *J. biol. Chem.* **234,** 472.

Axelrod, B. (1960). *In* Greenberg, D. M. Ed. *"Metabolic Pathways"* 2nd Ed. (Vol. 1). Academic Press, New York.

Baker, E. M., Sauberlich, H. E., and Wolfskill, S. J. (1961). *Fed. Proc.* **20,** 85.

Barker, J., and Mapson, L. W. (1950). *New Phytologist* **49,** 283.

Barker, J., and Mapson, L. W. (1952). *New Phytologist* **51,** 90.

Belkhode, M. L., and Nath, M. C. (1962). *Biochem. J.* **84,** 71.

Boyland, E., and Grover, P. L. (1961). *Biochem. J.* **81,** 163.

Bublitz, C. (1961). *Biochim. biophys. Acta* **48,** 61.

Bublitz, C., and Lehninger, A. L. (1959). *Biochim. biophys. Acta* **32,** 290.

Burns, J. J. (1957). *Nature, Lond,* **180,** 553.

Burns, J. J. (1960). *In* Greenberg, D. M. Ed. *"Metabolic Pathways"* 2nd Ed. (Vol. 1). Academic Press, New York.

Burns, J. J., and Evans, C. (1956). *J. biol. Chem.* **223,** 894.

Burns, J. J., Evans, C., and Trousof, N. (1954). *J. biol. Chem.* **227,** 785.

Burns, J. J., Evans, C., and Trousof, N. (1957). *J. biol. Chem.* **227,** 785

Burns, J. J., Fullmer, H. M., and Dayton, P. G. (1959a). *Proc. Soc. exp. Biol., N.Y.* **101,** 46

Burns, J. J., Kanfer, J., and Ashwell, G. (1959b). *Biochim. biophys. Acta* **34,** 46.

Burns, J. J., and Mosbach, E. H. (1956). *J. biol. Chem.* **221,** 107.

Burns, J. J., Mosbach, E. H., Schulenberg, S., and Reichenthal, J. (1955). *J. biol. Chem.* **214,** 504.

Burns, J. J., Peyser, P., and Moltz, A. (1956). *Science* **124,** 1148.

Caputto, R., McCay, P. B., and Carpenter, M. P. (1958). *J. biol. Chem.* **233,** 1025.

Carpenter, M. P., Kitabchi, A. E., McCay, P. B., and Caputto, R. (1959). *J. biol. Chem.* **234,** 2814.

Carpenter, M. P., McCay, P. B., Kitabchi, A. E., Trucco, R. E., and Caputto, R. (1961). *Fed. Proc.* **20,** 452.

Chang, Y., and Tung, L. (1958). *Vitaminy, Akad. Nauk. Ukr. S. S. R. Inst. Biochim.* **4,** 37.

Chatterjee, I. B., Chatterjee, G. C., Ghosh, N. H., Ghosh, J. J., and Guha, B. C. (1959a). *Sci. and Culture (India)* **24,** 340, 534.

Chatterjee, I. B., Chatterjee, G. C., Ghosh, N. K., Ghosh, J. J., and Guha, B. C. (1959b). *Naturwissenschaften,* **45,** 475.

Chatterjee, I. B., Chatterjee, G. C., Ghosh, N. C., Ghosh, J. J., and Guha, B. C. (1960a). *Biochem. J.* **74,** 193.

Chatterjee, I. B., Kar, N. C., Ghosh, N. C., and Guha, B. C. (1960b). *Arch. Biochem. Biophys.* **86,** 154.

Chatterjee, I. B., Kar, N. C., Ghosh, N. C., and Guha, B. C. (1961). *Ann. N. Y. Acad. Sci.* **92,** 36; *Nature, Lond.* **192,** 163.

Conney, A. H., and Burns, J. .J. (1959). *Nature, Lond.* **184,** 363.

Dakshinamurti, K., and Mistry, S. P. (1962). *Arch. Biochem. Biophys.* **99,** 254

Dayton, P. G. (1957). *Proc. Soc. exp. Biol., N.Y.* **94,** 286.

Evans, C., Conney, A. H., Trousof, N., and Burns, J. J. (1959). *Fed. Proc.* **18,** 223.

Evans, C., Conney, A. H., Trousof, N. and, Burns, J. J. (1960). *Biochim. biophys. Acta,* **41,** 9.

Feinberg, R. H., and Caputti, R. (1960). *Biochem. biophys. Res. Comm.* **3,** 110.

Feingold, D. S., Neufeld, E. F., and Hassid, W. Z. (1958). *Arch. Biochem. Biophys.* **78,** 401.

Finkle, B. J., Kelly, S., and Loewus, F. A. (1960). *Biochim. biophys. Acta,* **38,** 332.

Ginsberg, V., Weissbach, A., and Maxwell, E. S. (1955). *Biochim. biophys. Acta* **28,** 649.

Ginsberg, V., Dayton, P.G., and Eisenberg, F. (1957). *Biochim. biophys. Acta* **25,** 647

Ginsberg, V., Weissbach, A., and Maxwell, E. S. (1959). *Biochim. biophys. Acta* **28,** 649.

Gmelin, R., and Virtanen, A. I. (1961). *Ann. Acad. Sci. Fenn. A, II Chemica,* **107,**

Goodwin, T. W. (1960). "Recent Advances in Biochemistry". Churchill, London.

Grollman, A. P., and Lehninger, A. L. (1957). *Arch. Biochem. Biophys.* **69,** 458.

Gunn, O. B., Brown, H. D., and Burrell, R. C. (1945). *Plant Physiol.* **20,** 267.

Hamner, K. C., Bernstein, L., and Maynard, L. (1945). *J. Nutrit.* **29,** 85.

Harris, L. J., and Roy, S. N. (1933). *Biochem. J.* **27,** 580.

Hester, J. B. (1941). *Science* **93,** 401.

Hewitt, E. J., Agarwala, S. C., and Jones, E. W. (1950). *Nature, Lond.* **166,** 119.

Hickman, J., and Ashwell, G. (1956). *J. Amer. chem. Soc.* **78,** 6209.

Hollman, S., and Touster, O. (1957). *J. biol. Chem.* **225,** 87.

Horowitz., H. H., Doerschuk, A. P., and King, C. G. (1952). *J. biol. Chem.* **199,** 193.

Horowitz, H. H., and King, C. G. (1953). *J. biol. Chem.* **200,** 125.

Isherwood, F. A., Chen, Y. T., and Mapson, L. W. (1954). *Biochem. J.* **56,** 1

Isherwood, F. A., and Mapson, L. W. (1961). *Ann. N. Y. Acad. Sci.* **92,** 3.

Isherwood, F. A., and Mapson, K. W. (1962). *Ann. Rev. Plant. Physiol.* **14,** 329.

Isherwood, F. A., Mapson, L. W., and Chen, Y. T. (1960). *Biochem. J.* **76,** 157.

Ishikawa, S., and Noguchi, K. (1957). *J. Biochem. Tokyo* **44,** 465.

Jackson, G. A. D., Wood, R. B., and Prosser, M. V. (1961). *Nature, Lond.* **191,** 282.

Kanfer, J., Burns, J. J., and Ashwell, G. (1959). *Biochim. biophys. Acta* **31,** 556.
Kar, N. C., Chatterjee, I. B., Ghosh, N. C., and Guha, B. C. (1962). *Biochem. J.* **84,** 16.
Kawada, M., and Yamada, K. (1961). *J. Biochem. Tokyo,* **50,** 419.
Kawada, M., Yamada, K., Kagawa, K., and Mano, Y. (1961). *J. Biochem., Tokyo* **50,** 74.
Kennaway, E. L., and Daff, M. E. (1946). *Brit. J. exp. Pathol.* **27,** 63.
Key, J. L. (1962). *Plant. Physiol.* **37,** 349.
Kitabchi, A. E., McCay, P. B., Carpenter, M. P., Feinberg, R. H., Trucco, R. E., and Caputto, R. (1959). *Biochem. biophys. Res. Comm.* **1,** 216.
Kutáček, M., Procházka, Ž., and Grunberger, D. (1960). *Nature, Lond.* **187,** 61.
Kutáček M., Proházka, Ž., and Veres, K. (1962). *Nature, Lond.* **194,** 393.
Lehninger, A. (1959). *Proc. 4th Int. Cong. Biochem.* **11,** 17.
Loewus, F. A. (1963). *Phytochemistry,* **2,** 109.
Loewus, F. A., and Jang, R. (1958). *J. biol. Chem.* **232,** 505, 521.
Loewus, F. A., Jang, R., and Seegmiller, C. G. (1956). *J. biol. Chem.* **222,** 649.
Loewus, F. A., Jang, R., and Seegmiller, C. G. (1958). *J. biol. Chem.* **232,** 533,
Loewus, F. A., Kelly, S., and Hiatt, H. H. (1960). *J. biol. Chem.* **235,** 937.
Loewus, F. A., and Kelly, S. (1961). *Nature, Lond.* **191,** 1059.
Longenecker, H. E., Fricke, H. H., and King, C. G. (1940). *J. biol. Chem.* **135,** 497.
Mano, Y., Yamada, K., Suzuki, K., and Shimazono, N. (1959). *Biochim. biophys. Acta* **34,** 563.
Mapson, L. W. (1955). *Vitam. & Horm.* **13,** 71.
Mapson, L. W., and Breslow, E. (1958). *Biochem. J.* **68,** 395.
Mapson, L. W., and Cruickshank, E. M. (1947). *Biochem. J.* **41,** 194.
Mapson, L. W., Cruickshank, E. M., and Chen, Y. T. (1949). *Biochem. J.* **45,** 171.
Mapson, L. W., and Isherwood, F. A. (1956). *Biochem. J.* **64,** 13.
Mapson, L. W., Isherwood, F. A., and Chen, Y. T. (1954). *Biochem. J.* **56,** 1.
Mapson, L. W., and Walker, S. (1948). *Brit. J. Nutrit.* **2,** 1.
McCollum, J. P. (1944). *Proc. Soc. Hort. Sci* **45,** 382.
McCay, P. B., Carpenter, M. P., Kitabchi, A. E., and Caputto, R. (1959). *Arch. Biochem. Biophys.* **82,** 472.
Mineseta, T., Yamaguchi, K., and Yamamoto, K. (1959). *Proc. Japan. Acad.* **35,** 405.
Mituda, H. (1938). *J. agric. chem. Soc. Japan* **14,** 1228.
Phillips, P. H., Lindquist, N. S., and Boyer, P. D. (1941). *J. Dairy Sci.* **24,** 977.
Procházka, Z., Sanda, V., and Sorm, F. (1957). *Coll. Czech. Comm.* **22,** 33.
Rabinowitz, J. C. (1959). *Ann. Rev. Microbiol.* **13,** 441.
Roy, R. N., and Guha, B. C. (1958). *Nature, Lond.* **182,** 319, 1689.
Roy, S. C., Roy, S. K., and Guha, B. C. (1946). *British J. exp. Pathol.* **27,** 36.
Rudra, M. N. (1938). *Nature, Lond.* **141,** 203.
Rudra, M. N. (1939). *Nature, Lond.* **144,** 868.
Salmon, L. L., and Stubbs, D. W. (1961). *Biochem. biophys. Res. Comm.* **4,** 239.
Sastry, K. S., and Sarma, P. S. (1955). *Biochem. J.* **62,** 451.
Smith, A. M., and Gillies, J. (1940). *Biochem. J.* **34,** 1312.
Smith, E.E.B., and Mills, G. T. (1954). *Biochim. biophys. Acta,* **13,** 386.
Somers, G. F., Kelley, W. C., and Hamner, K. C. (1948). *Arch. Biochem. Biophys.* **18,** 59.
Strominger, J., Kalckar, H. M., Axelrod, J., and Maxwell, E. S. (1954). *J. Amer. chem. Soc.* **76,** 6411.

Storey, I. D. E., and Dutton, G. J. (1955). *Biochem. J.* **59,** 279.

Stubbs, D. W., and Salomon, L. L. (1962). *Fed. Proc.* **21,** 472.

Sugawara, T. (1939). *Japan J. Bot.* **10,** 325.

Sure, B., Theis, R. M., and Harrelson, R. T. (1939). *J. biol. Chem.* **129,** 245

Takahashi, T., Mitsumoto, M., and Kayamori, H. (1960). *Nature, Lond.* **188,** 411; *J. agric. chem. Soc. Japan* **34,** 788, 958.

Takahashi, T., Mitsumoto, M., and Kayamori, H. (1961). *J. agric. chem. Soc. Japan* **35,** 51.

Takahashi, T., and Mitsumoto, M. (1961). *Biochim. biophys. Acta* **51,** 410.

Touster, O., Mayberry, R. H., and McCormick, D. B. (1957). *Biochim. biophys. Acta,* **25,** 196.

Touster, O., and Hollman, S. (1961). *Fed. Proc.* **20,** 84.

Ul Hassan, M., and Lehninger, A. L. (1956). *J. biol. Chem.* **223,** 123.

Winkelman, J., and Lehninger, A. L. (1958). *J. biol. Chem.* **233,** 794.

Yamada, K. (1959). *J. Biochem. Tokyo* **46,** 361, 529.

Yamada, K., Ishikawa, S., and Shimazono, N. (1959). *Biochim. biophys. Acta* **32,** 253.

Yamada, K., Suzuki, K., Mano, Y., and Shimazono, N. (1961). *J. Biochem. Tokyo* **50,** 374.

Yamaguchi, K. (1959). *Shionogi Kenkyusho Nemp.* **9,** 59.

Chapter 12

ESSENTIAL FATTY ACIDS

I. Introduction

Burr and Burr (1929) were first to report a deficiency disease in rats brought upon by the absence of fat from the diet; they also showed that linoleic acid (I) in small amounts protected against and cured this condition (Burr and Burr, 1930). Subsequent work indicated that two other polyethenoid fatty acids, γ-linolenic acid (II) and arachidonic acid (III), showed high activity in curing all aspects of essential fatty acid (EFA) deficiency. α-Linolenic acid (IV) actively promotes growth of animals on a EFA-deficient diet,

$$CH_3(CH_2)_4CH=CHCH_2CH=CH(CH_2)_7COOH$$

(I)

$$CH_3(CH_2)_4CH=CHCH_2CH=CHCH_2CH=CH(CH_2)_4COOH$$

(II)

$$CH_3(CH_2)_4CH=CHCH_2CH=CHCH_2CH=CHCH_2CH=CH(CH_2)_3COOH$$

(III)

$$CH_3CH_2CH=CHCH_2CH=CHCH_2CH=CH(CH_2)_7COOH$$

(IV)

but does not cure certain dermal pathological states. As arachidonic acid is the most active of these acids (see Deuel, 1957) and as mammals can convert linoleic acid into linolenic acid and arachidonic acid (see p. 236), only linoleic acid is essential in the strict sense of the term. Presumably, also, arachidonic acid is the biologically active factor.

The best sources of essential fatty acids are vegetable oils such as safflower oil (78% linoleic acid), soyabean oil (58% linoleic acid) and maize oil (39% linoleic acid) (see Deuel, 1957; Hilditch, 1956, for full details).

II. BIOSYNTHESIS

A. *In Micro-organisms*

(i) *Oleic acid*

(a) *Fungi, Actinomycetes and Algae.* Bloch and his colleagues (Bloomfield and Bloch, 1960; Lennarz and Bloch, 1960) have obtained preparations from yeast which, in the presence of oxygen, Coenzyme A, ATP and NADPH, convert palmitic acid (16-C) into palmitoleic acid, and stearic acid (18-C) into oleic acid. Because of the requirement for O_2 and NADPH it was first postulated that the reaction involved a hydroxy acid (scheme 1), and this was supported by the observation that both 9-hydroxystearic acid and 10-hydroxystearic acid can replace oleic acid as an essential growth factor for yeasts growing anaerobically (Bloomfield and Bloch, 1960). However, it has recently been observed that the particulate enzyme from yeast which desaturates stearoyl–CoA and palmitoyl-CoA does not act on 9-hydroxystearic acid or 10-hydroxystearic acid or their CoA derivates (Light *et al.*, 1962). The hydroxy acids are converted into the corresponding acetoxy acids, which are probably the active growth factors, because they will effectively replace oleic acid.   A similar reaction was observed in the actinomycete *Mycobacterium phlei* (Lennarz *et al.*, 1962), and in the blue-green alga *Anabaena variabilis* as well as in a second mould, *Penicillium chrysogenum* (unpublished work quoted by Lennarz *et al.*, 1962).

$$CH_3(CH_2)_7CH_2CH_2(CH_2)_7COSCoA \xrightarrow[H_2O \quad NADP]{O_2 \quad NADPH_2} CH_3(CH_2)_7\overset{OH}{\underset{|}{C}}H.\overset{H}{\underset{|}{C}}H(CH_2)_7COSCoA \xrightarrow{H_2O}$$

$$CH_3(CH_2)_7CH=CH(CH_2)_7COSCoA \qquad (1)$$

However, this mechanism may not be a general reaction in fungi because Ballance and Crombie (1961) found that in *Trichoderma viride* acetate is incorporated effectively into palmitic (16-C) and oleic acid (18-C) but not into stearic acid (18-C) which, according to the scheme just discussed is the precursor of oleic acid.

(b) *Eubacteria.* Neither anaerobic *(Clostridium butyricum, Cl. kluyveri, Lactobacillus plantarum)* nor aerobic *(Escherichia coli, Sarcina* sp.) forms can desaturate stearic acid to oleic acid (Goldfine and Bloch, 1961). They do, however, synthesize oleic acid from both octanoic acid and decanoic acid by chain elongation and the

scheme outlined in (2) has been proposed to account for the experimental observations (Scheuerbrandt *et al.*, 1961). Some support
for this idea has recently been briefly reported (Baronowsky *et
al.*, 1962).

$$CH_3(CH_2)_6COOH \xrightarrow{\;C-2\;} CH_3(CH_2)_7CH_2COOH \xrightarrow{\;C-2\;} CH_3(CH_2)_7CH_2CHOHCH_2COOH$$

$$CH_3(CH_2)_7CH{=}CH(CH_2)_7COOH \xleftarrow{\;3\times C_2\;} CH_3(CH_2)_7CH{=}CHCH_2COOH \xleftarrow{\;H_2O\;} \tag{2}$$

(ii) *Linoleic and linolenic acids*

Yuan and Bloch (1961) have demonstrated the conversion of
oleic acid into linoleic acid in extracts from *Torulopsis utilis*, a
yeast which is known to produce considerable amounts of linoleic
acid. Once again the expected hydroxy intermediate ricinoleic acid
(12-hydroxy-Δ^9-octadecenoic acid) was not encountered. Evidence
for this conversion has also been obtained with *Trichoderma viride*
(Ballance and Crombie, 1961). Oxygen is required for the reaction
(Yuan and Bloch, 1961).

In *Penicillium javanicum*, on the other hand, the specific activity of linoleic acid was greater than that of oleic acid when [U-^{14}C]
acetate was the substrate, but the situation was reversed when
[U-^{14}C]sucrose was the substrate (Coots, 1961, 1962). Furthermore,
when [U-^{14}C]glucose was used no precursor-product relationship
between oleic acid and linoleic acid could be demonstrated in
Tricholoma nudum (Leegwater *et al.*, 1961).

The occurrence of γ-linolenic acid in fungi is limited; a recent
survey suggests that it occurs rather exclusively in the order Muco-
rales of the class Phycomycetes (R. Shaw, personal communication). No information is known about the formation of γ-linolenic
acid in fungi. Arachidonic apparently does not occur in fungi.

B. *In Higher Plants*

In 1954 Simmons and Quackenbush incubated soyabean preparations with [^{14}C]sucrose and found that radioactivity appeared in
oleic, saturated, linoleic and linolenic acids in that order. These
observations suggested that oleic acid was the primary product in
C-18 fatty acid synthesis. Gibble and Kurtz (1956) showed that
all fatty acids, both saturated and unsaturated, were synthesized

from acetate; stepwise degradation of the labelled linoleic and linolenic acids indicated that the distribution of the carbon atoms from acetate followed the conventional pattern. A little later Kurtz and Miramon (1958) found that in preparations from flax seedlings, the saturated acids and oleic acid were synthesized normally in the absence of biotin, whilst linoleic acid and linolenic acid synthesis was inhibited. This strongly suggested that two separate biosynthetic pathways were in operation; in the first the saturated acids and oleic acid were not being synthesized via the malonyl-CoA pathway, whilst in the second pathway linoleic and linolenic acids were.

The important work of Stumpf and his colleagues has also clearly demonstrated the existence of two pathways of fatty acid synthesis in preparations from avocado mesocarp, although they seem to be different in detail from those just mentioned. Particles from this tissue will synthesize both saturated and unsaturated fatty acids from acetate or acetyl-CoA (Mudd and Stumpf, 1961), but only saturated fatty acids from malonyl-CoA (Barron and Stumpf, 1962). Biotin appears to be concerned in the synthesis of both saturated and unsaturated fatty acids from acetate; the addition of avidin inhibits the incorporation of [^{14}C]acetate into both groups but increases the relative amounts in the unsaturated acids (oleic) compared with the saturated acids (palmitic acid). This does not support the conclusion that stearic acid is converted into oleic acid and this view is further substantiated by the direct observation that neither [1-^{14}C]stearoyl-CoA, [1-^{14}C]stearate nor [1-^{14}C]-10-hydroxystearate is converted into unsaturated acids. Similarly neither palmitic nor stearic acid gives rise to oleic acid in isolated leaves (James, 1963).

Oleic acid can, however, arise from [^{14}C]octanoic, [^{14}C]decanoic and [^{14}C]dodecanoic acids in isolated leaves and the position of the label indicates *in toto* incorporation of these acids (James, 1963). The situation in plants in general is, therefore, very reminiscent of that in the anaerobic bacteria studied by Bloch (see previous section), and the system in leaves, in particular, is very similar to that observed in *Cl. butyricum* (Scheuerbrandt *et al.*, 1961) except that *Cl. butyricum* will not utilize dodecanoic acid.

Stumpf and James (1963) have shown that the incorporation of [^{14}C]acetate into fatty acids (mainly palmitic and oleic) of isolated lettuce chloroplasts takes place optimally in the presence of coenzyme A, Mn^{2+}, Mg^{2+}, CO_2 and NADP. Light stimulates the incorporation some two-fold probably owing to the provision of a continuous supply of ATP by photophosphorylation.

C. *In Animals*

It has been known since the classical work of Schoenheimer and Rittenberg (1936) and Bernhard and Schoenheimer (1940) that animal tissues can convert stearic acid into oleic acid but not into the polyunsaturated acids. Bernhard *et al.* (1959) later demonstrated that, similarly to the yeast system, an *in vitro* system from animals which desaturates stearate also requires ATP and oxygen. It is also clear from evidence to be discussed later in this section that linoleic acid can be converted into linolenic acid and arachidonic acid. Thus the metabolic block which makes animals dependent on an exogenous source of linoleic acid, is the failure to convert oleic acid into linoleic acid.

Mead *et al.* (1953) injected [1-^{14}C]acetate intraperitoneally into rats and subsequently isolated pure linolenic and arachidonic acid from the depot and organ fats. The linolenic acid was unlabelled but the arachidonic acid was strongly labelled with most of the activity in its carboxyl carbon. This strongly suggested that arachidonic acid was being formed from an 18-C acid by addition of a 2-C unit (acetate). The the most likely precursor would be linoleic acid. Steinberg *et al.* (1956) fed [1-^{14}C]linoleic acid to rats and found that the isolated arachidonic acid was labelled; 74·7% of the activity was in C-1 and 24·5% in C-3. Thus it appears that some linoleic acid had been degraded to 2-C units which had then been condensed with undegraded linoleic acid to yield arachidonic acid labelled in C-3 (from C-1 of linoleic acid) and C-1 (from C-1 of acetate arising from β-oxidation of linoleic acid). Klenk (1954, 1955) had previously come to the same conclusion from the results of experiments on liver slices.

Two possible pathways from linoleic acid to arachidonic acid are indicated in schemes 3 and 4.

Support exists for both possibilities, but direct enzymatic evidence is available only for scheme (4). The following facts support scheme (3) – (a): homolinoleic acid ($\Delta^{11,14}$-eicosadienoic acid) is biologically less active than linoleic acid; Karrer and Koenig (1943) reported it to be without activity and Thomasson (1953) found it to be only 40% as active as linolenic acid; (b) γ-linolenic acid is biologically as active as linoleic acid (Thomasson, 1953); (c) arachidonic acid was the only highly labelled fatty acid resulting from the injection of [1-^{14}C]methyl γ-linoleate into a rat, and when this was degraded only C-3 (C-1 of linoleic acid) was significantly labelled (97·4% of total labelling). On the other hand, powerful evidence in favour of scheme (4) is provided by Stoffel (1961) who obtained a microsomal enzyme which converts [2-^{14}C]homolinoleic acid, and [2-^{14}C]-γ-

homolinolenic acid ($\Delta^{8, 11, 14}$-eicosatrienoic acid) into arachidonic acid in the presence of oxygen and NADH or NADPH. This is a reaction very similar to that occurring in yeast (see p. 233).

$$CH_3(CH_2)_4CH=CH-CH_2-CH=CH(CH_2)_7COOH$$

Linoleic acid

$$CH_3(CH_2)_4CH=CHCH_2CH=CHCH_2CH=CH(CH_2)_4COOH$$

γ-Linolenic acid

$$CH_3(CH_2)_4CH=CHCH_2CH=CHCH_2CH=CH=CHCH_2CH=CHCH_2COOH \qquad (3)$$

CH$_3$COSCoA

CoASH

$$CH_3(CH_2)_4CH=CHCH_2CH=CHCH_2CH=CHCH_2CH=CHCH_2CH_2CH_2COOH$$

Arachidonic acid

$$CH_3(CH_2)_4CH=CH-CH_2-CH=CH(CH_2)_7COOH$$

Linoleic acid

CH$_3$COSCoA

CoASH

$$CH_3(CH_2)_4CH=CHCH_2CH=CH(CH_2)_9COOH \qquad (4)$$

Homolinoleic acid

$$CH_3(CH_2)_4CH=CHCH_2CH=CHCH_2CH=CH(CH_2)_6COOH$$

γ-Homolinolenic acid

$$CH_3(CH_2)_4CH=CHCH_2CH=CHCH_2CH=CHCH_2CH=CH(CH_2)_3COOH$$

Arachidonic acid

Whatever the exact mechanism involved it is clear that arachidonic acid is synthesized by chain elongation, a process which occurs in mitochondria; the steps in this process are outlined in reactions 5–8 (see e.g. Mercer, 1962.)

$$\text{OSCoA} + CH_3COSCoA \xrightarrow[\text{(?pyridoxal phosphate)}]{\text{Condensing enzyme}} RCOCH_23NSCoA + CoASH \qquad (5)$$

$$OCH_2COSCoA + NADH + H^+ \xrightarrow[\text{dehydrogenase}]{\beta\text{-Hydroxyacyl-CoA}} RCHOHCH_2COSCoA + NAD^+ \qquad (6)$$

$$\text{HOHCH}_2COSCoA \xleftarrow{\quad} \xrightarrow[\text{Hydrase}]{\text{Enoyl}} RCH=CHCOSCoA + H_2O \qquad (7)$$

$$\text{H}=CHCOSCoA + NADPH + H^+ \xrightarrow[\text{acyl-CoA reductase}]{\alpha\beta\text{-Unsaturated}} RCH_2CH_2COSCoA + NADP^+ \qquad (8)$$

238 THE BIOSYNTHESIS OF VITAMINS AND RELATED COMPOUNDS

Reiser *et al.* (1962) have recently reported a new pathway for the synthesis of linoleic acid by laying hens, which convert *cis*-2-octenoic acid into linoleic acid; the mechanism involved would appear to be chain elongation.

The earlier reports of a relationship between pyridoxal deficiency and EFA deficiency (Birch and György, 1936; Sherman *et al.*, 1950) is now rationalized by the participation of pyridoxal phosphate in reaction 5. It will be recalled that the synthesis of saturated fatty acids up to 18-C atoms long proceeds, not according to reactions 5–8, but via the malonyl-CoA, biotin-dependent pathway (see Mercer, 1962).

REFERENCES

Ballance, P. E., and Crombie, M. W. (1961). *Biochem. J.* **80**, 170.
Baronowsky, P. E., Lennarz, W. J., and Bloch, K. (1962). *Fed. Proc.* **21**, 288.
Barron, E. J., and Stumpf, P. K. (1962). *J. biol. Chem.* **237**, PC613.
Bernhard, K., and Schoenheimer, R. (1940). *J. biol. Chem.* **133**, 707.
Bernhard, K., von Bulow-Koster, J., and Wagner, H. (1959). *Helv. chim. Acta* **42**, 152
Bloomfield, D. K., and Bloch, K. (1960). *J. biol. Chem.* **235**, 337.
Birch, T. W., and György, P. (1936). *Biochem. J.* **30**, 304.
Burr, G. O., and Burr, M. M. (1929). *J. biol. Chem.* **82**, 345.
Burr, G. O., and Burr, M. M. (1930). *J. biol. Chem.* **86**, 587.
Coots, R. H. (1961). *Fed. Proc.* **20**, 273.
Coots, R. H. (1962). *J. Lipid Res.* **3**, 84.
Deuel, H. J. Jr. (1957). "The Lipids", vol. III. Interscience, New York.
Gibble, W. P., and Kurtz, E. B. Jr. (1956). *Arch. Biochem. Biophys.* **64**, 1.
Goldfine, H., and Bloch, K. (1961). *J. biol. Chem.* **236**, 2596.
Hilditch, T. P. (1956). "The Chemical Constitution of Natural Fats". 3rd Ed. Chapman, and Hall, London.
James, A. T. (1963). *Biochim. biophys. Acta* **70**, 9.
Karrer, P., and Koenig, H. (1943). *Helv. chim. Acta* **26**, 619.
Klenk, E. (1954). *Naturwissenschaften*, **41**, 68.
Klenk, E. (1955). *Hoppe-Seyl. Z.* **302**, 268.
Kurtz, E. B. Jr., and Miramon, A. (1958). *Arch. Biochem. Biophys.* **77**, 514.
Leegwater, D. C., Craig, B. M., and Spencer, J. F. T. (1961). *Canad. J. Biochem. Physiol.* **39**, 1325.
Lennarz, W. J., and Bloch, K. (1960). *J. biol. Chem.* **235**, PC26.
Lennarz, W. J., Scheuerbrandt, G., and Bloch. K. (1962). *J. biol. Chem.* **237**, 664.
Light, R. J., Lennarz, W. J., and Bloch, K. (1962). *J. biol. Chem.* **234**, 1493.
Mead, J. F., Steinberg, G., and Howton, D. R. (1953). *J. biol. Chem.* **205**, 683. 664.
Mercer, E. I. (1962). *Ann. Rep. chem. Soc.* **58**, 353.
Mudd, M. B., and Stumpf, P. K. (1961). *J. biol. Chem.* **236**, 2602.
Reiser, R., Murty, N. L., and Rakoff, H. (1962). *J. Lipid Res.* **3**, 56.
Scheuerbrandt, G., Goldfine, H., Baronowsky, P. E., and Bloch, K. (1961). *J. biol. Chem.* **236**, PC70.
Schoenheimer, R., and Rittenberg, D. (1936). *J. biol. Chem.* **113**, 505; **114**, 381.

Sherman, H., Compling, L. M., and Harris, R. S. (1950). *Fed. Proc.* **9,** 371.

Simmons, R.O., and Quackenbush, F. W. (1954). *J. Amer. chem. Soc.* **31, 441.**

Stumpf, P. K., and James. A. T. (1963). *Biochim. biophys. Acta* **70,** 20.

Steinberg, G., Salton, W. H. Jr., Howton, D. R., and Mead, J. F. (1956). *J. biol. Chem.* **220,** 257.

Stoffel, W. (1961). *Biochem. biophys. Res. Comm.* **6,** 270.

Thomasson, H. J. (1953). *Rev. Vitamin Res.* **25,** 1.

Yuan, C., and Bloch. K. (1961). *J. biol. Chem.* **236,** 1277.

CHAPTER 13

VITAMINS D AND RELATED COMPOUNDS

I. INTRODUCTION

The existence of a lipid material which cured rickets was first indicated by the experiments of Mellanby in 1921 when he showed that rickets in puppies was a deficiency disease and that it could be cured by cod liver oil. Treatment of cod liver oil by bubbling oxygen through it destroyed its anti-xerophthalmic properties but left its anti-rachitic properties unharmed (McCollum *et al.*, 1922). This served to indicate the presence of at least two factors in cod liver oil — factor A (vitamin A — anti-xerophthalmic) and the anti-rachitic factor, vitamin D. It was soon shown that vitamin D was present in the unsaponifiable fraction of cod liver oil and that it was closely related chemically to cholesterol (I) (Zucker *et al.*, 1922).

Parallel investigations indicated that irradiation of certain foods increased their vitamin D activity, and later investigations indicated that it was the sterol components of the foodstuffs which were activated. Eventually this led to the isolation of ergosterol (II) from yeast as a pro-vitamin D and its conversion on irradiation into the

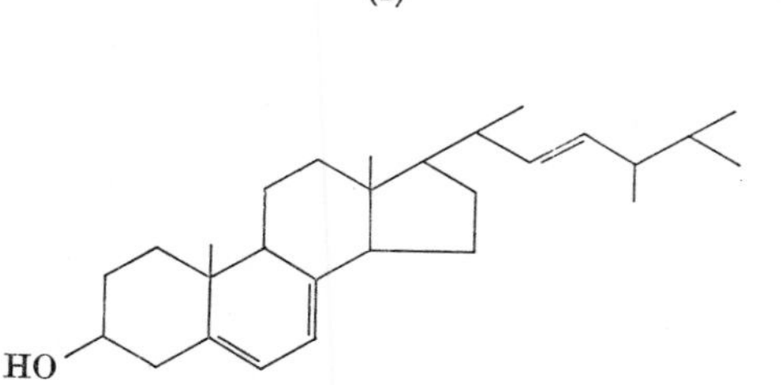

(I)

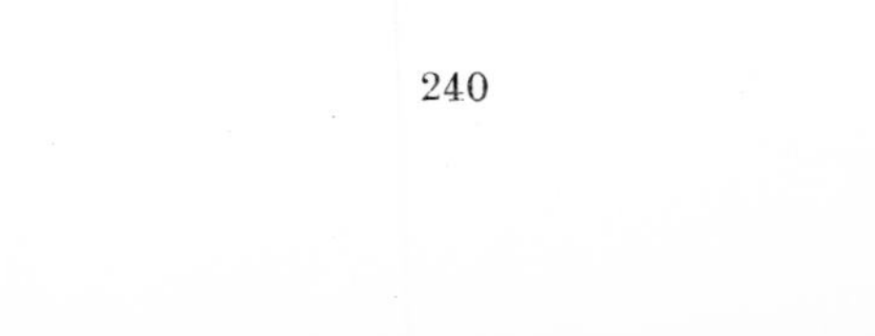

(II)

240

active vitamin D_2 (ergocalciferol) (III) [See Rosenberg (1945) and
Bills (1954) for details]. Then followed the discovery of 7-dehydro-
cholesterol (IV) as a minor component of 'cholesterol' in animals
which was converted by ultraviolet light, in the same way as ergosterol, into the biologically active vitamin D_3 (cholecalciferol) (V)
(Waddell, 1934; Windaus et al., 1935). A third provitamin D (Dm)
has been obtained from the sterols of the ribbed mussel (Modiolys
demissius) (Petering and Waddell, 1951); it appears to be a single
substance but its structure is still unknown.

In the following sections it will become clear that the formation
of ergosterol and 7-dehydrocholesterol follow the same biosynthetic
pathway until a very late stage; this is indeed true for all steroids.
The biosynthesis of cholesterol, which is very fully documented and
from which 7-dehydrocholesterol is formed, will first be considered;
the specific problems concerned with ergosterol biosynthesis will
then be considered in relation to the background information on
cholesterol synthesis.

Although the conversion of provitamins D into the vitamins D
is essentially a photochemical and not a biochemical problem, this
chapter will close with a short discussion on the mechanism of the
reactions involved.

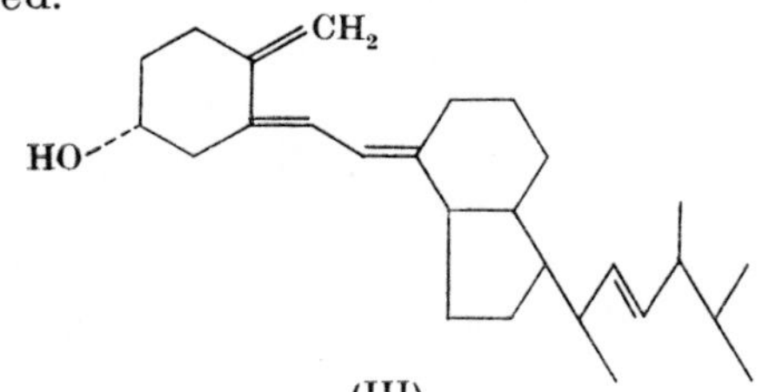

(III)

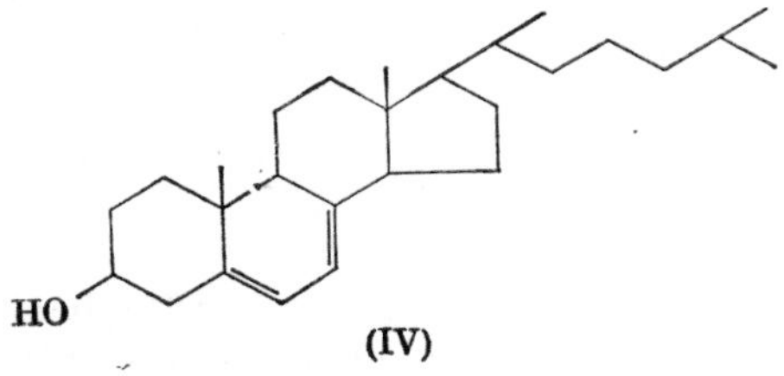

(IV)

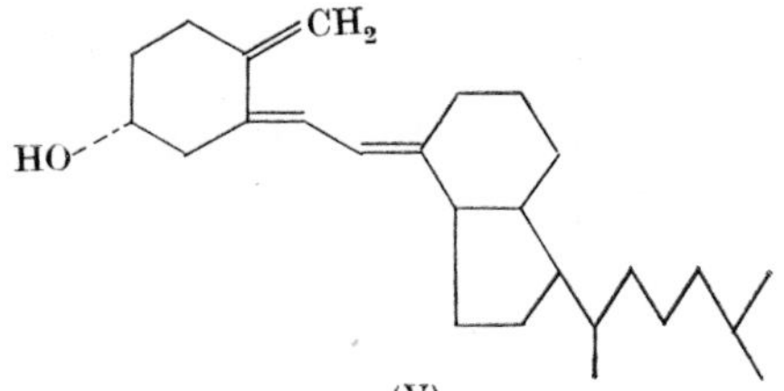

(V)

II. CHOLESTEROL BIOSYNTHESIS

A. *Squalene as a Precursor of Cholesterol*

The modern phase of the attack on the problem of cholesterol biosynthesis began with the now classical observations of Rittenberg and Schoenheimer (1937) and Bloch and Rittenberg (1942). These investigators demonstrated by the use of D_2O and CD_3COOH that cholesterol could be synthesized from small molecules. When ^{14}C materials became available, it was not long before Wuersch *et al.* (1952) demonstrated that in rat liver slices [1-^{14}C]- and [2-^{14}C] acetate were effectively incorporated into cholesterol and that the pattern of labelling in the side chain was as indicated in VI. This

(VI)   (VII)

suggested that an isoprenoid repeating unit labelled as in (VII) was concerned in the formation of cholesterol and that biogenetically it was closely related to the terpenes. These observations led to the revival of the view which Sir Robert Robinson put forward in 1934 that the 30-C triterpene squalene (VIII) is the immediate precursor of cholesterol. Langdon and Bloch (1953) soon showed that [^{14}C] acetate was incorporated into squalene by rats and this was confirmed by *in vitro* experiments on rat liver slices and preparations from hens' ovaries (Popják, 1954), and also in experiments with perfused pig livers (Schwenk *et al.*, 1955a, b). Langdon and Bloch (1953) then fed [^{14}C] squalene, biosynthesized from [^{14}C] acetate, to rats and, in spite of its poor absorption from the intestinal tract, it was converted into cholesterol to the extent of 10–15%. Squalene is also effectively incorporated into cholesterol in liver homogenates (Tchen and Bloch, 1957) prepared according to the method of Bucher (1953). A carbon by carbon degradation of [^{14}C]squalene formed from [2-^{14}C]acetate by liver slices, indicated that at least 90% of the activity was located in the expected positions, that is in w, w' and y (VII) of the isoprenoid residues (Cornforth and Popják, 1954). The small amount of labelling which appeared in the other carbon atoms was probably due to a limited degree of randomization of C-2 of acetate via the tricarboxylic acid cycle.

Partial degradation of [^{14}C]cholesterol (I) indicated that C–7, C–13, C–18 and C–19 arose from C-2 of acetate and that C–10 originated from C–1 of acetate (Bloch, 1953; Woodward and Bloch, 1953). This strongly suggested that there was a centre of symmetry about C-11 and C-12 and Woodward and Bloch (1953) put forward the view that squalene is folded according to (VIII) before

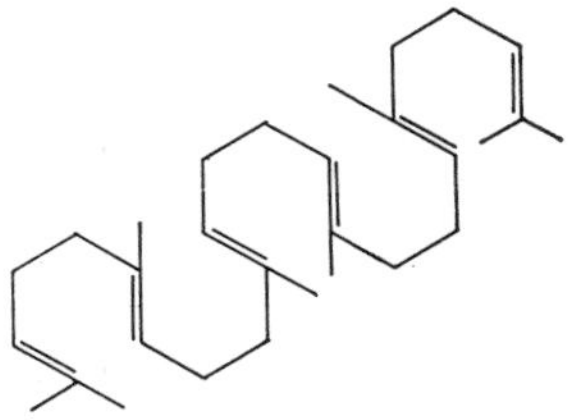

(VIII)

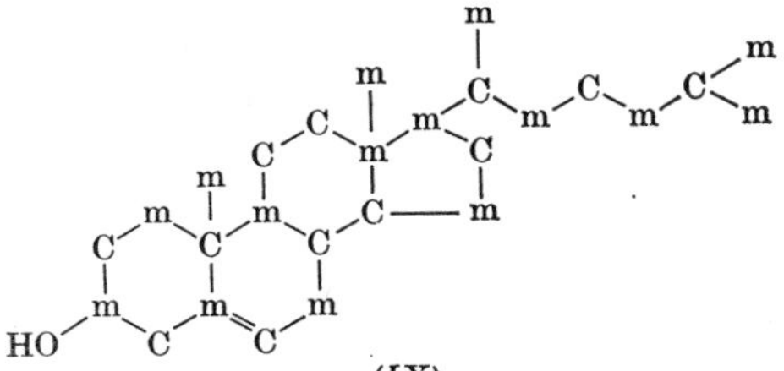

(IX)

being converted into cholesterol. This view implies (a) that only all-*trans* squalene would be a precursor of steroids; (b) the distribution of methyl and carboxyl carbons of acetate in cholesterol as indicated in (IX); (c) that, following two 1,2-methyl shifts, from C–14 to C-13 and from C–8 to C-14 (sterol numbering)*, lanosterol (X) would be formed and would be an intermediate in the conversion of squalene into cholesterol. All three assumptions have been completely justified by later experiments. In the first place Maudgal and Bloch (quoted by Bloch, 1959) synthesized [14C] all-*trans* squalene by the unambigous method of Dicker and Whiting (1956) and found that it was cyclized to lanosterol as quickly as natural [14C]squalene biosynthesized from [14C] acetate; *cis*-isomers, on the other hand, were inactive. In the second place Cornforth and Popják and their colleagues (Cornforth *et al.*, 1953, 1956, 1957a, b, 1958) have devised an elegant carbon by carbon degradation of the cholesterol ring system (see Fig. 1 for flow diagram) and used it to show that the pattern of incorporation of [1-14C]- and [2-14C] acetate into cholesterol by liver slices was identical with that forecast by Woodward and Bloch. In the third place Clayton and Bloch

* One 1–3 methyl shift would result in the same labelling pattern, but this does not occur (see p. 247).

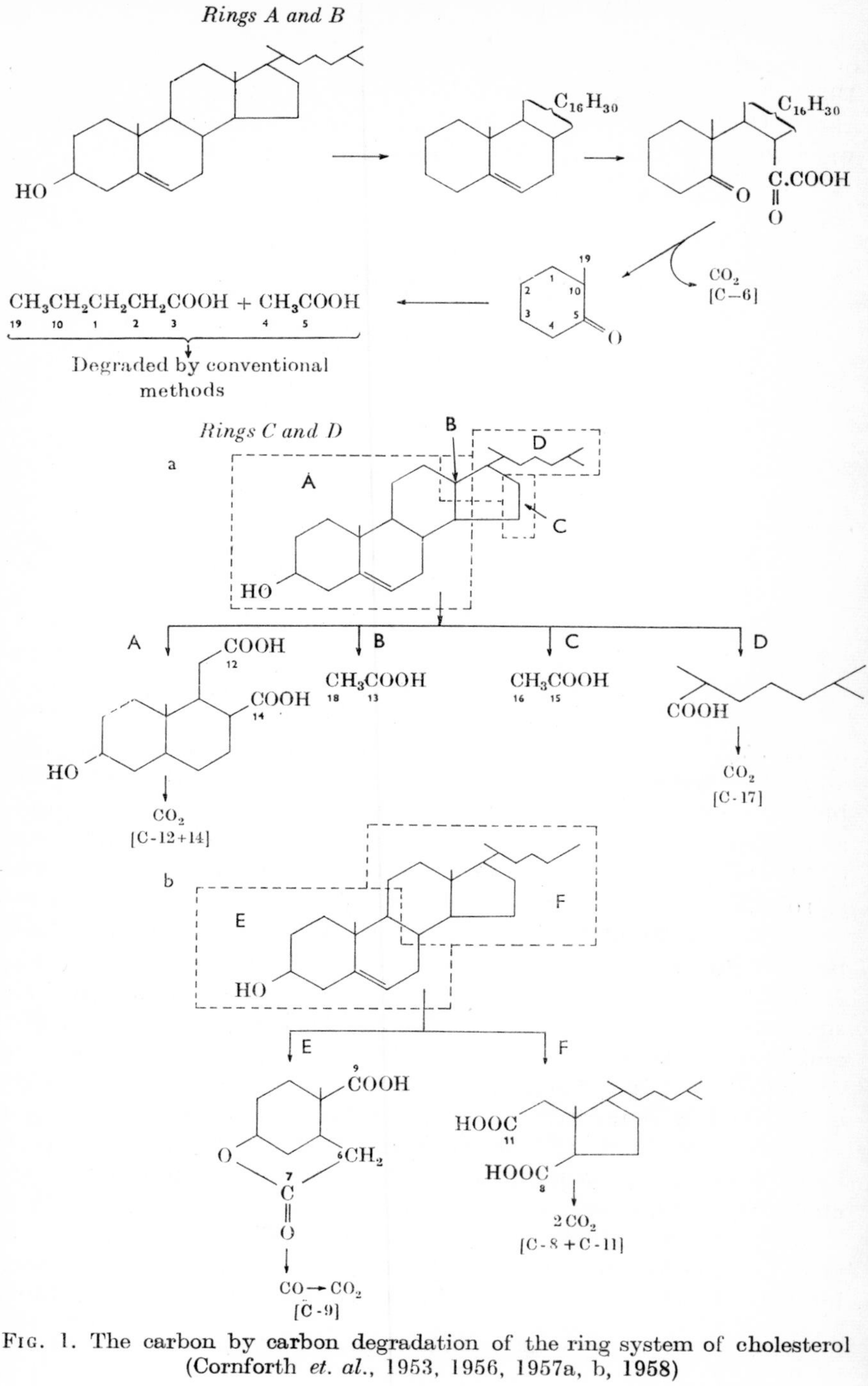

Fig. 1. The carbon by carbon degradation of the ring system of cholesterol (Cornforth *et. al.*, 1953, 1956, 1957a, b, 1958)

(1956) showed that [^{14}C]lanosterol was synthesized along with agnosterol (XI), a possible artifact from, [^{14}C]acetate in rat liver homogenates and Schneider *et al.* (1957) demonstrated the *in vivo*

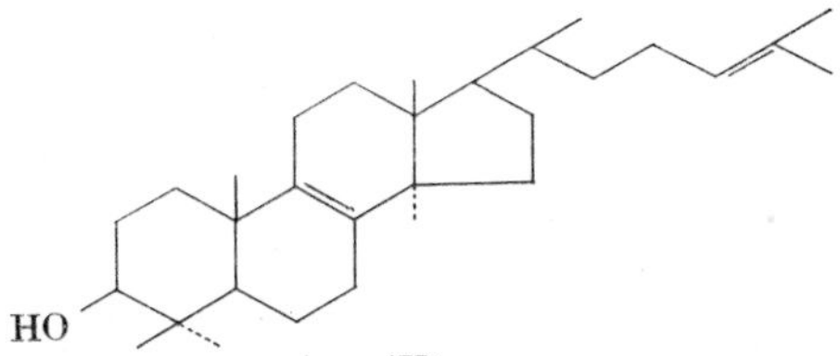

(X)

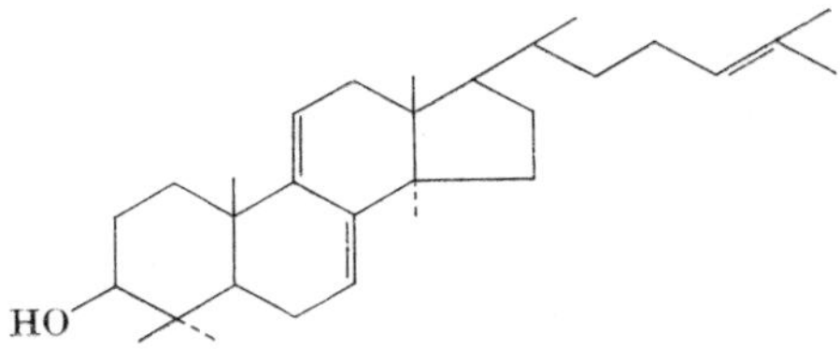

(XI)

formation of [^{14}C]lanosterol from injected [^{14}C]acetate in the liver and intestine of rats. The kinetic studies in the latter investigation indicated that lanosterol was a precursor of cholesterol; ten minutes after injection of [^{14}C]acetate one third of the activity in the unsaponifiable fraction of the intestine is found in squalene, lanosterol and an associated sterol. In later samples (75 min. after injection) the bulk of the activity was in the cholesterol fraction. Direct evidence of the precursor activity of lanosterol was obtained when Clayton and Bloch (1956) isolated [^{14}C]cholesterol from liver homogenates incubated with [^{14}C]lanosterol.

B. *Mechanism of Squalene Cyclization*

The cyclization of squalene is considered to begin with an electrophilic attack by an oxidant formally represented as OH$^+$. This results in a forward cyclization which leads to an electron deficiency at C-20 [(1) Fig. 2] and the production of a transient carbonium ion. This leads to lanosterol by a backward rearrangement [(2), Fig. 2] in which (a) one hydrogen moves to C-20 and one to C-17, (b) one methyl group moves to C-13 and one to C-14, and (c) the hydrogen at C-9 is expelled as a proton (Ruzicka, 1953; Tchen and Bloch, 1957; Cornforth *et al.*, 1959a).

When the conformational isomerization, or "folding", of the squalene molecule required for the formation of lanosterol is considered then it would appear that it has a chair-boat-chain folding (Fig. 3). This folding allows the squalene to exist on the enzyme surface in such a way that the π electrons in the double bonds are co-planar and close together (Ruzicka, 1953, 1959). The type of carbonium ion postulated as the intermediate between squalene and la-

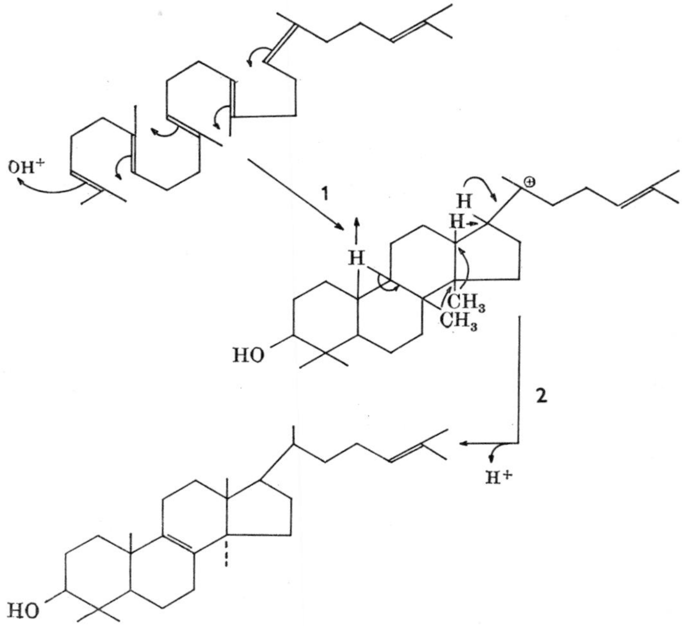

FIG. 2. Probable mechanism for cyclization of squalene to lanosterol (Ruzicka, 1953; Tchen and Bloch, 1957; Cornforth *et al.*, 1959a)

nosterol is unique, in that all other tetra- and penta-cyclic triterpenoid can be formally derived from two other carbonium ions which are also indicated in Fig. 3. (Arigoni, 1959).

Direct experimental proof of the details of the cyclization of squalene to lanosterol became available following the preparation of rat liver homogenates which would carry out the cyclization but which would not convert acetate into squalene or lanosterol into cholesterol (Tchen and Bloch, 1957). The mechanism outlined in Fig. 2 requires that neither H^+ nor OH^- be incorporated from water but that "activated molecular oxygen" (i.e. OH^+) is necessary. Tchen and Bloch (1957) demonstrated that cyclization of squalene in the presence of D_2O or $H_2{}^{18}O$ did not result in the incorporation of either D or ^{18}O into lanosterol; however, the process had an absolute requirement for oxygen which, as demonstrated by experiments with $^{18}O_2$ in the gas phase, was incorporated into lanosterol. The enzyme system concerned, which may be a multiplex rather than a simple enzyme, has been termed squalene oxidocyclase I. It is particulate and requires NADPH specifically; it thus falls into the class of oxidases termed by Mason (1957) "mixed function oxidases". In these reactions one atom of oxygen appears in the substrate and one in water. Tchen and Bloch consider that other squalene cyclizing enzymes will be discovered, probably in plants.

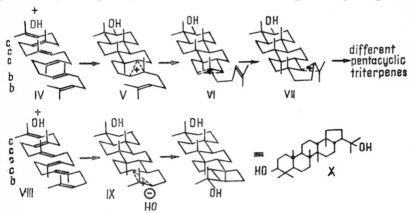

FIG. 3. General scheme for cyclization of squalene (Arigoni, 1959)

The mechanism outlined in Fig. 2 also requires two 1,2-methyl shifts rather than one 1,3-methyl shift. Bloch and his colleagues (Maudgal et al., 1958) and Cornforth and Popják and their associates (Cornforth et al., 1959a,b) have ingeniously demonstrated the correctness of this assumption. Here only the experiments of Maudgal et al., (1958) will be described in detail, those of Cornforth et al. (1959a,b) are, however, based on the same principle. Two species of geranylacetone were synthesized from geranyl chloride and a mixture of [3-^{13}C]- and [4-^{13}C]acetoacetic ester (Fig. 4): on condensation these in turn gave rise to a mixture of four species of all-trans squalene. This specimen was then converted into lanosterol by the liver system of Tchen and Bloch (1957). The lanosterol synthesized was then oxidized by the Kuhn–Roth procedure and the distribution of ^{13}C between the carbons of the acetic acid determined in the mass spectrograph after conversion of the acetic acid into ethylene. The possibilities arising from two 1–2 methyl shifts and one 1–3 methyl shifts are indicated in Fig. 4. Doubly labelled ethylene (mass 30) can only arise if 1–2 shifts are involved in the transformation. This species of ethylene was detected and it was present in approximately the expected proportions (1 in 24). It should be emphasized that only heavy isotopes are applicable to this type of approach.

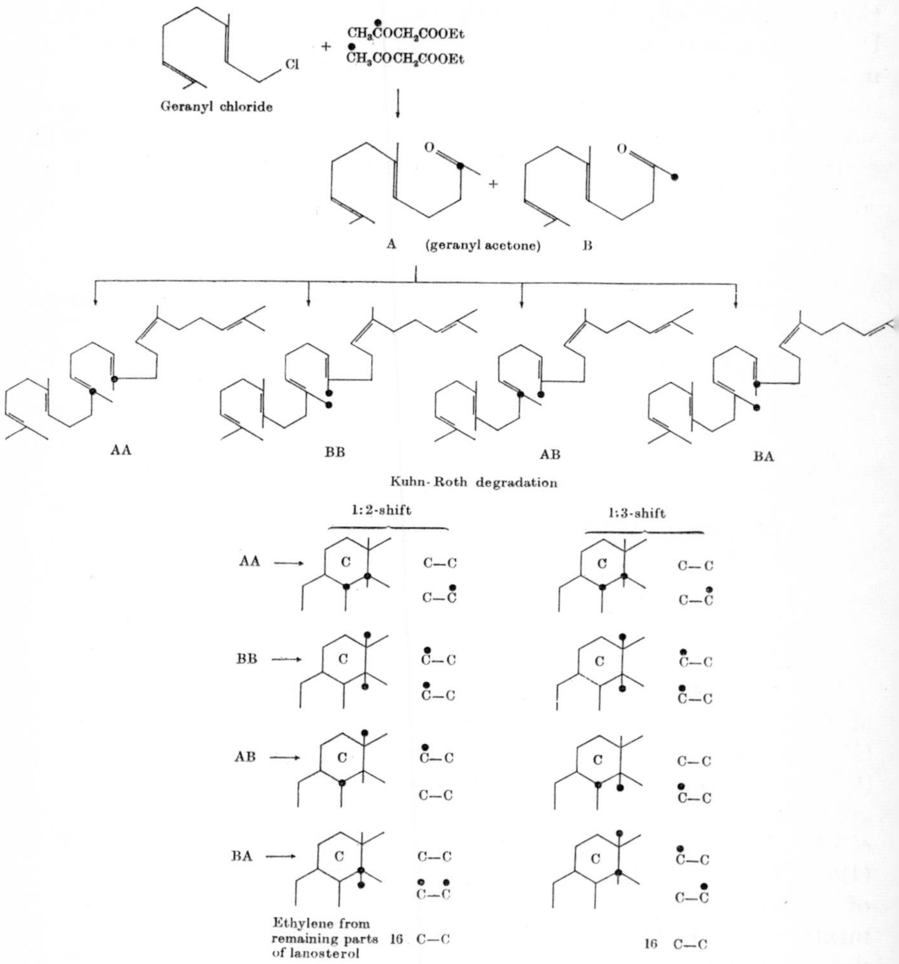

FIG. 4. Procedure for distinguishing between 1-2 and 1-3 shifts in cyclization of squalene (Maudgal *et al.*, 1958)

C. *Conversion of Lanosterol into Cholesterol*

The overall conversion of lanosterol into cholesterol involves the removal of three angular methyl groups together with the saturation of the double bond at the junction of ring C and D and the formation of a double bond between C-5 and C-6. The removal of the three angular methyl groups was followed by Olson *et al.* (1957) who

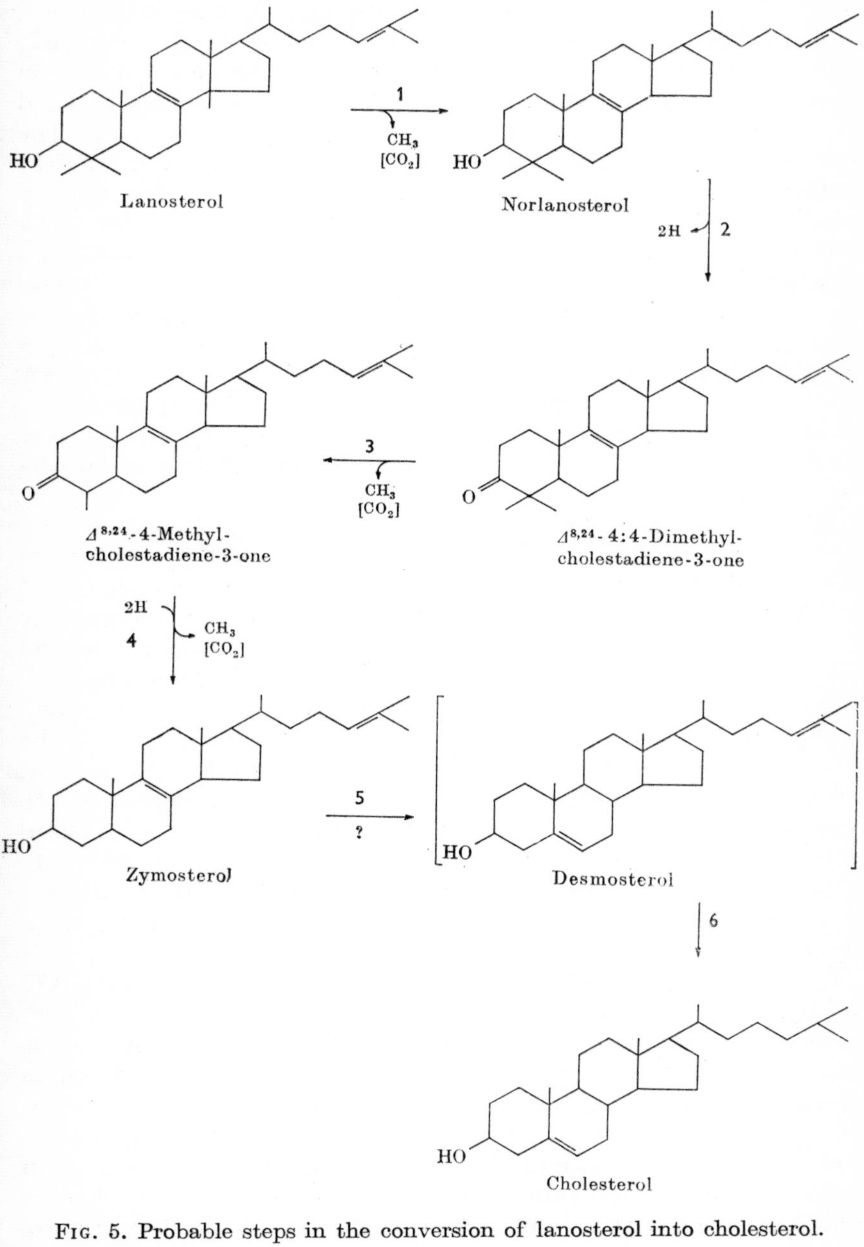

FIG. 5. Probable steps in the conversion of lanosterol into cholesterol.

showed that the carbons of all three appeared as CO_2. There was no indication of liberation of these carbon atoms at a lower oxidation level; on the other hand there were indications that carboxyl groups had been formed. Both NADPH and O_2 were mandatory, indicating a direct attack on the CH_3 group by "active oxygen"; indeed because of the absence of hydrogen on the adjacent carbon atoms, preliminary dehydrogenation is ruled out. The detailed steps in the conversion are probably those indicated in Fig. 5. The first reaction is the removal of the angular methyl group at C-14 to form norlanosterol (Gautschi and Bloch, 1957). It has already been concluded that the angular methyl group is oxidized to a carboxyl group before removal, and certainly the double bond between C-8 and C-9 would facilitate decarboxylation. However, the chemical decarboxylation of β-unsaturated acids would be accompanied by a migration of the double bond to between C-8 and C-14. Possible reasons why this does not happen in the present case are, (a) steric hindrance would arise if the double bond migrated and (b) the lack of a proton on the enzyme surface near C-9 which would not permit a simultaneous β-protonation and decarboxylation (Tchen, 1960).

The existence of ketonic intermediaties in the path from lanosterol to cholesterol was suggested by paper chromatographic examination of the reaction mixture and confirmed by the observation that [3α-T]lanosterol and [3α-T]norlanosterol lose their label completely when they are transformed into cholesterol. As (a) [3α-T]zymosterol retains its label on conversion into cholesterol; (b) $\Delta^{8,24}$-4,4-dimethyl-cholestadien-3-one is as effective as norlanosterol (the corresponding alcohol) as a cholesterol precursor; and (c) lanostadienone (the ketone corresponding to lanosterol) is not a cholesterol precursor, Bloch (1959) concluded that the sequence from norlanosterol to zymosterol is as indicated in Fig. 5; that is the hydroxyl is oxidized to the keto level at the 4,4-dimethylcholestadiene stage, probably to facilitate the removal of the *gem* methyl groups by decarboxylation, and then regenerated after their removal. It is not known whether the α- or β-methyl group on C-4 is first removed.

The steps from zymosterol to cholesterol are not well characterized and it is possible that the final reactions in the extra-hepatic synthesis of cholesterol may be different from those in the liver. It is clear, however, that dihydrozymosterol (double bond in side chain saturated) is not an intermediate. Under conditions which allow the active conversion of zymosterol into cholesterol (Schwenk *et al.*, 1955b; Johnston and Bloch, 1957), dihydrozymosterol is an ineffective precursor; under certain conditions, however, it does show some activity (Johnston and Bloch, 1957). Desmosterol

(Fig. 5) is probably on the pathway because, after injection of [^{14}C]acetate into chick embryos, it can be isolated with a much higher specific activity than that of the accompanying cholesterol (Stokes *et al.*, 1956). These results all indicate that the saturation of the side chain double bond is a very late step, if not the final one, in the conversion of lanosterol into cholesterol.

It should, however, be borne in mind that the naturally occurring lathosterol (Δ^7-cholestenol, XII) and 7-dehydrocholesterol (IV) can also be converted into cholesterol (Davidson *et al.*, 1957; Glover *et al.*, 1952). However, as the 7-dehydrocholesterol-cholesterol transformation is reversible, 7-dehydrocholesterol need not be a normal precursor of cholesterol. As is more likely, it may normally

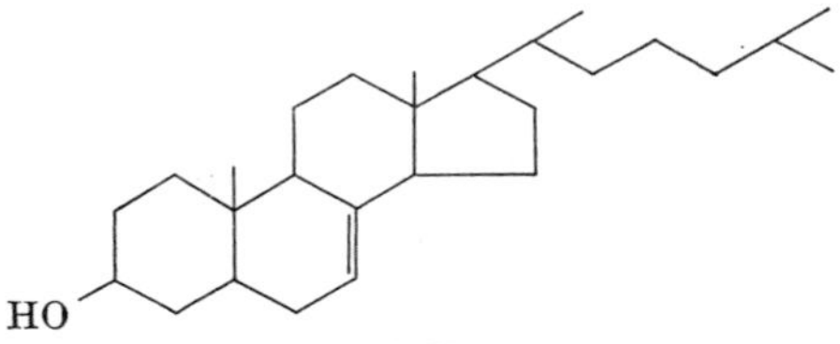

(XII)

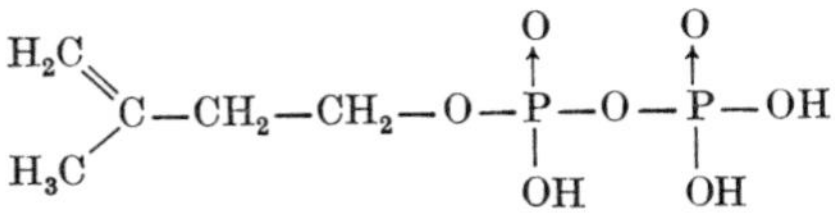

(XIII)

be produced from cholesterol as a precursor of cholecalciferol (see p. 261). The position of lathosterol remains doubtful.

D. *The Formation of Squalene*

The stages from squalene to cholesterol have now been considered in detail; the present section will be concerned with the formation of squalene from the basic 5-C building unit, isopentenyl pyrophosphate (XIII) and the synthesis of the building unit itself.

The observed labelling pattern in cholesterol and other terpenoids biosynthesized in the presence of [^{14}C]acetate early led to the view that three molecules of acetate combined to form a C-6 compound which lost one C-atom to yield "active isoprene" (Reaction 1)

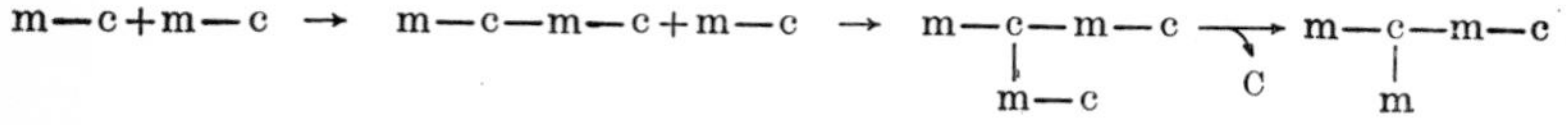

Rudney (1959), Ferguson and Rudney (1959) and Lynen *et al.* (1958a) have demonstrated that the 6-C compound formed by purified liver and yeast enzyme systems is β-hydroxy-$\bar{\beta}$-methylglutaryl-CoA (HMG-CoA) (reaction 2). The enzymes concerned are *β-ketothiolase* [acyl-CoA: acetyl-CoA acyltransferase] (A, reaction 2) and *HMG-CoA condensing enzyme* [3-hydroxy-3-methylglutaryl-CoA acetoacetyl-CoA-lyase (CoA-acetylating)] (B, reaction 2).

$$2\,CH_3COSCoA \xrightarrow[CoASH]{A} CH_3COCH_2COSCoA \xrightarrow[CoASH\ B]{CH_3COSCoA} CH_3C(OH)CH_2COSCoA \quad (2)$$
$$\underset{CH_2COOH}{|}$$

The latter enzyme, which is similar to the citrate condensing enzyme in that the methyl group of acetyl-CoA undergoes an aldol condensation with the keto group of the acceptor molecule with the simultaneous liberation of CoASH, has been obtained in a high state of purity from yeast; but the animal enzyme, on the other hand, which occurs in the microsomal cell fraction, becomes very unstable on attempted purification (Rudney and Ferguson, 1957; Rudney, 1959; Ferguson and Rudney, 1959; Lynen *et al.*, 1958b). Recently Brodie *et al.* (1962) have shown that malonyl-CoA is incorporated into HMG-CoA by a pathway which appears to be identical to the first stages in fatty acid synthesis. An enzyme system from pigeon liver which in the presence of acetyl-CoA, malonyl CoA and NADPH synthesizes fatty acids, will, in the absence of NADP, synthesize HMG-CoA. This important observation is being investigated further. HMG-CoA can also arise during the metabolism of leucine (scheme 3) which involves the biotin-dependent fixation of CO_2 (Coon *et al.*,

$$
\begin{array}{l}
\underset{H_3C}{\overset{H_3C}{>}}CHCH_2CHNH_2COOH \xrightarrow[\text{amination}]{\text{trans-}} \underset{H_3C}{\overset{H_3C}{>}}CHCH_2CCOOH \\
\qquad\qquad\qquad\qquad\qquad\qquad\qquad\qquad\qquad\qquad \underset{O}{\overset{\|}{\ }}
\end{array}
$$

CoASH, CO₂

$$
\underset{H_3C}{\overset{H_3C}{>}}C{=}CHCOSCoA \xleftarrow[\ \ NADP\ ]{NADPH_2} \underset{H_3C}{\overset{H_3C}{>}}CHCH_2COSCoA \qquad (3)
$$

CO₂

$$
\underset{H_2CCOOH}{\overset{H_3C}{>}}C{=}CHCOSCoA \xrightarrow{H_2O} \underset{H_2CCOOH}{\overset{H_3C}{>}}C(OH)CH_2COSCoA
$$

1959). Confusion has arisen over HMG as a precursor of steroids. [^{14}C]-HMG-CoA is incorporated into steroids in yeast and liver systems (Popják, 1959a) whereas free [^{14}C]-HMG is only insignificantly incorporated (Tavormina et al., 1956; Dituri et al., 1957). This is due to the absence of an HMG-activating enzyme, converting HMG into HMG-CoA, from yeast and liver. However, it should be noted that [^{14}C]-HMG is incorporated into β-carotene and ergosterol in both intact cells and cell-free systems of the mould *Phycomyces blakesleeanus* (Chichester et al., 1959; Yokoyama et al., 1960, 1962) and into terpenoid material in some bacteria (Kodicek, personal communication); it will also function in the same way as mevalonate as the acetate-replacing factor in *Lactobacilli* (Thorne and Kodicek, 1962). The ability of HMG to "dilute out" the incorporation of [^{14}C]acetate into cholesterol (Isler et al., 1959) appears not to be an isotope dilution effect but to be the result of HMG acting as an anti-metabolite for the cholesterol-synthesising system (Wright, 1957). This is a clear example of an important hazard which can be encountered in isotope dilution experiments (see also Popják, 1958).

HMG-CoA is then converted into mevalonic acid as indicated in scheme (4). It appears that the reduction of HMG-CoA to mevalonic acid (MVA) in yeast requires NADP as hydrogen acceptor and proceeds without the formation of free mevaldic acid (XIV); the enzyme concerned is *HMG-CoA reductase* [mevalonate-NADP oxidoreductase (acylating CoA)] (Durr et al., 1959; Ferguson et al., 1959; Lynen

$$\underset{CH_2COOH}{\overset{H_3C}{\diagdown}}C(OH)CH_2COSCoA \xrightarrow[\text{CoASH}]{2NADPH_2 \quad 2NADP} \underset{CH_2COOH}{\overset{H_3C}{\diagdown}}C(OH)CH_2CH_2OH \quad (4)$$

$$\underset{CH_2COOH}{\overset{H_3C}{\diagdown}}C(OH)CH_2CHO$$

(XIV)

et al., 1959a). Experiments with [1-^{14}C]-and [2-^{14}C]-HMG-CoA indicate that it is the carboxyl group carrying the CoA residue which is reduced to the primary alcohol group of MVA (Durr et al., 1959). In spite of the absence of free mevaldic acid in this reaction, enzymes catalyzing the conversion of HMG-CoA into mevaldic acid *(mevaldic acid dehydrogenase)* and mevaldic acid into MVA (MVA dehydrogenase) [mevalonate: NADP oxidoreductase] have also been reported to be present in yeast (Lynen et al., 1959b). The first is present in the particulate material and the second in the supernatant fraction of yeast homogenates; both are NADP-dependent. In animal tissues only the reaction converting mevaldic acid into mevalonate has been detected; this has been achieved in homogenates treated with ribonuclease to block cholesterol synthesis (Wright et al., 1957), and in dialysed preparations from pig liver, heart and kidney (Coon et al., 1959; Schlesinger, 1959). It appears unsettled whether NAD or NADP is the cofactor involved. Both reduction reactions are relatively irreversible and lead to the quantitative formation of mevaldic acid and mevalonate, respectively. This gives rise to the situation that mevalonate has "substantially no metabolic future except as a source of isoprenoids" (Popják and Cornforth, 1960), and it is relevant to note at this point that considerable difficulty was encountered in demonstrating the conversion of [^{14}C]acetate into MVA in liver tissues, presumably owing to its rapid conversion into sterols. For example, Popják (1959b) added [^{14}C]acetate and excess unlabelled MVA to active liver homogenates and found that the MVA isolated after incubation was unlabelled; however, when a partial system [liver microsomes and the soluble enzyme fraction precipitating between 40 and 80% saturation with $(NH_4)_2SO_4$] was incubated with [^{14}C]acetate, ATP, Mg^{2+}, CoASH, NADPH and reduced glutathione, [^{14}C]-MVA was obtained (Witting et al., 1959).

Popják and Cornforth (1960) have suggested a mechanism for the reduction of HMG-CoA to MVA without the intermediation of free mevaldic acid, (scheme 5). In this scheme reduction of the carbonyl group in HMG-CoA is preceded by CoA exchange with an SH group of the enzyme, leaving HMG attached to the enzyme as a thiol ester. This would probably resist dissociation especially if the oxygen atom were also bound, for example, by co-ordination with a metallic cation. Such bonding would also increase the electronic deficit on the acetal carbon and facilitate its acceptance of another proton from NADPH. If the final step, the dissociation of the enzyme-MVA complex were not readily reversible then the overall reaction would be essentially irreversible. If mevaldate were added to the enzyme system then it would be taken up rapidly.

This would also explain why, in animal tissues conversion of HMG-CoA to mevaldic acid has not been demonstrated. However, as mentioned earlier it has been demonstrated in yeast extracts.

It should be noted that at this stage the type of biosynthetic reaction changes. All the steps leading to MVA involve CoASH which ensures an increased electron deficit at a carbonyl carbon. From MVA onwards coenzyme A is not required but the intermediates exist in the form of pyrophosphates.

The conversion of MVA into isopentenyl pyrophosphate occurs according to reaction (6). *Mevalonic kinase* [ATP: mevalonate 5-phosphotransferase], which catalyses the formation of MVA

$$
\begin{array}{ccc}
\underset{\text{CH}_2\text{COOH}}{\overset{\text{H}_3\text{C}}{\diagdown}}\!\!\text{C(OH)CH}_2\text{CH}_2\text{OH} & \xrightarrow[\text{ATP}\quad\text{ADP}]{\textbf{A}} & \underset{\text{CH}_2\text{COOH}}{\overset{\text{H}_3\text{C}}{\diagdown}}\!\!\text{C(OH)CH}_2\text{CH}_2\text{O}\text{P}
\end{array}
$$

$$\textbf{B}\quad\Big\langle\begin{array}{l}\text{ATP}\\ \text{ADP}\end{array}\qquad\qquad (6)$$

$$
\begin{array}{ccc}
\underset{\text{H}_3\text{C}}{\overset{\text{H}_2\text{C}}{\diagdown\!\!\diagup}}\!\!\text{CCH}_2\text{CH}_2\text{O}\text{P}-\text{P} & \xleftarrow[\text{CO}_2\quad\text{P}_\text{i}]{\overset{\text{ADP}\quad\text{ATP}}{\textbf{C}}} & \underset{\text{CH}_2\text{COOH}}{\overset{\text{H}_3\text{C}}{\diagdown}}\!\!\text{C(OH)CH}_2\text{CH}_2\text{O}\text{P}-\text{P}
\end{array}
$$

5-phosphate (step A, scheme 6) has been purified 200-fold from yeast (Tchen, 1957); it is also present in the soluble fraction of liver homogenates (Witting et al. 1959) and has been partly purified from pig liver (Levy and Popják, 1959). There are some differences between the enzymes isolated from liver and yeast and these are summarized in Table 1. *Phosphomevalonate kinase* [ATP: 5-phosphomevalonate phosphotransferase] (B, scheme 6) has been purified from pig liver (Levy and Popják, 1960; Hellig and Popják, quoted by Popják and Cornforth, 1960) and from yeast autolysates (Bloch et al., 1959; Henning et al., 1959). With both enzymes an equilibrium is established (Bloch et al., 1959; Levy and Popják, 1960), the K_m for the liver enzyme being $3\cdot0\times10^{-4}$M. The enzymatic decarboxylation of 5-pyrophosphomevalonate to isopentenyl pyrophosphate (C, scheme 6) is catalysed by the enzyme *5-diphosphomevalonic anhydrodecarboxylase*, which has been purified from yeast (de Waard et al., 1959), and pig liver (Hellig and Popják, 1961).

$$
\begin{array}{ccc}
\underset{\text{CH}_2\text{COOH}}{\overset{\text{H}_3\text{C}}{\diagdown}}\!\!\text{C(OH)CH}_2\text{O}-\text{P}-\text{P} & \xrightarrow[]{\text{ATP}\quad\text{ADP}} & \underset{\text{CH}_2-\text{C}-\text{O}^-}{\overset{\text{H}_3\text{C}}{\diagdown}}\!\!\text{C}-\text{CH}_2\text{CH}_2\text{O}-\text{P}-\text{P} & \xrightarrow[\text{CO}_2\ \text{P}_\text{i}]{} & \underset{\text{H}_2\text{C}}{\overset{\text{H}_3\text{C}}{\diagdown\!\!\diagup}}\!\!\text{CCH}_2\text{CH}_2\text{O}-\text{P}-\text{P} \quad (7)
\end{array}
$$

TABLE 1. Comparison of Mevalonic Kinase from Yeast and Liver (Popják and Cornforth, 1960)

	Yeast enzyme	Liver enzyme
Cation requirement	Mn^{2+} required specifically, although Mg^{2+} at high concs. is effective	high concs. of Mg^{2+} required: Mn^{2+} effective at low concs., inhibitory at high concs.
	Ca^{2+} ineffective	Ca^{2+} effective
Coenzyme	ATP, or UTP, or CTP or GTP	ATP only
Other factors required	none	Cysteine or glutathione
Action of inhibitors	inhibited by p-chloromercuribenzoate	Not inhibited by p-chloromercuribenzoate
	—	Not inhibited by iodoacetamide
Stereospecificity	Acts only on (+)-MVA	Acts only on (+)-MVA
Substrate specificity		does not act on MVA lactone or the α, β, and β, γ unsaturated analogues
Michaelis constant	—	$5 \cdot 0 \times 10^{-5} M$

The liver enzyme has a high affinity for its substrate ($K_m = 5\cdot0 \times 10^{-7} M$). The reaction requires ATP and Mn^{2+} and the mechanism proposed for the reaction (scheme 7) suggests the formation of a labile phosphate ester, 5-pyrophospho-3-phosphomevalonate and will not allow the uptake of D^+ into the terminal methylene group when the reaction is carried out in the presence of D_2O; stepwise elimination of CO_2 and water (or $H_2PO_4^-$) would entail D^+ uptake. Uptake of D^+ at this stage cannot occur as will be seen later when the formation of squalene is discussed. Although the labile phosphate ester has not been isolated, experiments with [^{18}O]mevalonate pyrophosphate have provided evidence for an ester link with the tertiary hydroxyl group of mevalonate (Lindberg et al., 1962).

The next steps (scheme 8) lead to the formation of farnesyl phosphosphate and do not require ATP. The initiating reaction (A, scheme 8) is the isomerization of isopentenyl pyrophosphate to dimethylallyl pyrophosphate in the presence of an enzyme *isopentenyl pyrophosphate isomerase* [isopentenyl pyrophosphate Δ^3–Δ^2-isomerase] which has been purified from yeast (Lynen *et al.*, 1959a, b; Agranoff *et al.*, 1959). The suggested mechanism of the

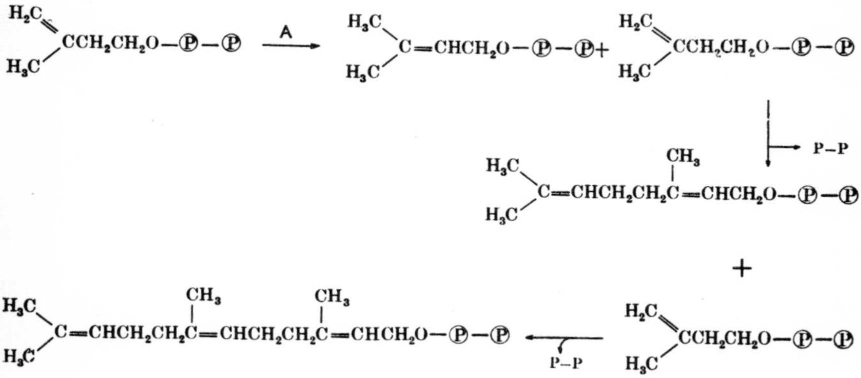

$$
\begin{array}{l}
\text{H}_2\text{C} \\
\quad\!\!\!\!\!\backslash \\
\quad\quad\text{CCH}_2\text{CH}_2\text{O}-\text{P}-\text{P} \xrightarrow{\ \text{A}\ } \\
\quad\!\!\!\!\!/ \\
\text{H}_3\text{C}
\end{array}
\begin{array}{l}
\text{H}_3\text{C} \\
\quad\!\!\!\!\!\backslash \\
\quad\quad\text{C}=\text{CHCH}_2\text{O}-\text{P}-\text{P}+ \\
\quad\!\!\!\!\!/ \\
\text{H}_3\text{C}
\end{array}
\begin{array}{l}
\text{H}_2\text{C} \\
\quad\!\!\!\!\!\backslash \\
\quad\quad\text{CCH}_2\text{CH}_2\text{O}-\text{P}-\text{P} \\
\quad\!\!\!\!\!/ \\
\text{H}_3\text{C}
\end{array}
$$

$$
\begin{array}{l}
\text{H}_3\text{C} \quad\quad\quad\quad\quad\quad\quad\quad\text{CH}_3 \\
\quad\!\!\!\!\!\backslash \quad\quad\quad\quad\quad\quad\quad\quad\quad\ | \\
\quad\quad\text{C}=\text{CHCH}_2\text{CH}_2\text{C}=\text{CHCH}_2\text{O}-\text{P}-\text{P} \quad (8) \\
\quad\!\!\!\!\!/ \\
\text{H}_3\text{C}
\end{array}
$$

$$+$$

$$
\begin{array}{l}
\text{H}_3\text{C} \quad\quad\quad\text{CH}_3 \quad\quad\quad\text{CH}_3 \\
\quad\!\!\!\!\!\backslash \quad\quad\quad\quad | \quad\quad\quad\quad\ | \\
\quad\quad\text{C}=\text{CHCH}_2\text{CH}_2\text{C}=\text{CHCH}_2\text{CH}_2\text{C}=\text{CHCH}_2\text{O}-\text{P}-\text{P} \xleftarrow[\ \text{P}-\text{P}\ ]{} \\
\quad\!\!\!\!\!/ \\
\text{H}_3\text{C}
\end{array}
\begin{array}{l}
\text{H}_2\text{C} \\
\quad\!\!\!\!\!\backslash \\
\quad\quad\text{CCH}_2\text{CH}_2\text{O}-\text{P}-\text{P} \\
\quad\!\!\!\!\!/ \\
\text{H}_3\text{C}
\end{array}
$$

isomerization of isopentenyl pyrophosphate is that envisaged in scheme 9 (Lynen *et al.*, 1958a); this type of reaction which is similar to the Willgerodt reaction for the migration of an olefinic double bond (King and McMillan, 1946), is assumed to be operative in this case because isopentenyl pyrophosphate isomerase is the only enzyme concerned in cholesterol synthesis which is sensitive to iodoacetamide. An alternative mechanism (scheme 10) has been proposed by Popják and Cornforth (1960). Similar results have been obtained with a soluble preparation from liver (Popják, 1959).

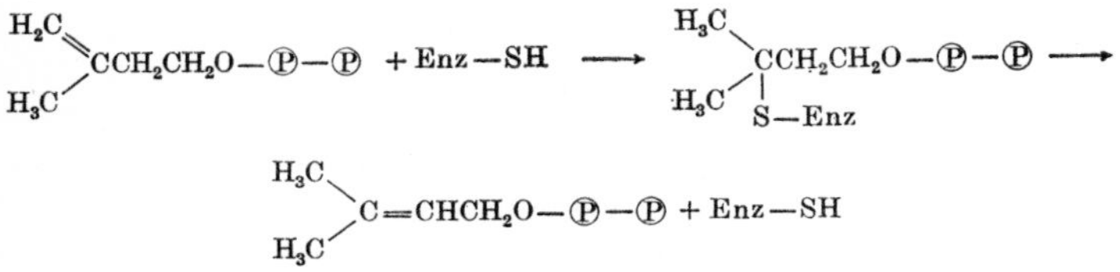

$$
\begin{array}{l}
\text{H}_2\text{C} \\
\quad\!\!\!\!\!\backslash \\
\quad\quad\text{CCH}_2\text{CH}_2\text{O}-\text{P}-\text{P} + \text{Enz}-\text{SH} \longrightarrow \\
\quad\!\!\!\!\!/ \\
\text{H}_3\text{C}
\end{array}
\begin{array}{l}
\text{H}_3\text{C} \\
\quad\!\!\!\!\!\backslash \\
\quad\quad\text{CCH}_2\text{CH}_2\text{O}-\text{P}-\text{P} \longrightarrow \\
\quad\!\!\!\!\!/ \quad | \\
\text{H}_3\text{C} \quad\ \text{S}-\text{Enz}
\end{array}
$$

$$
\begin{array}{l}
\text{H}_3\text{C} \\
\quad\!\!\!\!\!\backslash \\
\quad\quad\text{C}=\text{CHCH}_2\text{O}-\text{P}-\text{P} + \text{Enz}-\text{SH} \\
\quad\!\!\!\!\!/ \\
\text{H}_3\text{C}
\end{array} \quad (9)
$$

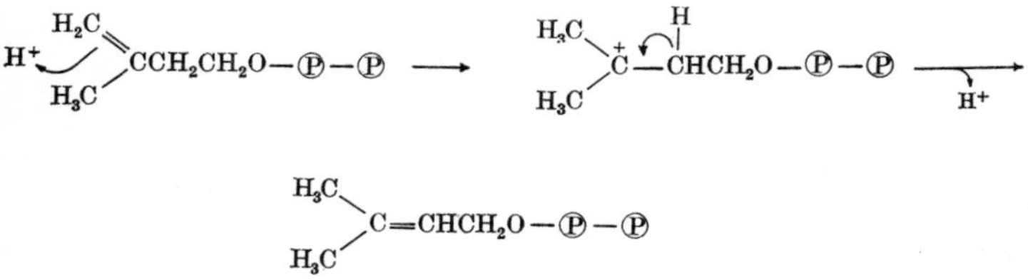

$$
\begin{array}{l}
\text{H}_2\text{C} \\
\quad\!\!\!\!\!\backslash\!\!\!\!\nearrow \\
\text{H}^+ \quad\quad\text{CCH}_2\text{CH}_2\text{O}-\text{P}-\text{P} \longrightarrow \\
\quad\!\!\!\!\!/ \\
\text{H}_3\text{C}
\end{array}
\begin{array}{l}
\quad\quad\quad\ \text{H} \\
\text{H}_3\text{C} \quad + \quad\frown \\
\quad\!\!\!\!\!\backslash\ \ \text{C}-\text{CHCH}_2\text{O}-\text{P}-\text{P} \xrightarrow[\ \text{H}^+\ ]{} \\
\quad\!\!\!\!\!/ \\
\text{H}_3\text{C}
\end{array}
$$

$$
\begin{array}{l}
\text{H}_3\text{C} \\
\quad\!\!\!\!\!\backslash \\
\quad\quad\text{C}=\text{CHCH}_2\text{O}-\text{P}-\text{P} \\
\quad\!\!\!\!\!/ \\
\text{H}_3\text{C}
\end{array} \quad (10)
$$

Dimethylallyl pyrophosphate then acts as starter for polymer growth by condensing with isopentenyl pyrophosphate in the presence of *farnesyl pyrophosphate synthetase* (Agranoff *et al.*, 1959) to form geranyl pyrophosphate which, under the influence of the same enzyme, condenses with a further molecule of isopentenyl pyrophosphate to yield farnesyl pyrophosphate (scheme 8). A mechanism for the condensation (scheme 11) has been suggested by Popják and Cornforth (1960). It should be noted that no reductive steps are involved in these reactions.

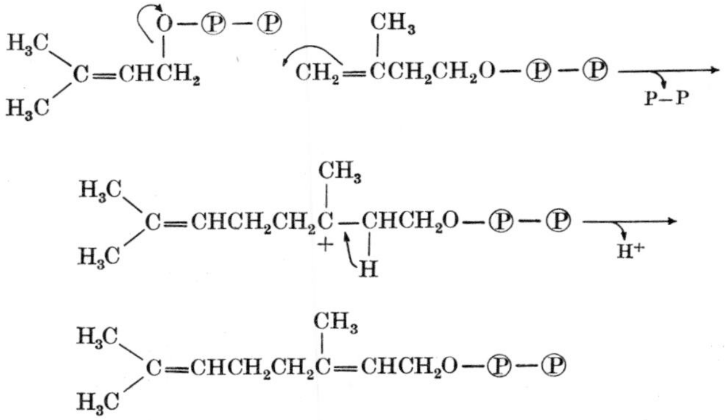

$$
\begin{aligned}
& \underset{\substack{\text{H}_3\text{C} \\ \text{H}_3\text{C}}}{\diagup}\!\!\!\!\!\overset{\displaystyle}{\diagdown}\,\text{C}=\text{CHCH}_2 \qquad \overset{\text{O}-\text{P}-\text{P}}{\underset{}{\Big|}} \quad \overset{\text{CH}_3}{\underset{}{\Big|}} \\
& \qquad\qquad\qquad\qquad \text{CH}_2=\text{CCH}_2\text{CH}_2\text{O}-\text{P}-\text{P} \xrightarrow{\;\;\text{P}-\text{P}\;\;}
\end{aligned}
$$

$$
\underset{\substack{\text{H}_3\text{C} \\ \text{H}_3\text{C}}}{\diagup}\!\!\!\!\!\overset{\displaystyle}{\diagdown}\,\text{C}=\text{CHCH}_2\text{CH}_2\overset{\overset{\text{CH}_3}{\Big|}}{\underset{\underset{\text{H}}{\overset{+}{\Big|}}}{\text{C}}}\!-\text{CHCH}_2\text{O}-\text{P}-\text{P} \xrightarrow{\;\;\text{H}^+\;\;} \tag{11}
$$

$$
\underset{\substack{\text{H}_3\text{C} \\ \text{H}_3\text{C}}}{\diagup}\!\!\!\!\!\overset{\displaystyle}{\diagdown}\,\text{C}=\text{CHCH}_2\text{CH}_2\overset{\overset{\text{CH}_3}{\Big|}}{\text{C}}\!=\text{CHCH}_2\text{O}-\text{P}-\text{P}
$$

Two molecules of farnesyl pyrophosphate are then converted anaerobically into one molecule of squalene by a particulate yeast enzyme system and NADPH (Lynen *et al.*, 1958a, b) and by liver microsomes in the presence of NADPH and ascorbate (Popják, 1959). The mechanism of the conversion has not yet been completely defined but a great advance was made by Popják *et al.* (1961) who found (a) that each molecule of squalene formed from [5-D_2]-mevalonate contained eleven atoms of deuterium instead of the theoretically possible 12 [Rilling and Bloch (1959) reported that only ten atoms were taken up in their yeast system, but this was due to an analytical error (Childs and Bloch, 1962)]; (b) that the labelling in the centre of the squalene molecule was asymmetrical (–CDH–CD$_2$–); (c) that in the liver microsomal system no tritium was incorporated into squalene formed from farnesyl pyrophosphate in the presence of T_2O; (d) in the same system, up to 0·8 g. atom of tritium was added to the central carbon atoms of squalene from [T]NADPH; (e) synthetic [1-T: 2-^{14}C] *trans-trans* farnesyl pyrophosphate is converted by the same system into squalene with a T:^{14}C ratio of 0·76 when the ratio of the starting materials was taken to be 1·0; this indicates the loss of one hydrogen atom from C-1 of *one* farnesyl pyrophosphate molecule during the synthesis of squalene; similar results were obtained with synthetic

[1-D: 2-^{14}C]-*trans-trans* farnesyl pyrophosphate (Popják *et al.*, 1962).

From these observations it is clear that: (1) the last step involves an asymmetrical process in the sense that one of the two participating farnesyl pyrophosphate molecules is subjected to different

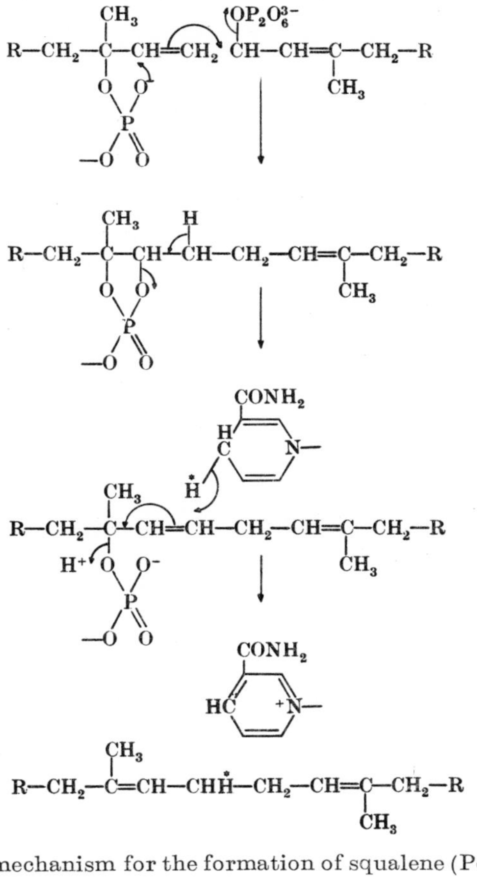

FIG. 6. Probable mechanism for the formation of squalene (Popják *et al.*, 1962).

reactions from those of the other; and (b) NADPH is not concerned with the synthesis of a double bond, because this would involve the uptake of a proton from water together with the transfer of H$^-$ from NADPH. The exchange of one hydrogen attached to C-1 of one of the precursors with H$^-$ of NADPH is stereospecific (Popják *et al.*, 1962). The process conferring asymmetry on the reaction may be the isomerization of one molecule of farnesyl pyrophosphate to nerolidyl pyrophosphate (XV), because **Popják** (1959) found an acid-labile derivative, probably nerolidyl pyrophosphate in liver preparations which were synthesizing farnesyl pyrophosphate. The isomerization could take place by a nucleophilic mechanism (reaction 12) similar to that already described for the isomerization of isopentenyl pyrophosphate to dimethylallyl pyrophosphate (p. 257), and Popják and Cornforth (1960) have postulated the occurrence of an isomerase for this reaction; proof of its existence

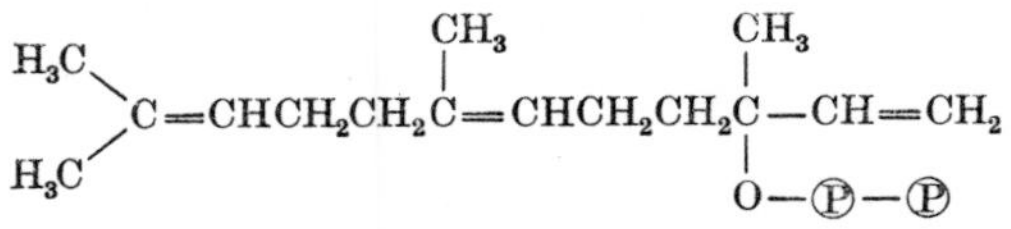

(XV)

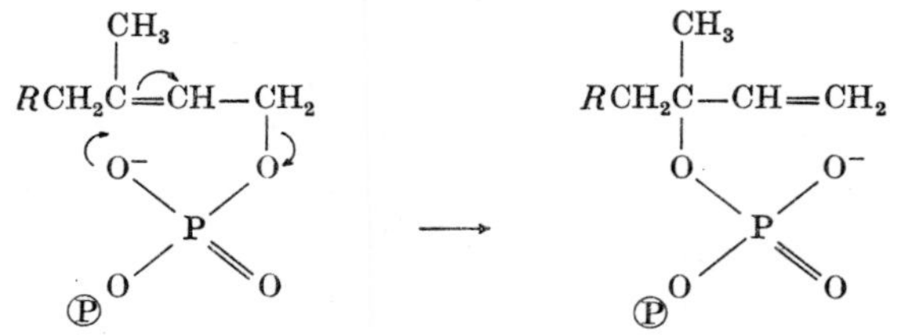

has not yet been reported. The first suggestion for the mechanism for the condensation of farnesyl pyrophosphate and nerolidyl pyrophosphate put forward by Cornforth and Popják (1959) involved dehydro-squalene (XVI) as the first 30 C compound formed. Their

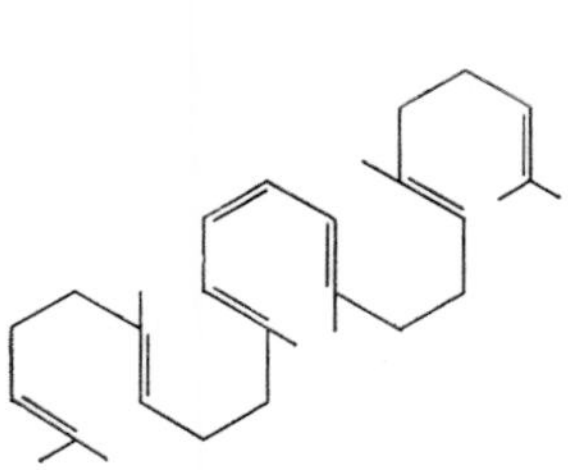

(XVI)

recent work (Popják et al., 1961) has shown that this idea was incorrect in this case, but the basic idea may hold with slight variations for carotenoid biosynthesis (see p. 284). The most favoured latest view of Popják et al. (1961) is indicated in Fig. 6; other possibilities are given in their paper. In this scheme it is assumed that the condensation is facilitated by the phosphate anion in nerolidyl pyrophosphate and that the cyclic phosphate ester is the first "stable" product. Johnson and Bell (1960) have postulated a similar intermediate for the condensation of 5-C units leading to farnesyl pyrophosphate. The transfer of one hydride ion from NADPH which would not exchange with H^+ or D^+ (Vennesland and Westheimer, 1954), and the necessary allylic rearrangement could then take place simultaneously.

III. FORMATION OF PROVITAMINS D

A. *7-Dehydrocholesterol*

Glover *et al.* (1952) showed that cholesterol fed to animals was converted into 7-dehydrocholesterol as it crossed the intestinal tract. In some animals, e.g. the guinea-pig, it represents a considerable part of the total intestinal sterol (about 25%), but occurs only as traces in the intestine of other animals such as rat, pig, ox and sheep. A soluble NADP-dependent *7-dehydrocholesterol reductase* has been purified from rat liver homogenates (Dempsey, 1962). Considerable amounts of 7-dehydrocholesterol is present in the skin of rats (Idler and Baumann, 1952) but it is not known whether it is synthesized there or is transported there from the intestine. Cod livers are rich in 7-dehydrocholesterol (Cook, 1958). Axenic insects (*Eurycotis floridiana* and *Blattella germanica*) do not convert cholesterol into 7-dehydrocholesterol (Clayton and Edwards, 1962).

B. *Ergosterol*

There is no doubt that the general pattern just outlined for the formation of cholesterol holds also for ergosterol biosynthesis. In 1951 Ottke *et al.* showed that at least 26 of the 28 carbon atoms of ergosterol arose from acetate in a *Neurospora* mutant which could not convert pyruvate or any other metabolite into acetate, and Hanahan and Wakil (1952) and Klein and Lipmann (1953) showed, by use of a coenzyme A-requiring yeast, that acetyl-CoA was the 2-C unit utilized. Furthermore, ergosterol synthesized by yeast derived C-11, 12, 23 and 25 from the carboxyl C carbon of acetate (Hanahan and Wakil, 1953; Dauben and Hutton, 1956; Dauben *et al.*, 1959), which is in accord with the folding of squalene to yield lanosterol (Fig. 2: p. 246), and squalene is synthesized by yeast (Schwenk *et al.*, 1954, 1955a, b; Johnston and Bloch, 1957;

Amdur *et al.*, 1957) as are lanosterol and zymosterol (Schwenk *et al.*, 1955b; Kodicek, 1959).

The first indication that squalene was a precursor came from the work of Schwenk *et al.* (1954, 1955a) which showed that squalene synthesized by yeast from [^{14}C]acetate had a higher specific activity than the ergosterol formed under the same conditions. Direct conversion of [^{14}C]squalene into ergosterol in yeast was first demonstrated by Corwin *et al.* (1956), although there was obviously considerable degradation of the squalene to 2-C units, which was very marked when homogenates were used. Alexander *et al.* (1957, 1958) confirmed the observation with squalene, and also showed that lanosterol but not zymosterol was a precursor of ergosterol.

We move now to the source of the extra carbon (C-28) atom and the point on the biosynthetic chain at which it is inserted. Hanahan and Wakil (1953) showed that it did not arise from acetate whilst Danielsson and Bloch (1957) showed that it could arise from formate. Alexander and Schwenk (1958) took the problem a stage further by showing that [^{14}C-T-methyl]methionine gave rise to ergosterol with the same ^{14}C:T ratio in C-28 as that originally existing in the methionine. They also showed that the incorporation of the methyl group of methionine is not inhibited by aminopterin, which inhibits enzymes concerned with 1-C transfers mediated by tetrahydrofolic acid (see e.g. Goodwin, 1960), whilst the incorporation of [^{14}C]formate is strongly inhibited. Their conclusion that the 1-C transfer involved in ergosterol biosynthesis takes place at the methyl level of oxidation and is mediated by methionine is confirmed by the later work of Parks (1958) who showed that "active methionine" (S-adenosylmethionine) is the methyl donor in this reaction. The nature of the methyl acceptor is not yet known, but as [^{14}C]lanosterol and not [^{14}C]zymosterol is converted into ergosterol by yeast preparations, it must be either lanosterol itself or a sterol intermediate between it and zymosterol.

IV. The Activation of Provitamins D

Full details of the early work on the physico-chemical and organo-chemical aspects of the photoactivation of provitamins D are to be found in Sebrell and Harris (1954). Ultraviolet light of wavelengths covering that region of the spectrum in which ergosterol and 7-dehydrocholesterol absorb will bring about a complex series of chemical changes in which ergocalciferol and cholecalciferol are not the end products. The changes involved were studied, some years ago, in detail by Windaus *et al.* (1932) and the mechanism proposed by these investigations for the ergosterol transformation is indicated in Scheme 13. The structures of lumisterol$_2$ and tachysterol$_2$ are known (XVII, XVIII). Corresponding compounds have been derived from 7-dehydrocholesterol on ultraviolet irradiation. However, more recent work by Havinga *et al*, (1955a), Verloop *et al*. (1957), Rappoldt and Havinga, (1960) and by Velluz *et al*. (1955) have indicated certain inadequacies in this scheme. For example, lumisterol$_2$ and tachysterol$_2$ are not obligatory intermediates in the formation of ergocalciferol, and some at least of the reactions are reversible and a new intermediate, previtamin D (XIX) is involved. The most probable reaction scheme

$$\text{Ergosterol} \rightarrow \text{lumisterol}_2 \rightarrow \text{tachysterol}_2 \rightarrow \text{D}_2 \qquad (13)$$

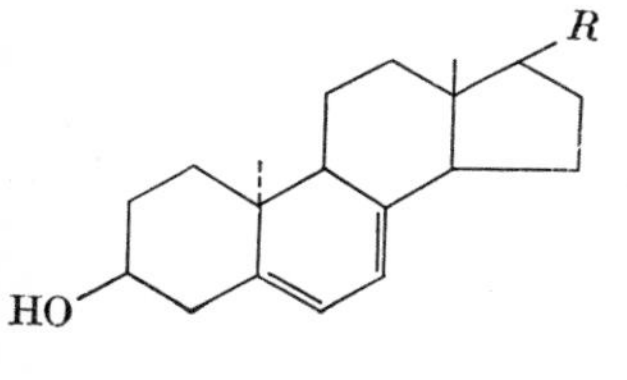

(XVII) 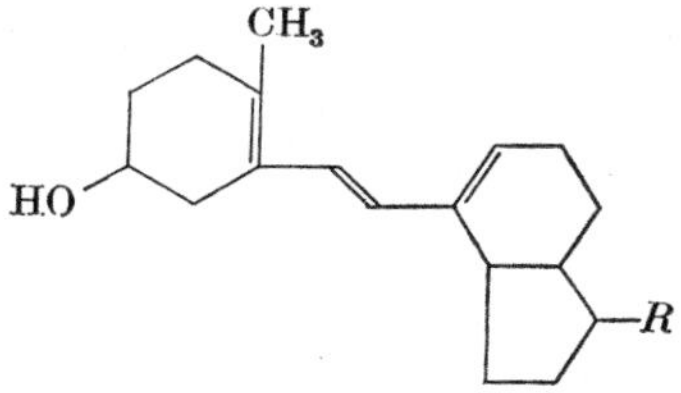   (XVIII)

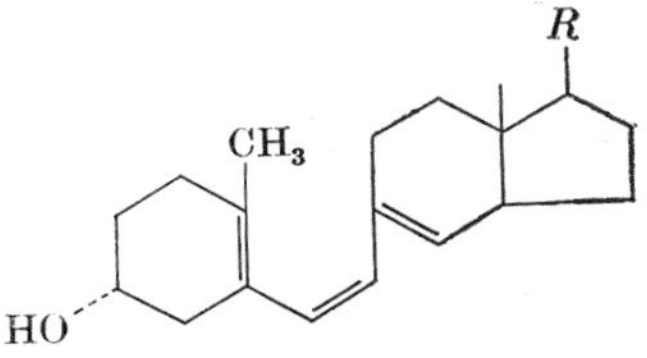

(XIX)

is indicated in Fig. 7 (Havinga *et al*., 1955a, b). This system, which may be oversimplified, appears to hold both for the ergosterol → ergocalciferol and 7-dehydrocholesterol → cholecalciferol transformations (Havinga *et al*., 1955). On absorbing a quantum of light the provitamin D becomes activated (starred in Fig. 7); it can then return to its ground state by transformation into lumisterol, tachysterol or vitamin D. The intermediate in the formation of vitamin D is previtamin D. It has recently been shown that previtamin D$_2$ and tachysterol$_2$ (XVIII) are *cis/trans* isomers (Koevoet *et al*., 1955). This also indicates the close spatial relationship between previtamin D and vitamin D (Verloop *et al*., 1955).

The situation becomes more complicated on prolonged illumination of the reaction mixture, because lumisterol itself is activated and is transformed into tachysterol and previtamin D, whilst activated tachysterol is also converted into previtamin D (Havinga *et al.*, 1955).

Lumisterol

$h\nu$ ⇅

$$\text{Pro-vitamin D} \overset{h\nu}{\rightleftharpoons} \text{pro-vitamin D* } \rightleftharpoons \text{tachysterol}$$

$h\nu$ ⇅

Previtamin D $\rightleftharpoons$ vitamin D

Fig. 7. Action of ultraviolet radiation on Lumisterol.

A somewhat similar scheme to that proposed by Havinga *et al.* (1955) has been put forward by Velluz *et al.* (1955).

The synthesis of vitamin D *in situ* in the skin of various animals has also been demonstrated (Beckemeier and Pfennigsdorf, 1959; Beckemeier, 1958; Cruickshank and Kodicek, 1955). The reported values per sq. cm. of skin are 30–100, 4–18, and 5–15 I. U. for the pig, human and rat respectively.

V. SOURCE OF VITAMINS D IN FISH

It would appear from all the previous discussions that the vitamins D are not biological materials in the sense that they do not arise in living systems as a result of enzymatic synthesis. There is no convincing evidence that they are synthesized by plants or by protists; and in all animals, except fish, the vitamin D activity can be ascribed to that present in the diet or that arising from irradiation of pro-vitamins D occurring in various exterior regions of the animals. However, fish still pose a problem of great biochemical interest, this is whether or not they can synthesize vitamin D. All fish liver oils contain vitamin D but some, e.g. the Percomorphi, accumulate relatively enormous amounts. A typical example is the tuna (*Rhunnus* spp.), the liver oil of which can contain up to 45,000 I. U. gram (see Sebrell and Harris, 1954). The vitamins D isolated also differ from genus to genus; for example, tuna liver oil contains ergocalciferol (vitamin D_2) and cholecalciferol (vitamin D_3) whilst halibut liver oil contains only cholecalciferol.

The first question is whether fish with high vitamin D levels can get sufficient in their diet to account for the amounts accumulated. The general opinion would appear to be that they do not, for only relatively small amounts of vitamins D are present in marine animals other than fish; zooplankton contain traces (Drummond and Gunther, 1934; Copping, 1934) and large invertebrates such as the squid, only about 6 I.U. per gram of body oil (Bills, 1927).

On the other hand, the view that fish could get sufficient pro-vitamins D in their diet has more to support it. Marine invertebrates have very high levels of pro-vitamins D, and the molluscs in particular are the best animal sources known (see Sebrell and Harris, 1954). The sterols of the ribbed mussel, for example contain 37% of pro-vitamins D; this should be compared with a figure of about 0·1% for the pro-vitamins D in the sterols of the vitamin D-accumulating fish.

If one assumes that fish such as the halibut and tuna obtain sufficient dietary provitamin D, then one has to decide whether the vitamin which they accumulate arises by irradiation or by an enzymatic transformation. It is generally agreed that activating rays from sunlight can penetrate clear sea water to a depth of about one metre and thus although photoconversion could occur in the smaller plankton, it is unlikely to be significant for fish or the larger invertebrates, many species of which do not inhabit this region of the sea. An interesting exception is the basking shark, *Cetorhinus maximus*, which spends considerable periods at the surface feeding on plankton and small fish; however, its liver oil is exceedingly low in vitamin D (Schmidt-Nielsen and Schmidt-Nielsen, 1930); similar observations have been made on the common goldfish *(Carassius auratus)* which feeds in shallow pools (C. E. Bills, unpublished work, quoted in Sebrell and Harris, 1954).

All the information so far reported leads naturally to the view that fish can carry out a biological conversion of pro-vitamins D into vitamins D. The results of early experiments designed to test this view have all been essentially negative; for example, laboratory goldfish dosed with ergosterol either intramuscularly or orally did not convert any into vitamin D (Hess *et al.*, 1932), and experiments in which cod livers were incubated with ergosterol were also negative (Hess *et al.*, 1929).

It is hoped that this important problem will soon be re-examined with modern techniques; however, the long delay in reinvestigation is indicative of the great technical difficulties involved.

VI. THE STEROL REQUIREMENTS OF INSECTS

It has been clear for some time from nutritional studies that a variety of insects have a specific requirement for cholesterol (see e.g. Gilmour, 1960). It is also clear that the reason for various contradictory reports can be traced to the sterol-synthesizing ability of the symbiotic micro-organisms. Investigations into the biochemistry of this interesting nutritional requirement have recently been reported. Clark and Bloch (1959) have shown that axenic larvae of the beetle *Dermestres vulpinus* cannot convert [^{14}C]acetate into squalene or cholesterol, and similar results were obtained with adult *Periplaneta americana* (Louloudes *et al.*, 1961) and *Calliphora erythrocephala* (Sedee, 1961). [2-^{14}C]Mevalonate is also not converted into sterols in male and female house flies (Kaplanis *et al.*, 1961).

Although it can be concluded that the insects so far examined have no ability to convert mevalonate into cholesterol via squalene, it should be noted that some unsaponifiable material is synthesized (Clark and Bloch, 1959).

REFERENCES

Agranoff, B. W., Eggerer, H., Henning, U., and Lynen, F. (1959). *J. Amer. chem. Soc.* **81**, 1255.
Alexander, G. J., Gold, A. M., and Schwenk, E. (1957). *J. Amer. chem. Soc.* **79**, 2967.
Alexander, G. J., Gold, A. M., and Schwenk, E. (1958). *J. biol. Chem.* **232**, 599.
Alexander, G.J., and Schwenk, E. (1958). *J. biol. Chem.* **232**, 611.
Amdur, B. H., Rilling, H., and Bloch, K. (1957). *J. Amer. chem. Soc.* **79**, 2646 2647.
Arigoni, D. (1959). *In* "The Biosynthesis of Terpenes and Sterols", ed. by G. E. W. Wolstenholme and M. O'Connor. Churchill, London.
Atkins, W. R. G., and Poole, H. H. (1933). *Trans. Roy. Soc. (London)* **B222**, 129.
Beckemeier, H. (1958). *Acta Biol. Med. Ger.* **1**, 756 (1958).
Beckemeier, H., and Pfenningsdorf, G. (1959). *Hoppe-Seyl. Z.* **214**, 120, 125.
Bills, C. E. (1927). *J. biol. Chem.* **72**, 751.
Bills, C. E. (1945). *In* "The Vitamins", ed. by W. E. Sebrell and R. S. Harris, Vol. 2, 132. Academic Press, New York.
Bloch, K. (1953). *Helv. chim. Acta* **36**, 1611.
Bloch, K. (1959). *In* "Biosynthesis of Terpenes and Sterols," ed. by G. E. W. Wolstenholme and M. O'Connor, p. 4. Churchill, London.
Bloch, K., and Rittenberg, D. (1952). *J. biol. Chem.* **145**, 625.
Bloch, K., Chaykin, S., and Phillips, A. H. (1959). *Fed. Proc.* **18**, 193.
Brodie, J. D., Wasson, G. W., and Porter, J. W. (1962). *Biochem. biophys. Res. Comm.* **8**, 76.
Bucher, N. L. R. (1953). *J. Amer. chem. Soc.* **75**, 498.
Chichester, C. O., Yokoyama, H., Nakayama, T. O. M., Lukton, A., and Mackinney, G. (1959). *J. biol. Chem.* **234**, 598.
Childs, C. R. Jr., and Bloch, K. (1962). *J. biol. Chem.* **237**, 62.
Clark, A. J., and Bloch, K. (1959). *J. biol. Chem.*, **234**, 2589, 2583, 2578.
Clayton, R. B., and Bloch, K. (1956). *J. biol. Chem.* **218**, 305, 319.
Clayton, R. B., and Edwards, A. M. (1962). *Fed. Proc.* **21**, 297.
Cook, R. P. Ed. (1958). "Cholesterol". Academic Press, New York.
Coon, M. J., Kupiecki, F. P., Dekker, E. E., Schlesinger, M. J., and del Campillo, A. (1959). *In* "The Biosynthesis of Terpenes and Sterols, ed. by G. E. W. Wolstenholme and M. O'Connor. p. 62. Churchill, London.
Copping, A. M. (1934). *Biochem. J.* **28**, 1516.

Cornforth, J. W., Cornforth, R. H., Horning, M. G. Pelter, A., and Popják, G. (1959a). *In* "The Biosynthesis of Terpenes and Sterols", ed. by G. E. W. Wolstenholme and M. O'Connor, p. 119. Churchill, London.
Cornforth, J. W., Cornforth, R. H., Pelter, A., Horning, M. G., and Popják, G. (1958). *Proc. chem. Soc.* 112.
Cornforth, J. W., Cornforth, R. H., Pelter, A., Horning, M. G., and Popják, G. (1959b). *Tetrahedron*, **5**, 311.
Cornforth, J. W., Cornforth, R. H., Popják, G., and Gore, I. Y. (1957a). *Biochem. J.* **66**, 10P.
Cornforth, J. W., Gore, I. Y., and Popják, G. (1957b). *Biochem. J.* **65**, 94.
Cornforth, J. W., Hunter, G. D., and Popják, G. (1953). *Biochem. J.* **54**, 590, 597.
Cornforth, J. W., and Popják, G. (1954). *Biochem. J.* **58**, 403.
Cornforth, J. W., and Popják, (1959). *Tetrahedron Letters*, **19**, 29.
Cornforth, J. W., Popják, G., and Gore, I. Y. (1956). Proc. 2nd Int. Conference Biochem. Prob. Lipids, p. 216. Butterworth, London.
Corwin, L. M., Schroeder, L. J., and McCullough, W. G. (1956). *J. Amer. chem. Soc.*, **78**, 1372
Cruickshank, E. M., and Kodicek, E. (1955). *Proc. Nutrit. Soc. Eng. Scot.* **14**, VIII.
Danielsson, H., and Bloch, K. (1957). *J. Amer. chem. Soc.* **79**, 500.
Dauben, W. G., and Hutton, T. W. (1956). *J. Amer. chem. Soc.* **78**, 2647.
Dauben, W. G., Hutton, T. W., and Boswell, G. A. (1959). *J. Amer. chem. Soc.* **81**, 403.
Davidson, A. G., Bulit, E. G., and Frantz, I. D. Jr. (1957). *Fed. Proc.* **16**, 169.
Dempsy, M. E. (1962). *Fed. Proc.* **21**, 299.
de Waard, A., Phillips, A. H., and Bloch, K. (1959). *J. Amer. chem. Soc.* **81**, 2913.
Dicker, D. W., and Whiting, M. C. (1956). *Chem. & Ind. (Rev.)* 351.
Dituri, F., Rabinowitz, J. L., Hullin, R. P., and Gurin, S. (1957). *J. biol. Chem.* **229**, 826.
Drummond, J. C., and Gunther, E. R. (1934). *J. exp. Biol.* **11**, 203.
Durr, I. F., Rudney, H., and Ferguson, J. J. Jr. (1959). *Fed. Proc.* **18**, 219.
Ferguson, J. J. Jr., Durr, I. F., and Rudney, H. (1959). *Proc. nat. Acad. Sci.*, *Wash.* **45**, 499.
Ferguson, J. J. Jr., and Rudney, H. (1959). *J. biol. Chem.* **234**, 1072.
Gautschi, F., and Bloch, K. (1957). *J. Amer. chem. Soc.* **79**, 684.
Gilmour, D. (1960). "Biochemistry of Insects". Academic Press, New York.
Glover, M., Glover, J., and Morton, R. A. (1952). *Biochem. J.* **51**, 1.
Goodwin, T. W. (1960). "Recent Advances in Biochemistry". Churchill, London.
Hanahan, D. J., and Wakil, S. J. (1952). *Arch. Biochem. Biophys.* **37**, 167.
Hanahan, D. J., and Wakil, S. J. (1953). *J. Amer. chem. Soc.* **75**, 273.
Havinga, E., Koevoet, A. L., and Verloop, A. (1955). *Rec. Trav. chim. Pays-Bas.* **74**, 1230.
Hellig, H., and Popják, G. (1961). *Biochem. J.* **80**, 41P.
Henning, U., Moslein, E. M., and Lynen, F. (1959). *Arch. biochem. Biophys.* **83**, 259.
Hess, A. F., Bills, C. E., and Honeywell, E. M. (1929). *J. Amer. med. Assn.* **92**, 226.
Hess, A. F., Bills, C. E. Weinstock, M., and Imboden, M. (1932). *Proc. Soc. exp. Biol.*, *N. Y.* **29**, 1227.
Idler, D. R. and Baumann, C. A. (1952). *J. biol. Chem.* **195**, 623.
Isler, O., Rüegg, R., Saucy, G., Würsch, J., Gey, K. F. and Pletscher, A. (1959). *In* "The Biosynthesis of Terpenes and Sterols", ed. by G. E. W. Wolstenholme and M. O'Connor. Churchill, London.

Johnson, W. S., and Bell, R. A. (1960). *Tetrahedron Letters*, Nos. 12, 27.
Johnston, J. D., and Bloch, K. (1957). *J. Amer. chem. Soc.* **79**, 1145.
Kaplanis, J. N., Dutky, R. C., and Robbins, W. E. (1961). *Ann. ent. Soc. Amer.* **54**, 114.
King, J. A., and McMillan, F. H. (1946). *J. Amer. chem. Soc.* **68**, 632
Klein, H. P., and Lipmann, F. (1953). *J. biol. Chem.* **203**, 95.
Kodicek, E. (1959) *In* "The Biosynthesis of Terpenes and Sterols", ed. by G. E. W. Wolstenholme and M. O'Connor, p. 773. Churchill, London.
Koevoet, A. L., Verloop, A., and Havinga, E. (1955). *Rec. Trav. chim. Pays-Bas.* **74**, 788.
Langdon, R., and Bloch, K. (1953). *J. biol. Chem.* **200**, 129, 135.
Levy, H. R., and Popják, G. (1959). *Biochem. J.* **72**, 35P.
Levy, H. R., and Popják, G. (1960). *Biochem. J.* **75**, 417.
Lindberg, M., Yuan, C., de Waard, A., and Bloch, K. (1962). *Biochemistry*, **1**, 182.
Louloudes, S. J., Kaplanis, J. N., Robbins, W. E., and Monrose, R. E. (1961). *Ann. ent. Soc. Amer.* **54**, 99.
Lynen, F., Agranoff, B. W., Eggerer, H., Henning, U., and Moslein, E. M. (1959a). *Angew. Chem.* **71**, 657.
Lynen, F., Eggerer, H., Henning, U., and Kessel, I. (1958a). *Angew Chem.* **70**, 783.
Lynen, F., Henning, U., Bublitz, C., Sorbo, B., and Kroplen-Rueff, L. (1958b). *Biochem. Z.* **330**, 269.
Lynen, F., Knappe, J., Eggerer, H., Henning, U., and Agranoff, B. W. (1959b). *Fed. Proc.* **18**, 278.
McCollum, E. V., Simmonds, N., Becker, J. E., and Shipley, P. G. (1922). *J. biol. Chem.* **191**, 765.
Maudgal, R. K., Tchen, T. T., and Bloch, K. (1958). *J. Amer. chem. Soc.* **80**, 2589.
Mason, H. S. (1957). *Advanc. Enzymol.* **19**, 79.
Olson, J. A. Jr., Lindberg, M., and Bloch, K. (1957). *J. biol. Chem.* **226**, 941.
Ottke, R. C., Tatum, E. L., Zabin, I., and Bloch, K. (1951). *J. biol. Chem.* **189**, 429.
Parks, L. W. (1958). *J. Amer. chem. Soc.* **80**, 2023.
Petering, H. G., and Waddell, J. (1951). *J. biol. Chem.* **191**, 765.
Popják, G. (1954). *Arch. Biochem. Biophys.* **48**, 102.
Popják, G. (1958). *Ann. Rev. Biochem.* **27**, 583.
Popják, G. (1959b). *Tetrahedron Letters*, **19**, 19.
Popják G. (1959a). *In* "The Biosynthesis of Terpenes and Sterols", ed. by G. E. W. Wolstenholme and M. O'Connor, p. 93. Churchill, London.
Popják, G., and Cornforth, J. W. (1960). *Advanc. Enzymol.* **22**, 281.
Popják, G., Cornforth, J. W., Cornforth, R. H., Ryhage, R., and Goodman, de W. S. (1962). *J. biol. Chem.* **234**, 56.
Popják, G., Goodman, de W. S., Cornforth, J. W., Cornforth, R. H., and Ryhage, R. (1961). *J. biol. Chem.* **236**, 1934.
Rappoldt, M. P., and Havinga, E. (1960). *Rec. Trav. chim. Pays-Bas* **79**, 369.
Rilling, H. C., and Bloch, K. (1959). *J. biol. Chem.* **234**, 1424.
Rittenberg, D., and Schoenheimer, R. (1937). *J. biol. Chem.* **121**, 235.
Rosenberg, H. R. (1945). "Chemistry and Physiology of Vitamins". Interscience, New York.
Rudney, H. (1959). *In* "The Biosynthesis of Terpenes and Sterols", ed. by G. E. W Wolstenholme and M. O'Connor, p. 75. Churchill, London.
Rudney, H., and Ferguson, J. J. Jr. (1957). *J. Amer. chem. Soc.* **79**, 558.
Ruzicka, L. (1953). *Experientia*, **9**, 357.
Ruzicka, L. (1959). *Proc. chem. Soc.* 341.
Schlesinger, M. J. (1959). *Fed. Proc.* **18**, 317.
Schmidt-Nielsen, S., and Schmidt-Nielsen, S. (1930). *Hoppe-Seyl. Z.* **189**, 229.
Schneider, P. B., Clayton, R. B., and Bloch, K. (1957). *J. biol. Chem.* **224**, 175.

Schwenk, E., Alexander, G. J., Stoudt, T. H., and Fish, C. A. (1955a). *Arch. Biochem. Biophys.* **55**, 274.

Schwenk, E. Alexander, G. J., Fish, C. A., and Stoudt, T. H. (1955b). *Fed. Proc.* **14**, 752.

Schwenk, E., Todd, D., and Fish, C. A. (1954). *Arch. Biochem. Biophys.* **49**, 187.

Sebrell, W. H. and Harris, R. S. (1954). "The Vitamins", Vol. II. Academic Press, New York.

Sedee, D. J. W. (1961). *Arch. Int. Physiol. Biochem.* **69**, 284.

Stokes W. M., Fish, C. A., and Hickey, F. C. (1956). *J. biol. Chem.* **220**, 415.

Tavormina, P. A., Gibbs, M. H., and Huff, J. W. (1956). *J. Amer. chem. Soc.* **78**, 4498.

Tchen, T. T. (1960). *In* "Metabolic Pathways", ed. by D. M. Greenberg, Vol. 1, p. 389. Academic Press, New York.

Tchen, T. T., and Bloch, K. (1957). *J. biol. Chem.* **226**, 921.

Thorne, K. J. I., and Kodicek, E. (1962). *Biochim. biophys. Acta*, **59**, 273.

Velluz., L., Amiard, G., and Goffinet, B. (1955). *C. R. Acad. Sci. Paris* **240**, 2076, 2156.

Vennesland, B., and Westheimer, F: H. (1954), *In* "The Mechanism of Enzyme Action", ed. by W. D. McElroy and B. Glass., p. 357. Johns Hopkins Press, Baltimore.

Verloop, A., Koevoet, A. L., and Havinga, E. (1955). *Rec. Trav. chim. Pays-Bas* **74**, 1125.

Verloop, A., Koevoet, A. L., and Havinga, E. (1957). *Rec. Trav. chim. Pays-Bas* **76**, 689.

Waddell, J. (1934). *J. biol. Chem.* **105**, 711.

Windaus, A., von Werder, F., Luttringhaus, A., and Fernholz, E. (1932). *Liebigs Ann.* **499**, 188.

Windaus, A., Lettré, H., and Schenck, F. (1935). *Liebigs Ann.* **520**, 98.

Witting, L. A., Knauss, H. J., and Porter, J. W. (1959). *Fed. Proc.* **18**, 353.

Woodward, R. B., and Bloch, K. (1953). *J. Amer. chem. Soc.* **75**, 2023.

Wright, L. D. (1957). *Proc. Soc. exp. Biol., N. Y.* **96**, 364.

Wright, L. D., Cleland, M., Dulta, B. N., and Norton, J. S. (1957). *J. Amer. chem. Soc.* **79**, 6572.

Wuersch, J., Huang, R. L., and Bloch, K. (1952). *J. biol. Chem.* **195**, 439.

Yokoyama, H., Chichester, C. O., and Nakayama, T. O. M., (1960). *Nature, Lond.* **185**, 687.

Yokoyama, H., Nakayama, T. O. M., and Chichester, C. O. (1962). *J. biol. Chem.* **237**, 681.

Zucker, T. F., Pappenheimer, A. M., and Barnett, M. (1922). *Proc. Soc. exp. Biol., N. Y.* **29**, 167.

CHAPTER 14

CAROTENOIDS AND VITAMIN A

I. INTRODUCTION

The full story of the discovery of vitamin A has been authoritatively discussed by Moore (1957) and here it is necessary only to outline the salient facts.

Hopkins (1912), McCollum and Davis (1913) and Osborne and Mendel (1914) all reported that the retardation of growth of rats on a synthetic diet could be cured by the addition of some fats (e.g. butter), but not others (e.g. almond oil). Important subsequent developments were (a) the discovery that the activity of "fat-soluble A" was exclusively present in the non-saponifiable matter of lipids (McCollum and Davis, 1914), and (b) the discovery that the anti-xerophthalmic factor (vitamin A) was chemically distinct from the anti-rachitic factor (vitamin D) (McCollum et al., 1922).

The continued examination of many materials indicated that sources of vitamin A existed in both plants and animals, but that whilst the yellow colour of plant materials (e.g. maize and carrots) appeared to be directly correlated with their vitamin A activity (Steenbock, 1919; Steenbock and Boutwell, 1920), this correlation did not exist in animal products (Stephenson, 1920). Steenbock et al. (1921) showed that crystalline carotene obtained from plant materials was vitamin A-active and this was confirmed by Moore (1929) who showed that the feeding of carotene to rats resulted in the appearance of vitamin A in the livers of these animals. The final steps in this part of the vitamin A-carotene story were (a) the elucidation of their structures (I, II) by Karrer and Kuhn and their colleagues (see Karrer and Jucker, 1950; Moore, 1957), and (b) the realization that vitamin A occurs only in animals (Moore, 1957). The structures of the two compounds made it certain that "carotene" (in effect β-carotene, I) was a provitamin A and was being converted by animals into vitamin A (II). This process is considered in detail on p. 299, but before this the carotenoids themselves must be considered. They are only synthesized *de novo* by higher plants and protista; animals do not have this ability, so that all

270

carotenoids found in animals as well as all the naturally occurring vitamin A are ultimately derived from the higher plants and

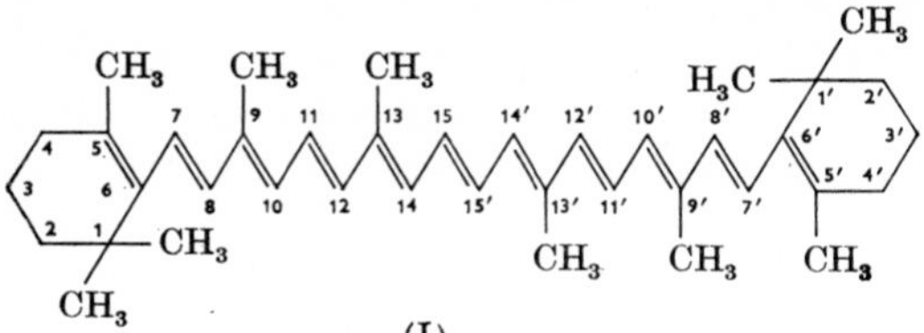

(I)

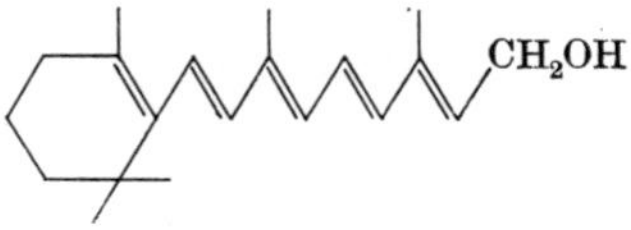

(II)

protista. It is important, therefore, to see where carotenoids are
found and how they are synthesized.

II. CAROTENOIDS

A. *Nature*

All naturally occurring carotenoids with minor exceptions (e.g.
crocetin and bixin) are tetraterpenoids; that is their structural ske-

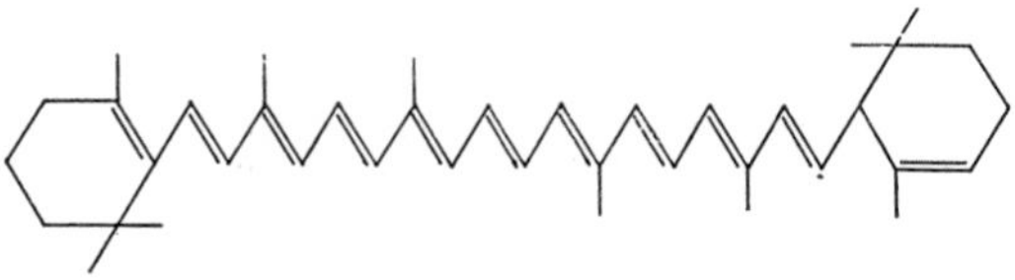

(III)

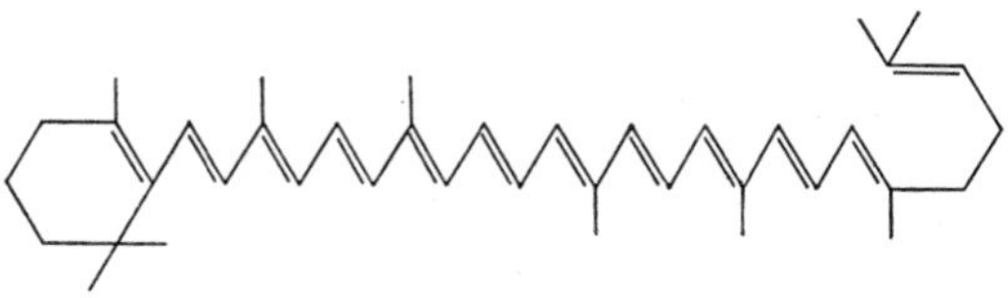

(IV)

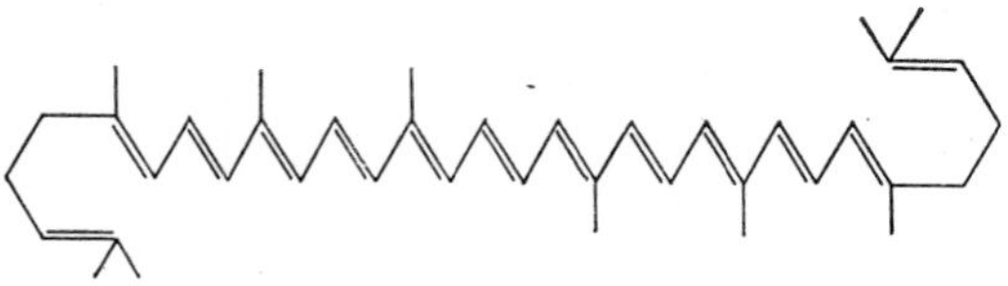

(V)

leton is made up of 8 isoprenoid (branched 5-C units), so arranged as if two 20-C units, formed by the head to tail condensation of 4 isoprenoid units, had joined tail to tail.

Carotenoids are divided into two groups: *carotenes*, which are hydrocarbons, and *xanthophylls*, which contain oxygen in the form of hydroxyl, methoxyl, carboxyl, oxo- or epoxy-groupings. The number of naturally occurring carotenoids is considerable (see Goodwin, 1952a, 1962a,b,c) but most are derivatives of either β-carotene (I), α-carotene (III), γ-carotene (IV) or lycopene (V).

B. *Distribution*

(i) *Higher plants*

(a) *Photosynthetic tissues.* All photosynthetic tissues of higher plants contain carotenoids which are concentrated in the grana of the chloroplasts. The major components vary little from one plant to another and are β-carotene, lutein (3,3'-dihydroxy-α-carotene) (VI), violaxanthin (5,6,5'6'-diepoxy-3-,3'-dihydroxy-β-carotene) (VII), and neoxanthin (3,3',5 (or 6) trihydroxy-6 (or 5) hydro-5',6'-epoxy-β-carotene (VIII); small amounts of α-carotene (III) cryptoxanthin (3-hydroxy-

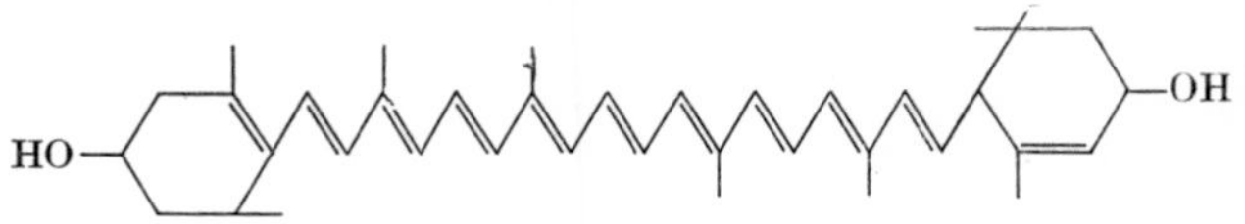

(VI)

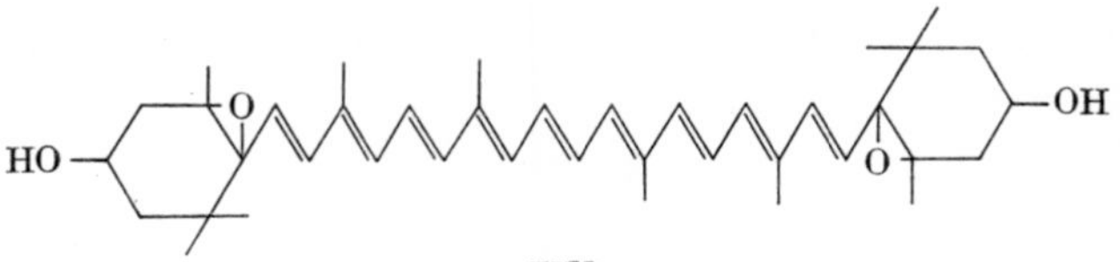

(VII)

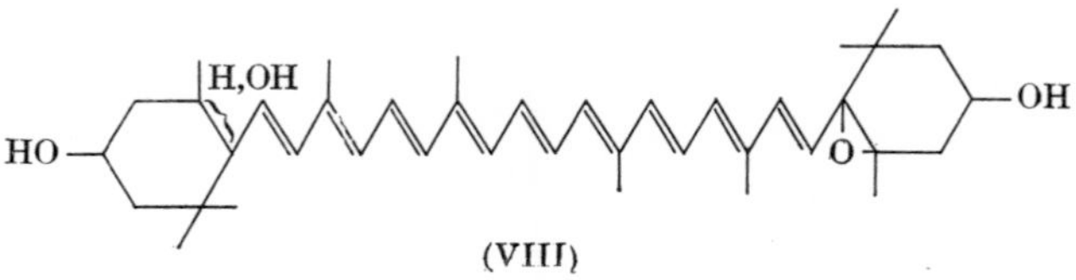

(VIII)

β-carotene) (IX), zeaxanthin (3,3'-dihydroxy-β-carotene) (X) and flavoxanthin (XI) are often encountered. The absence of acyclic carotenoids (lycopene derivatives) should be emphasized.

(b) *Fruit*. The distribution of carotenoids in fruit is spasmodic and un-predictable (Goodwin, 1952a, 1958, 1962b,c), but carotenogenic fruit

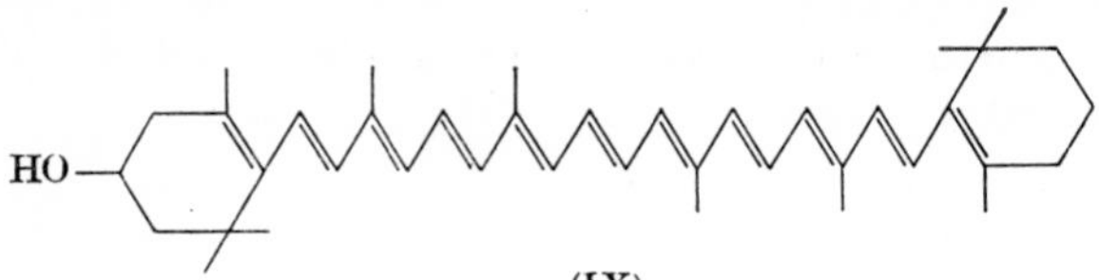

(IX)

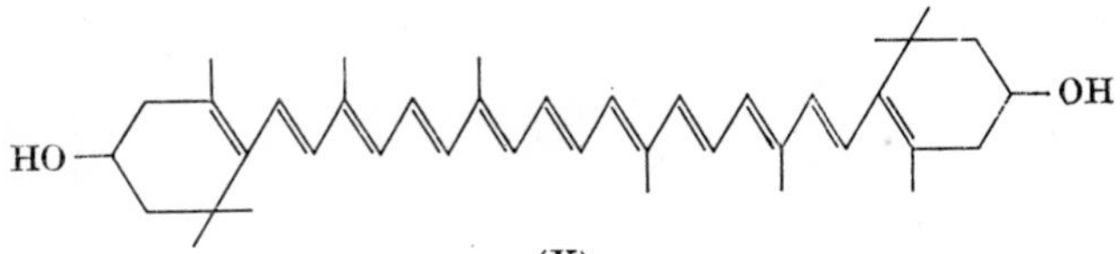

(X)

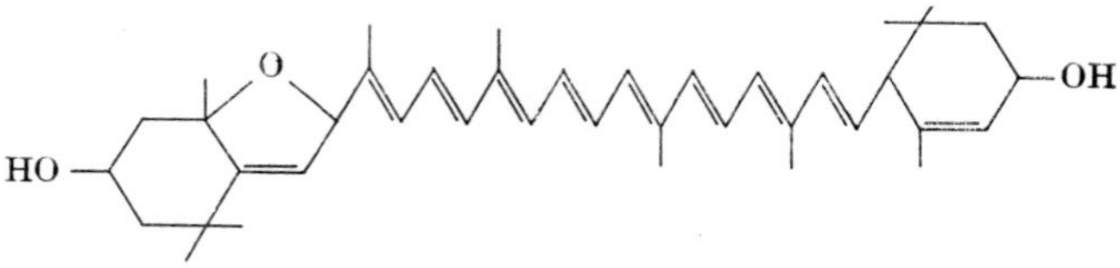

(XI)

can be divided into five main groups: (a) those which contain chlorophylls and relatively small amounts of the same carotenoids found in chloroplasts (e.g. *Sambucus nigra*); (b) those which syn-thesize acyclic pigments (e.g. tomato); (c) those which synthesize large amounts of β-carotene and/or its derivatives (e.g. red palm, yellow maize); (d) those which synthesize species-specific carote-noids (e.g. red peppers produce capsanthin (XII)); and (e) those which synthesize *cis* isomers* of carotenoids (e.g. *Pyracantha an-gustifolia*). Group (b) fruit are important from the biosynthetic

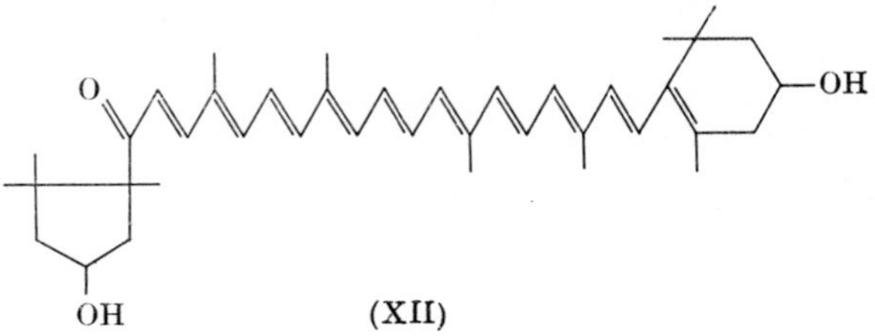

(XII)

point of view because many, e.g. tomatoes, contain the partly satu-rated derivatives of lycopene which are now known to be biosynthe-

---

* As indicated in formulae I, VII, IV, V, naturally occurring carotenoids have *trans* configurations around their double bonds; occasionally *cis* isomers are present; these are discussed on p. 305.

tic precursors of lycopene. These compounds phytoene, (XIII), phytofluene (XIV) ζ-carotene (XV), and neurosporene (XVI) were first proposed as precursors by Porter and Lincoln (1950) and this aspect will be discussed later. Their structures have been finally elucidated by Davis *et al.* (1961).

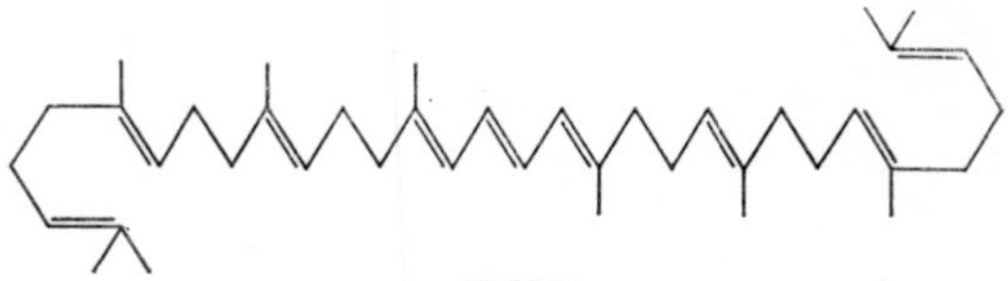

(XIII)

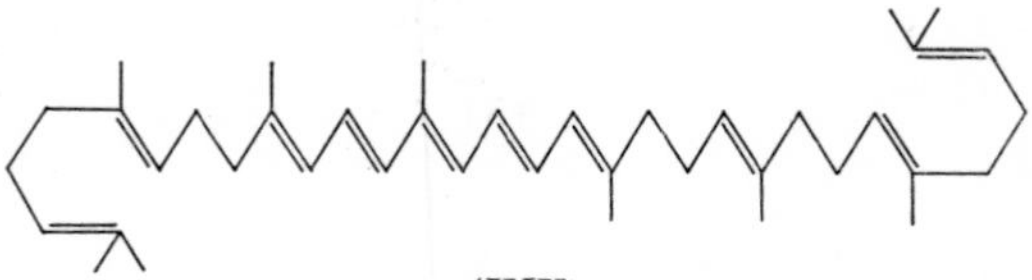

(XIV)

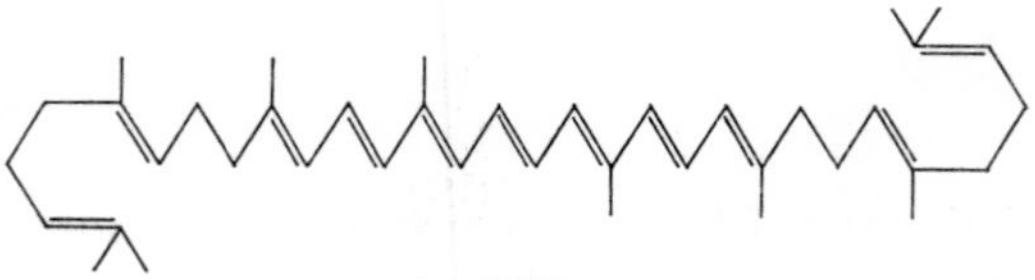

(XV)

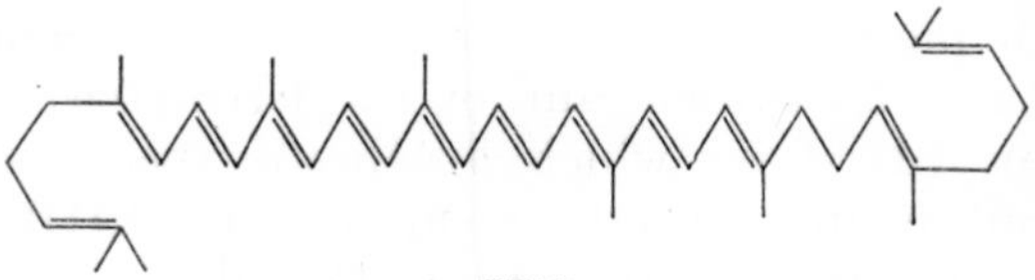

(XVI)

(c) Flower petals. The carotenoids of flower petals are characterized by (a) highly oxidized xanthophylls, in particular furanoid epoxides (e.g. flavoxanthin (XI) and auroxanthin (5,8,5′,8′-diepoxyzeaxanthin) (b) unique pigments such as eschscholtzxanthin (3,3′-dihydroxy-retro-β-carotene*) (XVII) and many of indeterminate structure,

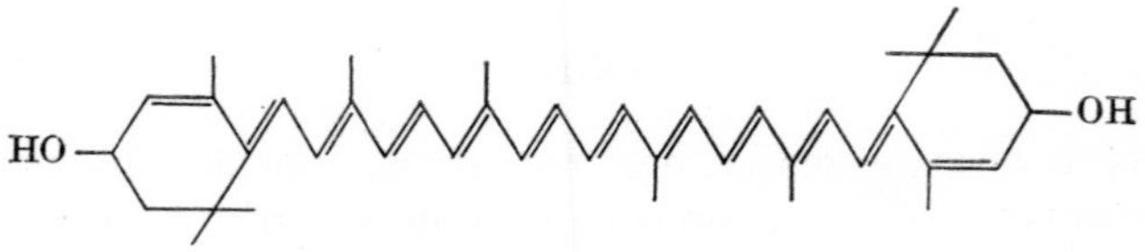

(XVII)

* Retro carotenoids contain the cyclohexylidene structure whilst normal carotenoids contain the cyclohexenyl structure.

such as taraxanthin; and (c) occasionally, in orange flowers when compared with yellow flowers, large amounts of carotenes (β-carotene and lycopene); occasionally the more saturated derivatives of lycopene are encountered (Goodwin, 1954a).

(d) *Roots*. Very few roots contain significant amounts of carotetoids, but in those that do (e.g. carrots and sweet potatoes) carotene preponderate (Goodwin, 1952a).

(ii) *Protista*

(a) *Algae*. As they are photosynthetic all algae contain carotenoids in their chloroplasts. The qualitative distribution of pigments in the various classes is complex and cannot be considered here. A summary of the available information, which has recently been discussed in detail (Goodwin, 1962a, b, c), is given in Table 1. All the pigments recorded in this Table appear to be derivatives of α- or β-carotene.

Some algae can under certain conditions accumulate extra-plastidic carotenoids. For example, the encysted flagellate *Trentepholia aurea* accumulates β-carotene (Heilbron, 1942) and the male and female gametes of *Ulva lactuca* contain comparatively high concentrations of γ-carotene (Haxo and Clendenning, 1953).

(b) *Photosynthetic bacteria*. All photosynthetic bacteria synthesize carotenoids which, together with bacteriochlorophyll, are concentrated exclusively in the chromatophores which are photoactive particles of 300-500 A diameter (Pardee *et al.*, 1952). The pigments present are all acyclic compounds which can be considered as derivatives of neuroporene. They are chloroxanthin (XVIII), rhodopin (XIX)*, 3,4-dehydrorhodopin (XX), P-481 (anhydrorhodovibrin) (XXI), rhodo-

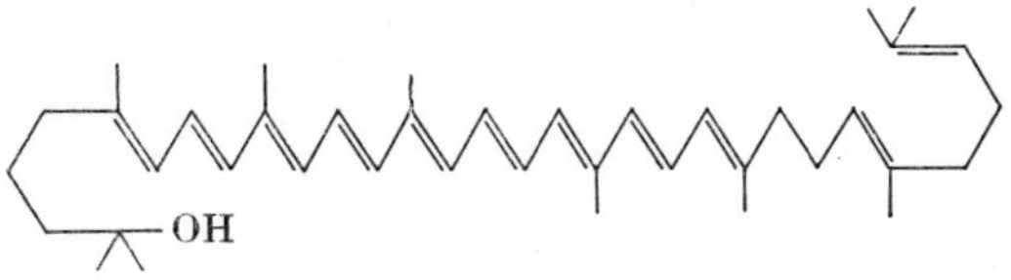

(XVIII)

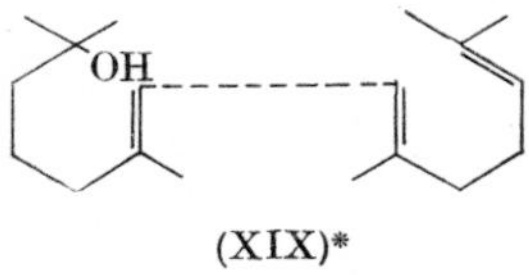

(XIX)* 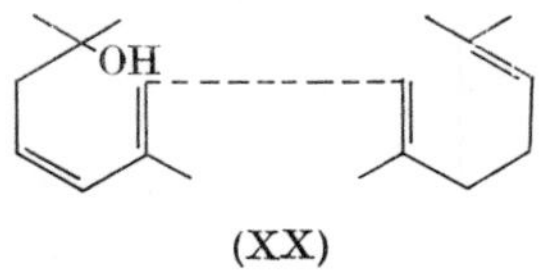   (XX)

* In formulae XIX → XXIV, the chromophore between C-6 and C-6′ is the same as that in β-carotene (I).

TABLE 1.

Major Carotenoid Distribution in Various Algal Classes[a,b]

(+ = present; - = absent; ? possibly present in traces)

	CHLOROPHYTA		PHAEOPHYTA				RHODO-PHYTA	PYRRO-PHYTA	EUG-LENO-PHYTA	ARCHE-PHYTA	CRYPTO-PHYTA
	Charophyceae[c]	Chlorophyceae	Xanthophyceae (Heterokontae)	Bacillariophyceae (Diatomophyceae)	Chrysophyceae	Phaeophyceae	Rhodophyceae	Dinophyceae	Euglenineae	Cyanophyceae	Cryptophyceae
Carotenes											
α-Carotene	-	-	-	-	-	-	+	-	-	-	+
β-Carotene	+	+	+	+	+	+	+	+	+	+	-
γ-Carotene	-	+[f]	-	-	-	-	-	-	-	-	-
ε-Carotene	-	?	-	+	-	-	-	-	-	+	-
Flavacene	-	-	-	-	-	-	-	-	-	+	-
Xanthophylls											
Echinenone	-	-	-	-	-	-	-	-	+	+?	-
Lutein	+++	+	-	-	-	+	+	-	-	-	-
Zeaxanthin	-	-	+?	-	-	-	-	-	+	+	+[g]
Violaxanthin	+	+	+?	-	-	+?	+?	-	-	-	-
Flavoxanthin	-	-	-	-	-	-	-	-	+	-	-
Neoxanthin	-	+	+?	-	-	+	-	-	+	-	-
Antheraxanthin	-	-	-	-	+	?	-	-	-	-	-
Fucoxanthin	-	-	-	++	++	+	-	-	-	-	-
Diatoxanthin	-	-	-	+	+	-	-	-	-	-	-
Diadinoxanthin	-	-	-	++	++	-	-	+	+	-	-
Dinoxanthin	-	-	-	-	-	-	-	+	-	-	-
Peridinin	-	-	-	-	-	-	-	+	-	-	-
Myxoxanthophyll	-	-	-	-	-	-	-	-	-	+	-
Siphonaxanthin	-	+[d]	-	-	-	-	-	-	-	-	-
Astaxanthin	-	+[e]	-	-	-	-	-	-	+[h]	-[h]	-
Oscillaxanthin	-	-	-	-	-	-	-	-	-	+	-

a Occasional variations from this general picture are discussed in the text. b No information exists on the carotenoids of the Chloromonadophyta (Chloromonadineae). c Only one species (*Chara fragilis*) studied; lycopene also reported present. d The main pigments of the Siphonales. e The main pigment (haematochrome) of many encysted forms; astaxanthin does not normally exist in green...

TABLE 2.

Carotenoid Distribution in Purple Photosynthetic Bacteria[a,b]

Organism	Lycopene	P 481 (Anhydrorhodovibrin)	Y	Spheroidenone (R)	Spirilloxanthin	3,4-Dehydrorhodopin	Rhodopin	Rhodovibrin (hydroxy P 481)	Hydroxy-Y	P 512	Hydroxy spheroidenone	Mono demethylated spirilloxanthin
Athiorhodaceae												
Rhodopseudomonas capsulatus	+	—	++	++	—	—	—	—	+	—	+	—
Rhodopseudomonas gelatinosa	?	—	++	++	+	—	—	—	+	+	+	—
Rhodopseudomonas palustris	+	+	—	—	++	+	+	+	—	—	—	+
Rhodopseudomonas spheroides	+	—	+	+	?	—	—	—	+	—	+	—
Rhodospirillum molischianum	+	—	—	—	—	—	+	+	—	—	—	—
Rhodospirillum photometricum	—	++	—	—	+	—	++	++	—	—	—	?
Rhodospirillum rubrum	++	++	—	—	+	—	++	++	—	—	—	+
Thiorhodaceae												
Chromatium spp.	+	+	—	—	+	—	+	?	—	—	—	—

a Symbols: +, present; —, absent; ?, possibly present in traces.
b See Jensen (1963) for new minor components.

vibrin (hydroxy P-481) (XXII), monodemethylated spirilloxanthin (XXIII), spirilloxanthin (XXIV), pigment Y (XXV) and spheroidenone (pigment R) (XXVI). These pigments have been discussed recently by Jensen *et al.* (1961). Their distribution in the photosynthetic bacteria is recorded in Table 2 (Goodwin, 1955, 1956; Goodwin and Land, 1956; Jensen *et al.*, 1961; Jensen, 1962).

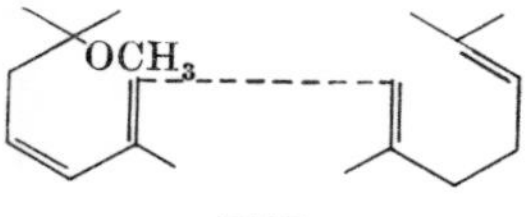

(XXI)

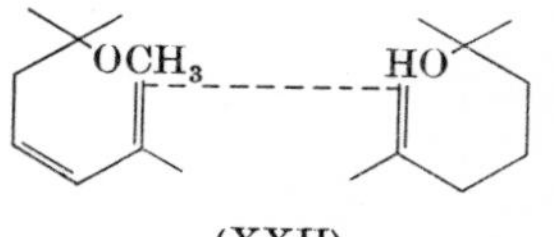

(XXII)

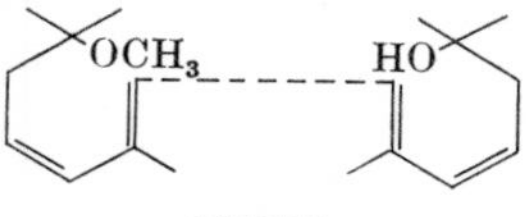

(XXIII)

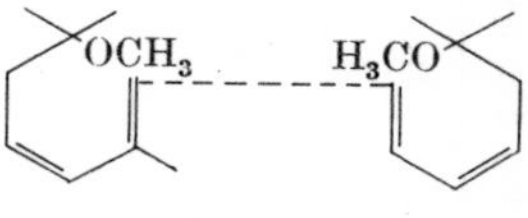

(XXIV)

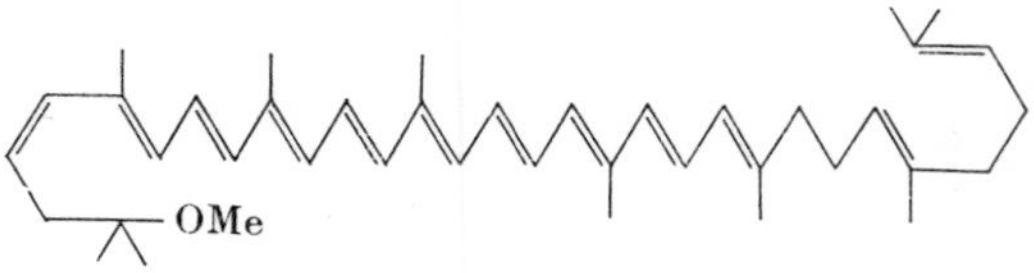

(XXV)

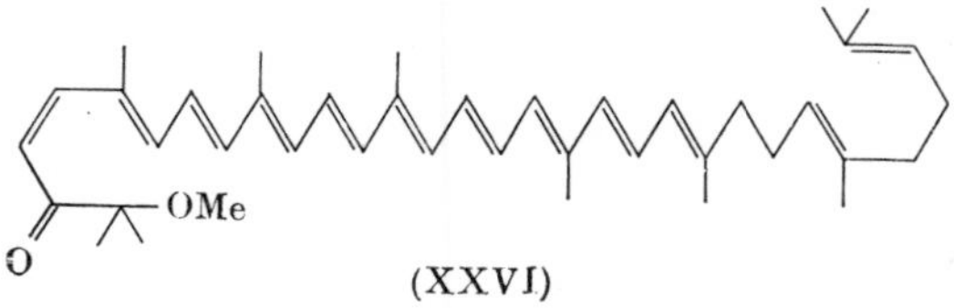

(XXVI)

(c) *Non-photosynthetic bacteria.* Carotenoids are not present in all non-photosynthetic bacteria and their distribution in those species which are carotenogenic appears to be totally capricious; the only clear generalization that can be made is that they are invariably absent from anaerobic organisms. Carotenogenic bacteria are characterized by the comparative absence of carotenes and the preponderance of highly oxygenated xanthophylls of indeterminate structure (for further details see Goodwin, 1952a, 1962a, c). Bacterial carotenoids often exist as protein complexes attached to the protoplast membrane (Mathews and Sistrom, 1959).

(d) *Fungi.* As in the case with the non-photosynthetic bacteria, carotenoid distribution in fungi is not universal and is apparently fortuitous. Three characteristics of fungal carotenoids are (a)

β-carotene is not universally present; (b) the characteristic xanthophylls of higher plants occur only very spasmodically, if at all, and
(c) specific fungal carotenoids are often acidic in nature (for further
details see Goodwin, 1962, a,b,c).

C. *Biosynthesis*

(i) *General nature of the process*

It is now well established that isopentenyl pyrophosphate formed
from acetate via mevalonate, is the basic 5-C unit for the synthesis
of many terpenoids and, in particular, steroids. The evidence for
this conclusion is described in the previous chapter (p. 255).

Isopentenyl pyrophosphate has also been shown to be the building unit for carotenoids (Varma and Chichester, 1962) and a considerable amount of evidence exists which indicates that it is synthesized from acetate conventionally via mevalonate (see p. 252).
For example, the incorporation of [1-^{14}C]- and [2-^{14}C]acetate into
β-carotene by *Mucor hiemalis* (Grob and Bütler, 1954, 1955, 1956),
Phycomyces blakesleeanus (Braithwaite and Goodwin, 1960; Good-

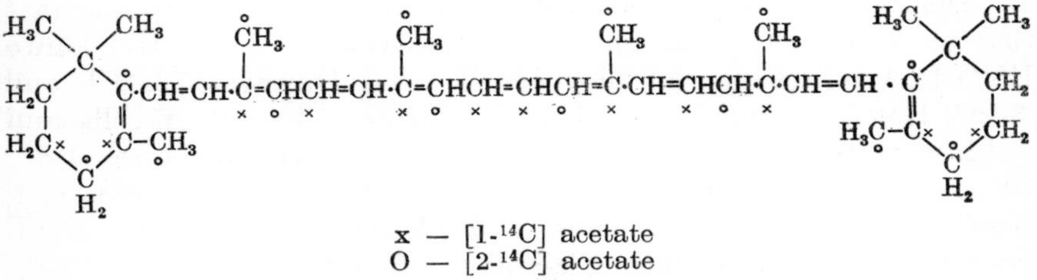

x — [1-^{14}C] acetate
O — [2-^{14}C] acetate

Fig. 1. The distribution of [1-^{14}C] and [2-^{14}C]acetate in β-carotene.

win, 1959a; Lotspeich *et al.*, 1959, 1961) and *Euglena gracilis* (Steele
and Gurin, 1960) follows a labelling pattern (Fig. 1) consistent
with the acetate → mevalonate pathway. Furthermore, mevalonate
has been shown to be actively incorporated into β-carotene by *P.
blakesleeanus* (Goodwin, 1959a; Yokoyama *et al.* 1960; Braithwaite
and Goodwin, 1957, 1960; Mackinney *et al.*, 1958), *Mucor hiemalis*
(Grob, 1959), *Blakeslea trispora* (Anderson *et al.*, 1960), *Neurospora crassa* (Krzeminski and Quackenbush, 1960), preparations
from a mutant of *Staphylococcus aureus* (Suzue, 1960), carrot root
preparations (Braithwaite and Goodwin, 1960; Modi and Patwa,
1961), leaves of *Hevea brasiliensis* (Barlow and Patrick, 1958)
and into lycopene in ripening tomatoes (Goodwin, 1959a; Braithwaite

and Goodwin, 1960; Shneour and Zabin, 1958; Purcell *et al.*, 1959). It is poorly incorporated into *Rhodospirillum rubrum* (Goodwin, 1959a,b; Davies and Goodwin, 1959) and *Euglena gracilis* (Steele and Gurin, 1960) and not incorporated at all into *Chlorella pyrenoidosa* (Anderson *et al.*, 1960). These observations may or may not be due to permeability barriers, but this explanation cannot be invoked to explain the lack of incorporation of [2-^{14}C]mevalonate into carotenoids in illuminated excised etiolated maize seedlings because the label is rapidly incorporated into the steroids of the seedlings (Goodwin, 1958). Mevalonate cannot penetrate the root system of maize seedlings (Goodwin, 1958).

Degradation of β-carotene produced by *P. blakesleeanus* and carrot root preparations (Goodwin, 1959a; Braithwaite and Goodwin, 1960) as well as *E. gracilis* (Steele and Gurin, 1960) in the presence of [2-^{14}C]mevalonate, showed that C-2 of mevalonate retained its individuality and appeared only in the 'backbone' of the molecule. Again, this is entirely analogous to the situation with steroids (p. 243).

The position of β-hydroxy-β-methylglutaric acid (HMG) as a carotenoid precursor remains equivocal. HMG-CoA is a precursor of steroids (Rudney, 1959) while free HMG is not (Tavormina *et al.*, 1956; Dituri *et al.*, 1957). This has been ascribed to the fact that an HMG-activating enzyme which would convert HMG into HMG-CoA is not present in yeast or liver. However, [2-^{14}C]- and [3-^{14}C]-HMG are incorporated into β-carotene by intact cells and cell-free preparations of *Phycomyces blakesleeanus* (Chichester *et al.*, 1959; Yokoyama *et al.*, 1960, 1962). On the other hand, it is efficiently absorbed into the cells of *Euglena gracilis* but not significantly incorporated into β-carotene (Steele and Gurin, 1960). The last observation raises the possibility of (a) a route of HMG metabolism different from that already known, which involves the formation of acetoacetate and acetyl-CoA, which could be incorporated into β-carotene or into other terpenoids, or (b) the non-metabolism of a compound which has been absorbed by *Euglena*. The latter conclusion would fit in with the alleged "animal" nature of this protozoon (see Hutner and Provasoli, 1951).

It was discovered some years ago that leucine stimulated carotenogenesis in *Phycomyces blakesleeanus* (Goodwin and Lijinsky, 1952). However, the failure of [2-^{14}C]leucine as well as [1-^{14}C] leucine to be incorporated into β-carotene (Chichester *et al.*, 1955) indicated that the conventional pathway leading to a C-5 unit such as isovaleryl-CoA or dimethylacrylyl-CoA (reaction 1), which was then incorporated into β-carotene, was not operating. This view has been justified by the fact that [^{14}C]dimethylacrylyl-CoA is not incorporated into carotenoids in ripening tomatoes and only slightly in *Chlorella pyrenoidosa* and *Blakeslea trispora* (Anderson et al., 1960). The free dimethylacrylic acid and other branched chain compounds e.g. isovaleric acid, were also very poorly incorporated

$$\begin{matrix} CH_3 \\ \diagdown \\ CH_3 \diagup \end{matrix} CHCH_2CHNH_2COOH \rightarrow \begin{matrix} CH_3 \\ \diagdown \\ CH_3 \diagup \end{matrix} CHCH_2\overset{O}{\underset{\parallel}{C}}COOH \rightarrow$$

$$\rightarrow \begin{matrix} CH_3 \\ \diagdown \\ CH_3 \diagup \end{matrix} CHCH_2COSCoA \rightarrow \begin{matrix} CH_3 \\ \diagdown \\ CH_3 \diagup \end{matrix} C{=}CHCOSCoA \qquad (1)$$

into β-carotene in *Euglena gracilis* (Steele and Gurin, 1960). Mackinney and his colleagues have investigated fully the incorporation of leucine labelled in different carbon atoms into β-carotene by *Phycomyces blakesleeanus* (Chichester et al., 1955, 1959; Wurhmann et al., 1957; Yokoyama et al., 1957; Varma et al., 1959). Their findings are consistent with the metabolism of leucine to HMG-CoA via a pathway involving CO_2 fixation which was elucidated by Coon and his colleagues (see Goodwin, 1960) (reaction 2).

$$\begin{matrix} H_3C \\ \diagdown \\ H_3C \diagup \end{matrix} CHCH_2CHNH_2COOH \xrightarrow[\text{amination}]{\text{trans-}} \begin{matrix} H_3C \\ \diagdown \\ H_3C \diagup \end{matrix} CHCH_2\overset{O}{\underset{\parallel}{C}}COOH$$

$$\begin{matrix} H_3C \\ \diagdown \\ H_3C \diagup \end{matrix} C{=}CHCOSCoA \leftarrow\!\!\!-\!\!\!-\!\!\!-\!\!\!- \begin{matrix} H_3C \\ \diagdown \\ H_3C \diagup \end{matrix} CHCH_2COSCoA$$

CoASH, 2 H, CO_2 (2)

$- CO_2$, ATP, AMP, P–P

$$\begin{matrix} H_3C \\ \diagdown \\ CH_2COOH \diagup \end{matrix} C{=}CHCOSoA \xrightarrow{\ H_2O\ } \begin{matrix} H_3C \\ \diagdown \\ CH_2COOH \diagup \end{matrix} C(OH)CH_2COSCoA$$

Furthermore it has been shown that $^{14}CO_2$ is incorporated into β-carotene by *Phycomyces blakesleeanus* in the presence of leucine but not in its absence (Goodwin, 1959b; Braithwaite and Goodwin, 1960; Chichester et al., 1959). However, a study of reaction 2 reveals that all the CO_2 fixed would become C-1 of mevalonic acid and thus be lost on incorporation into β-carotene. Randomization of C-1 and C-5 of HMG-CoA could occur as indicated in reaction 3 (the carbon arising from CO_2 is asterisked) and this label from $^{14}CO_2$ would appear in β-carotene.

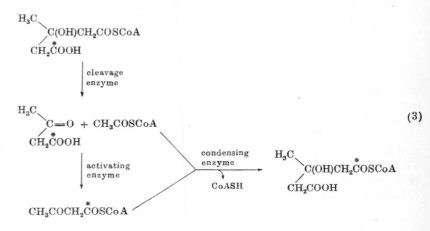

(3)

(ii) *The first 40-C compound formed*

Squalene the 30-C precursor of steroids is synthesized from two molecules of farnesyl pyrophosphate (15-C) (see p. 258). By analogy with this reaction the 40-C precursor of carotenoids would be lycopersene (XXVII), synthesized from two molecules of geranylgeranylpyrophosphate (20-C). In support of this view Grob *et al.*

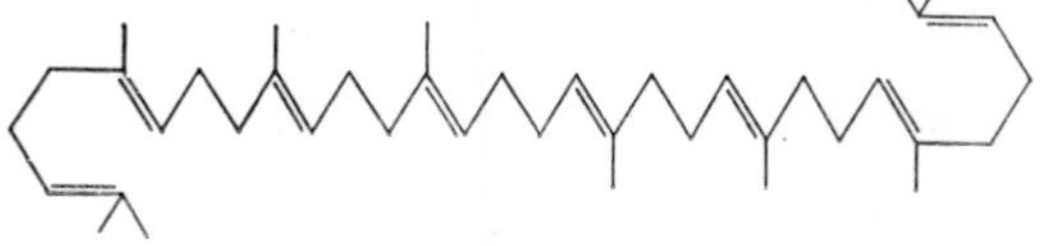

(XXVII)

(1961) have reported the enzymatic synthesis of geranylgeranyl pyrophosphate from isopentenyl pyrophosphate and the conversion of this compound into lycopersene by enzyme preparations from *Neurospora crassa*: furthermore, Grob and Boschetti (1962) also reported the presence of lycopersene in cultures of *Neurospora crassa* grown in the presence of diphenylamine, a specific inhibitor of carotenogenesis (see p. 284). On the other hand Anderson and Porter (1961, 1962) have obtained a system from carrot roots which converts terpenyl pyrophosphates (80—90% farnesyl pyrophosphate) into phytoene, but could not detect labelled lycopersene. In comparison with the formation of squalene which requires NADPH (see p. 259), phytoene synthesis required NADP; NADPH inhibits the reaction. [^{14}C]Farnesyl pyrophosphate is also incorporated into phytoene in preparations from *Phycomyces blakesleeanus*, but no mention was made of labelling of lycopersene (Yamamoto *et al.*, 1961). Furthermore, Davies *et al.* (1961, 1963) and Mercer *et al.*, (1963) have failed to find lycopersene in any carotenogenic system so far examined, and it does not accumulate in diphenylamine-inhibited cultures of the photosynthetic bacterium *Rhodospirillum rubrum* and the fungus *Neurospora crassa*. In addition Mercer *et al.* (1963) could not detect labelled lycopersene in systems, such as carrot root slices, which incorporate [^{14}C]mevalonate into phytoene. It is also absent from *Arum* spadix (Pennock *et al.*, 1962). Many mutants in which carotenoid synthesis is blocked accumulate either phytoene exclusively in amounts equivalent to the carotenoid present in the native strain, or preponderantly with traces of more saturated polyenes such as phytofluene, ζ-carotene and neurosporene (Table 3). Lycopersene has not been reported in

TABLE 3. Mutants which Produce only Phytoene

Organism	Reference
Chlorella vulgaris 5/871	Claes (1954, 1956, 1957, 1958)
Rhodopseudomonas spheroides blue-green	Griffiths *et al.* (1955)
Tomato *gh* (ghost)	Mackinney *et al.* (1956)
Staphylococcus aureus	Suzue (1960)
Maize	Anderson and Robertson (1960)

any of these mutants. The metabolic block in these mutants is obviously in the dehydrogenation of the fully formed polyene chain, and Jensen *et al.* (1961) suggest that the same enzyme is required for all steps. If this is so, there is no reason to suppose that the dehydrogenation of lycopersene, if it is formed, should not be carried out by the same enzyme; thus it, and not phytoene, should accumulate in these mutants. Other carotenoid-less mutants are known which do not accumulate any of the phytoene series, for example those obtained from *N. crassa* (Haxo, 1952) and *Corynebact. michiganese* (Saperstein *et al.*, 1954); one such strain of maize (Anderson and Robertson, 1960) has also been shown not to accumulate lycopersene (Griffiths *et al.*, 1962).

If phytoene (15, 15′-dehydrolycopersene) (XIII) is the first 40-C compound formed, the mechanism involved in its formation could

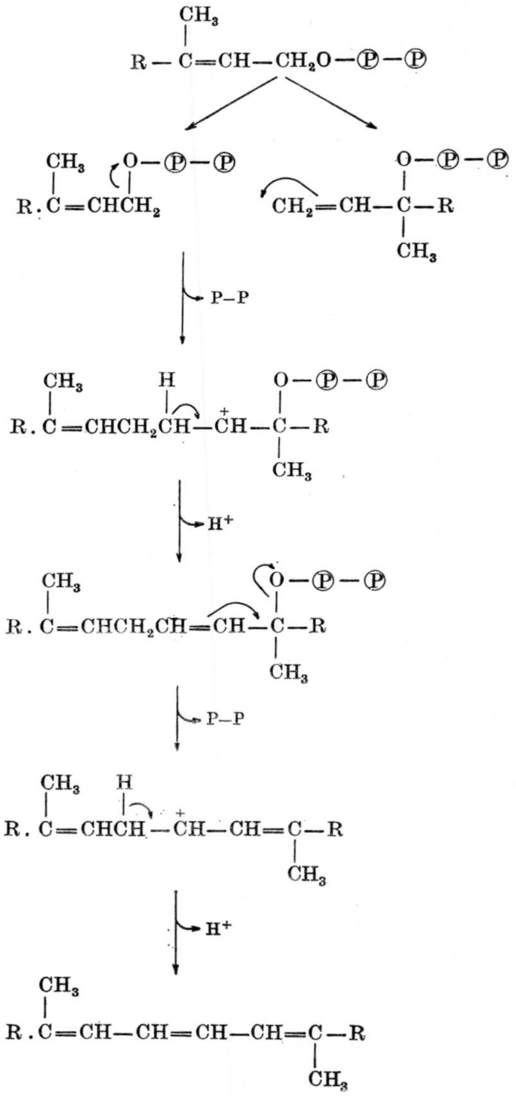

FIG. 2. Possible mechanism of conversion of geranylgeranyl pyrophosphate into phytoene (after Cornforth and Popják).

be that indicated in Fig. 2. Phytoene is a much more rigid molecule than lycopersene and its formation could account for the existence in Nature of carotenoids rather than polycyclic tetraterpenoids similar to the steroids.

(iii) *Conversion of phytoene into lycopene*

It now appears clear that phytoene and not lycopersene is the first 40-C compound formed, and there is very little doubt that phytoene is the precursor of lycopene and other acyclic carotenoids, such as spirilloxanthin, via the pathway indicated in reaction (4). This proposal was made some time ago on the basis

$$\text{Phytoene} \rightarrow \text{Phytofluene} \rightarrow \zeta\text{-Carotene} \rightarrow \text{Neurosporene} \rightarrow \text{Lycopene} \qquad (4)$$

of a study of the pigments of various tomato crosses (Porter and Lincoln, 1950), and it has now received support from recent experiments on the incorporation of [^{14}C]mevalonate into ripening tomatoes, the specific activities of the various components listed in reaction 4 were not inconsistent with the sequential pathway indicated (Anderson *et al.*, 1960). Furthermore, as indicated above, *Rhodospirillum rubrum* cultured in the presence of diphenylamine accumulates mainly phytoene but also small amounts of the other polyenes more saturated than lycopene; however, if such cells are washed free from diphenylamine resuspended in phosphate buffer and illuminated, then spirilloxanthin is rapidly synthesized (Goodwin and Osman, 1954). A kinetic study of the synthesis of spirilloxanthin under these conditions indicated that lycopene, and eventually spirilloxanthin, are produced sequentially via the phytoene series (Jensen *et al.*, 1958). The steps from lycopene to spirilloxanthin are discussed in detail on p. 291. Suzue (1961) has recently reported the conversion of phytoene into ζ-carotene (XV) by extracts of *Staph. aureus* and the conversion of phytoene into phytofluene by tomato plastids has been demonstrated by Beeler and Porter (1962).

(iv) *Formation of cyclic carotenoids*

It is now clear that squalene is almost certainly the precursor of all triterpenoids which are found in Nature (see p. 246); by analogy with this system it could be postulated that phytoene is the precursor of all carotenoids, both cyclic and acyclic. The evidence quoted in the previous section strongly supports the view that phytoene is the precursor of the acyclic lycopene. The key problem in the formation of cyclic carotenoids, such as β-carotene, is whether they are formed by the cyclization of lycopene or whether cyclization occurs prior to complete dehydrogenation of the polyene chain; for example cyclization could occur at the phytoene, phytofluene, ζ-carotene or neurosporene level.

The evidence in support of lycopene as a precursor of cyclic carotenoids has been considered in detail by Porter and Anderson (1962); it is necessary here only to emphasize the two main arguments.

In a tomato phenotype obtained by back-crossing a *Lycopersicon esculentum* x *L. hirsutum* hybrid to *L. esculentum*, the usual amount of lycopene is replaced by an equivalent amount of β-carotene, the synthesis of which is, like that of lycopene in commercial tomatoes, temperature-sensitive (Lincoln and Porter, 1950; Tomes *et al.*, 1954, 1956). The fact that the fruit of the F_1 generation of the high β-carotene strain contains more γ-carotene (a possible intermediate between β-carotene and lycopene) than do the fruit from the high lycopene strains suggests that lycopene might be the compound which cyclizes. It must, however, be admitted that this extra synthesis of β-carotene, which is controlled by one dominant gene B, is different from the temperature-insensitive synthesis in normal tomatoes.

More direct evidence was provided by Decker and Uehleke (1961) who found that isolated chloroplasts converted [^{14}C]lycopene into β-carotene; however, the same investigators report that β-carotene is converted into lycopene by tomato parenchyma.

If the phytoene series is concerned with the synthesis of cyclic carotenoids then the most likely candidate for the role of immediate precursor is neurosporene (XVI) (see reaction 4). Neurosporene is the branch point for the synthesis of the two types of pigments in the photosynthetic bacteria (p. 292) and two pigments have recently been isolated from maize α-zeacarotene (XXVIII) and β-zeacarotene (XXIX) (Rabourn and Quackenbush, 1959; Rüegg *et al.*, 1961), which could be formed by cyclization of one end of the neurosporene molecule. Pathways to α-carotene and β-carotene could then be envisaged is indicated in reaction (5). The structure of δ-carotene is (XXX).

$$\text{Neurosporene} \quad \begin{cases} \nearrow \beta\text{-zeacarotene} \rightarrow \gamma\text{-carotene} \rightarrow \beta\text{-carotene} \\ \searrow \alpha\text{-zeacarotene} \rightarrow \delta\text{-carotene} \rightarrow \alpha\text{-carotene} \end{cases} \qquad (5)$$

Claes (1958) isolated a mutant (5/520) of *Chlorella vulgaris* which, in the dark synthesizes some members of the phytoene series; anaerobic illumination of dark grown cells results in the synthesis of β-carotene and an unidentified pigment "X" simultaneously with the disappearance of members of the phytoene series. A comparison of the properties of "X" with those of β-zeacarotene suggests that they are identical; if this is rigorously proved then this may turn out to be the first demonstration of β-zeacarotene as

an intermediate in β-carotene synthesis. The possibility that cyclization occurs before the neurosporene stage has not yet received
experimental support. Contraindications come from some recent

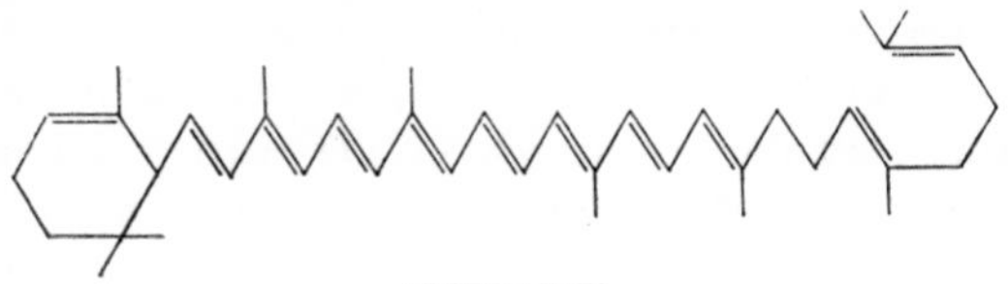

(XXVIII)

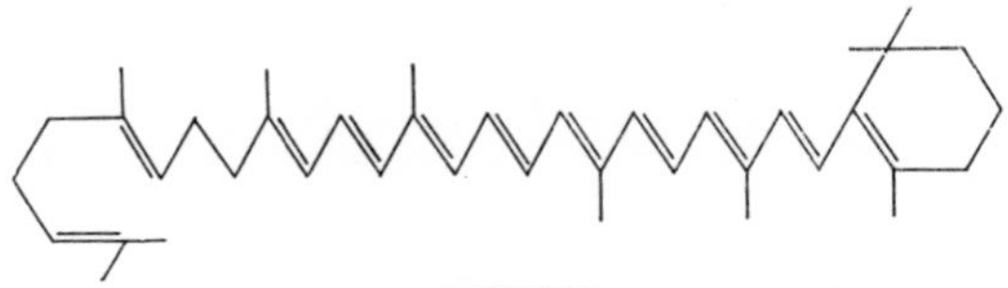

(XXIX)

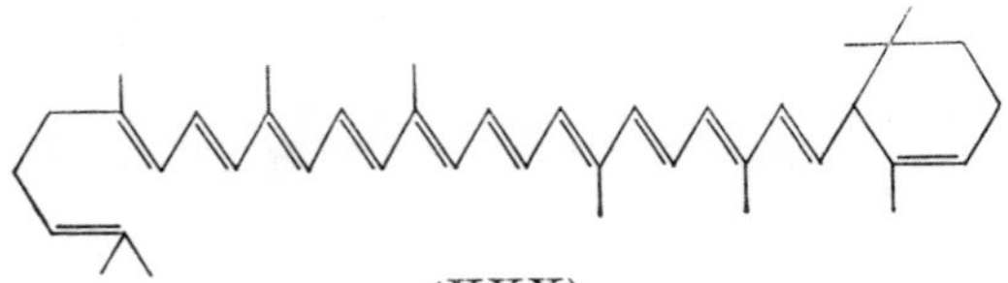

(XXX)

observations by B.H. Davies (unpublished) who could not find
"cyclic ζ-carotene" (XXXI) in diphenylamine-inhibited cultures of
Phycomyces blakesleeanus, which were accumulating large amounts
of the phytoene series including ζ-carotene and neurosporene.

In support of the view that lycopene is not the precursor of β-
carotene we have firstly the fact that if tomato fruit are ripened at
30° or higher, synthesis of lycopene and the more saturated polyene
precursors of lycopene is inhibited, whilst that of β-carotene is
unaffected (Goodwin and Jamikorn, 1952; McCollum, 1954). Secondly, a pink mutant of *Corynebacterium michiganese,* produces
only acyclic carotenoids [spirilloxanthin (XXIV) and lycopene
(V)]; an orange strain produces only cyclic carotenoids [β-carotene
(I), canthaxanthin (4,4′-dioxo-β-carotene) and cryptoxanthin (IX)]
whilst the wild strain produces both types (lycopene and cryptoxanthin) (Saperstein *et al.,* 1954); these observations combined with

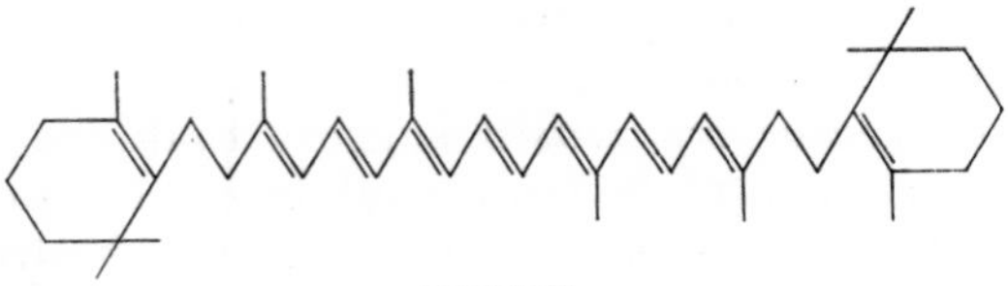

(XXXI)

the finding that a red back-mutant synthesizes only lycopene, suggest that there may be independent genetic control for the production of acyclic and cyclic carotenoids. Similarly, the carotenoid distribution in a series of mutants of *Rhodotorula mucilaginosa* indicate no direct biosynthetic relationship between acyclic and cyclic carotenoids (Villoutreix, 1960). For example, although the native strain contains mainly torularhodin (XXXII) and torulene (XXXIII), which are γ-carotene derivatives, a mutant has been obtained

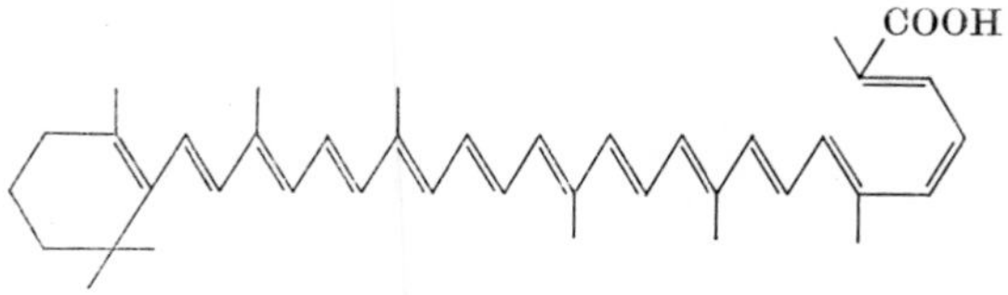

(XXXII)

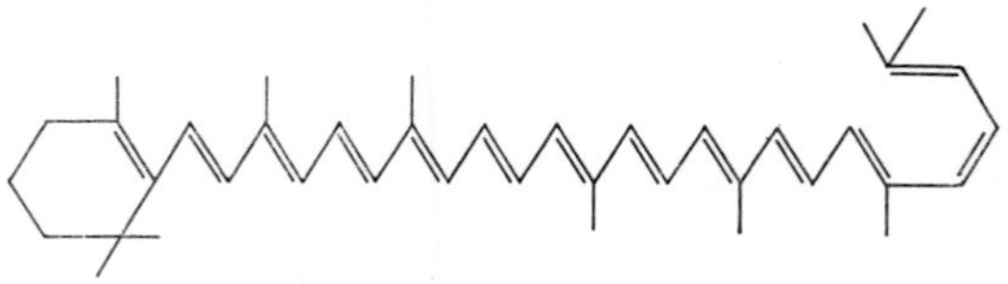

(XXXIII)

with its major pigment β-carotene, which is produced to almost the same extent as torularhodin in the native strain.

Thirdly, it has recently been found that the aquatic fungus *Rhizophlyctis rosea* synthesizes only lycopene during the early stages of growth, whilst mature cultures contain a mixture of lycopene and γ-carotene; kinetic studies indicated that γ-carotene synthesis began only after the lycopene level had reached a steady value. Furthermore, if [2-^{14}C]mevalonate was added to newly inoculated media and removed when lycopene synthesis had stopped, the γ-carotene subsequently synthesized was essentially unlabelled, whilst the lycopene was strongly labelled; conversely, if addition of [2-^{14}C]mevalonate was delayed until lycopene synthesis was completed, then the resulting γ-carotene was highly labelled and the lycopene unlabelled (Davies, 1961).

A final possibility which must be considered is that the phytoene series of polyenes are not precursors of cyclic carotenoids. The evidence is at present confusing. Experiments with *Phycomyces blakesleeanus* and *Neurospora crassa* suggest that they may not be precursors. Washed diphenylamine-inhibited cultures of *P. blakesleeanus* when resuspended in glucose, synthesized β-carotene but not apparently at the expense of the phytoene series (Goodwin,

1952b). However, if the diphenylamine-inhibited cultures of *P. bla-kesleeanus* are grown in the presence of [14C]mevalonate, then the β-carotene subsequently synthesized by washed suspensions is labelled, thus indicating that it is formed from an endogenous precursor (Braithwaite and Goodwin, 1960). Furthermore, if *Phycomyces blakesleeanus* is cultured in the presence of AMP (adenosine monophosphate) and diphenylamine, it accumulates the members of the phytoene series as well as normal amounts of β-carotene, although AMP alone has no effect on carotenogenesis (Goodwin *et al.*, 1953). From these observations it can be concluded that diphenylamine exerts two effects, firstly to inhibit β-carotene synthesis, and secondly to stimulate phytoene synthesis. This conclusion is supported by the view that in diphenylamine-inhibited cultures far more phytoene is produced than the amount of fully unsaturated carotenoid produced in normal cultures (Goodwin, 1959a; Olson, 1962). It is possible that in the early experiments of Goodwin (1952b) the amount of phytoene disappearing when β-carotene was being synthesized in washed resuspended mycelia was very small in relation to the amount present and consequently could not be detected. It will be recalled that Jensen *et al.* (1958) experienced the same problem with regard to phytoene in their experiments on spirilloxanthin synthesis in diphenylamine-inhibited cultures *Rhodospirillum rubrum*.

Other evidence which has been reported which suggests the phytoene is not a precursor of β-carotene includes (a) in *Neurospora crassa* grown in the presence of [14C]mevalonate, the specific activities of β-carotene and e.g. phytoene, do not follow a precursor/product relationship (Krezeminski and Quackenbush, 1960); (b) cells of *Rhodotorula mucilaginosa* when grown in the presence of 2-hydroxydiphenyl (which acts rather similarly to diphenylamine) are almost colourless, but they accumulate small amounts of the phytoene series with, rather unexpectedly, no phytofluene; if the colourless cells are washed and resuspended in phosphate buffer then the coloured carotenoids, β-carotene, torulene and torularhodin are synthesized, but not apparently from the phytoene series (Villoutreix, 1960).

(v) *Insertion of oxygen into carotenoids*

It will be recalled that during biosynthesis the first compound formed with an intact steroid nucleus contains a hydroxyl group at position 3 (lanosterol); the hydroxyl group is present because the cyclization of squalene is initiated by OH^+ attack (see p. 246).

All the evidence in the carotenoid field indicates that the oxygen functions, including hydroxyl groups, are added only at the end of the biosynthetic sequence.

Mutant 5/520 of *Chlorella vulgaris*, as already indicated (p. 286), synthesizes the phytoene series in the dark, and converts these into coloured carotenoids when illuminated anaerobically. If these cultures are now returned to the dark and allowed access to oxygen, xanthophylls are formed concomitantly with the disappearance of the carotenes (Claes, 1957, 1959). These observations indicate that the carotenes are the immediate precursors of the xanthophylls.

Isotope experiments with a deep red strain of *Mycobacterium phlei* indicate that myxoxanthophyll (a carotenoid of unknown constitution) is formed from hydrocarbon precursors, but the identity of the precursors is not yet established (Schlegel, 1958, 1959).

Exponentially growing cells of the photosynthetic bacterium *Rhodospirillum rubrum* contain mainly neurosporene, lycopene, rhodopin, P-481 (anhydrorhodovibrin) and rhodovibrin (van Niel *et al.*, 1956). If washed young cells are resuspended in phosphate buffer anaerobically in the light then there is a marked synthesis of spirilloxanthin accompanied by a concomitant disappearance of the pigments originally present (Jensen *et al.*, 1958; Sissins, 1956; Goodwin, 1959a); similar observations have been made with the sulphur photosynthetic bacterium *Chromatium* (Benedict *et al.*, 1961). All these results indicate that the pathway outlined in Fig. 3. is operative. All the intermediates in this scheme have now been isolated and their structures determined (Jensen, 1959, 1960, 1961; Jackman and Jensen, 1961). Further support for this pathway comes from the demonstration that young washed cells of *R. rubrum* when incubated anaerobically in phosphate buffer in the light and in the presence of [^{14}C]formate incorporate the label almost exclusively into the carbon of the methoxyl group of spirilloxanthin (Braithwaite and Goodwin, 1958).

Anaerobic cultures of the non-sulphur photosynthetic bacterium *Rhodopseudomonas spheroides* are yellowish-brown, but rapidly turn red on exposure to air (van Niel, 1947; Goodwin *et al.*, 1955). The colour change is due primarily to the conversion of a yellow pigment [pigment Y (XXV)] in the anaerobic cultures into the purple pigment [pigment R, spheroidenone (XXVI)] in the aerobic cultures by the insertion of oxygen into a carbonyl function at one end of the polyene chain (Goodwin *et al.*, 1956a; Davis *et al.*, 1961; Shneour, 1962). As brown and green mutants of *Rhodopseudomonas spheroides* accumulate chloroxanthin (Nakayama, 1958) which is 1-hydroxy-neurosporene (Davis *et al.*, 1961) the pattern of biosynthesis of

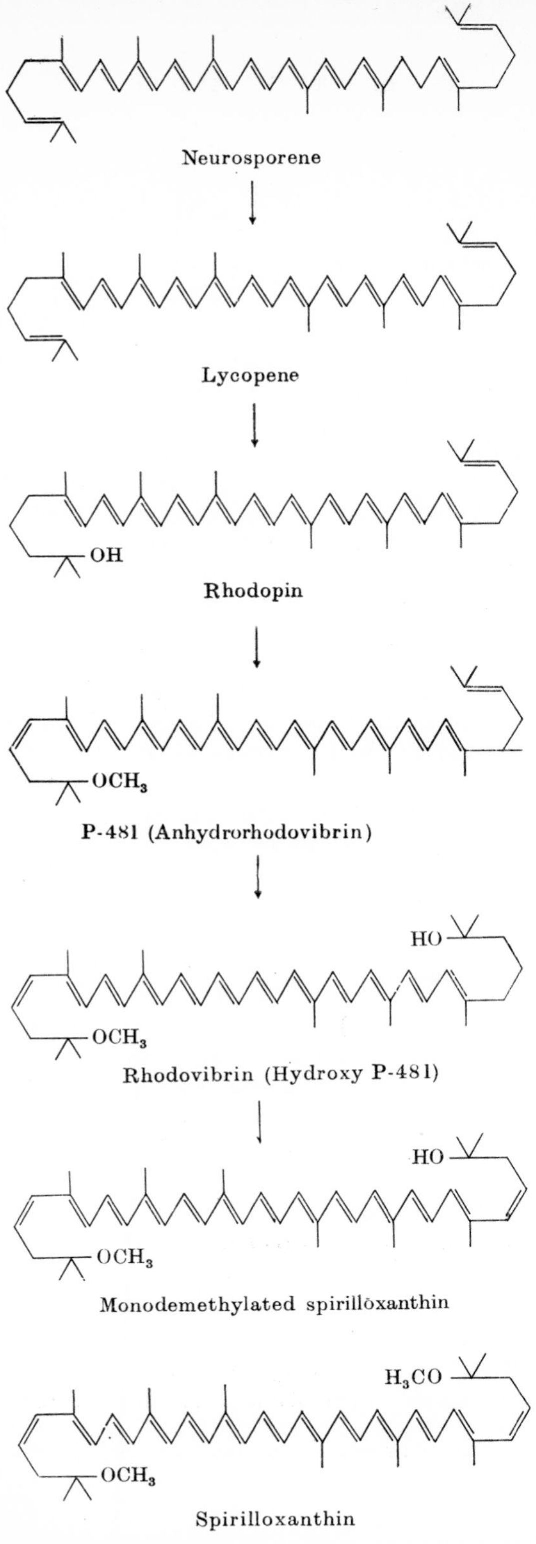

Neurosporene
Lycopene
OH
Rhodopin
OCH$_3$
P-481 (Anhydrorhodovibrin)
HO
OCH$_3$
Rhodovibrin (Hydroxy P-481)
HO
OCH$_3$
Monodemethylated spirilloxanthin
H$_3$CO
OCH$_3$
Spirilloxanthin

FIG. 3. The pathway of conversion of neurosporene into spirilloxanthin.

pigment Y and spheroidenone is almost certainly as indicated in reaction (6).

$$\text{Neurosporene} \rightarrow \text{chloroxanthin} \rightarrow \text{hydroxy Y} \begin{array}{c} \nearrow \text{hydroxy R} \\ \vdots \\ \searrow \\ \text{Y} \rightarrow \text{spheroidenone} \end{array} \qquad (6)$$

Epoxides of β-carotene, which are only minor components of fresh green leaves, accumulate at the expense of β-carotene in excised tomato leaves maintained in the dark in the absence of CO_2 (Glover and Redfearn, 1953). This suggests the direct oxidation of β-carotene to epoxides, is probably the first step in the complete degradation of the molecule, because on illuminating leaves previously kept in the dark, the epoxides soon disappear although β-carotene synthesis begins only after a lag period of about 24 hours. It has also been reported that in excised leaves kept aerobically in the dark the violaxanthin (VII) level increases with a concomitant loss of lutein (VI); on illumination in air the original pigments are restored (Sapozhnikov et al., 1959; Blass et al., 1959); more recent work, however, indicates that the relationship is between violaxanthin and zeaxanthin, with antheraxanthin (5,6-epoxy-β-zeaxanthin) as an intermediate. Yamamoto et al. (1962a) found the reactions indicated in (7) to occur with spinach leaves over a period of an hour. During this period no changes in the concentrations of β-carotene, lutein or neoxanthin were observed. Similar results were obtained with *Euglena* (Krinsky, 1962).

$$\text{Violaxathin} \underset{\text{dark, } O_2}{\overset{\text{light, } N_2}{\rightleftarrows}} \text{antheraxanthin} \underset{\text{dark, } O_2}{\overset{\text{light, } N_2}{\rightleftarrows}} \text{zeaxanthin} \qquad (7)$$

Yamamoto et al. (1962a,b) have recently shown with the aid of $^{18}O_2$ and $H_2{}^{18}O$ that the oxygen in the hydroxyl groups in the xanthophylls from *Chlorella* arise from $^{18}O_2$ and not from water; on the other hand water appears to supply the oxygen for the epoxy groups of violaxanthin and neoxanthin.

D. *General Factors Controlling Carotenoid Synthesis**

(i) *Higher plants*

(a) *Carbon sources.* Inhibition of photosynthesis in detached leaves, either by removal of CO_2 or by the addition of inhibitors such as hydroxylamine, also stops carotenoid biosynthesis; it is

---

* For fuller discussion of these topics see Goodwin (1959a, 1960).

restored by the addition of sucrose or glucose but not glycerol or pyruvate. This restoration is inhibited by fluoride (Bandurski, 1949). Carbon compounds other than CO_2 are poorly utilized for carotenoid synthesis; this is the case with acetate in isolated tomato leaves (Glover and Redfearn, 1953), with glutamine in maize seedlings (Roux and Husson, 1952) and acetate and mevalonate in illuminated excised maize seedlings (Goodwin, 1958).

(b) *Nitrogen sources*. Reports on the relative efficacy of NO_3^- and NH_4^+ in supporting carotenogenesis in higher plants are variable (see Goodwin, 1952a). These reports are not of necessity self-contradictory because in cress, the nature of the anion is important in assessing NH_4^+ activity; for example, ammonium phosphate, sulphate and chloride inhibited carotenogenesis whilst ammonium nitrate, bicarbonate, acetate and succinate were not inhibitory (Mapson and Cruickshank, 1947) (compare the effect on ascorbic acid synthesis, p. 226).

(c) *Light*. Small amounts of xanthophylls (primarily lutein) are synthesized by most monocotyledons germinated in the dark, but only traces of β-carotene are formed (Kay and Phinney,1956; Goodwin, 1958). In the case of a typical dicotyledon (dwarf bean) germinated in the dark, the first leaves contain the usual plastid carotenoids whilst the cotyledons synthesize mainly the furanoid epoxides chrysanthemaxanthin and auroxanthin (Goodwin and Phagpolngarm, 1960).

On illumination of etiolated seedlings, there is a rapid synthesis of the plastid carotenoids as the chloroplasts are formed and become fully functional (Goodwin, 1958). High light intensity reduces carotenogenesis in leaves (Seybold and Egle, 1938), the optimum intensity in the case of isolated bean leaves being 600 ft c. (Bandurski, 1949). It has been claimed that high light intensities favour the synthesis of zeaxanthin and violaxanthin, apparently at the expense of β-carotene and lutein, in maize leaves (Moster and Quackenbush, 1952). The optimal intensity of infra-red radiation (725 mμ) for carotenogenesis in bean and maize seedlings is 450 μW/cm². (Withrow *et al.*, 1953).

If 4-day etiolated maize seedlings are exposed to red light (660 mμ) for 5 minutes and returned to darkness then, on examination 24 hr later they are found to contain more carotenoids than the control seedlings kept continuously in the dark. This phenomenon is not observed if, following red light treatment, the seedlings are exposed to far red light (760 mμ) for five minutes (Cohen and Goodwin, 1962); this indicates that this is a phytochrome-mediated response (see Hendricks and Borthwick, 1959). Similar effects are observed with pea (Goodwin and Henshall, 1962) and dwarf bean seedlings (unpublished work quoted by Mego and Jagendorf, 1961).

(d) *Temperature*. A detailed investigation of the effect of temperature on carotenoid synthesis in tomato leaves in relation to the dark/light periodicity to which the plants are normally subjected has been carried out by Bandurski *et al.* (1953). If the night temperature is maintained at 17° and the phototemperature varied, then carotenoid synthesis is considerably decreased as the temperature is lowered, so that a phototemperature of 4° is physiologically equivalent to darkness. At a constant phototemperature (17°) variations in the nycto-temperature have little effect on carotenogenesis, although at higher temperatures the leaves are lighter coloured owing to changes in the anatomy of the leaf.

In leaves it is claimed that low temperatures favour the formation of zeaxanthin at the expense of β-carotene (Moster and Quackenbush, 1952).

The profound effect of temperature on carotenoid synthesis in tomatoes has already been discussed (p. 287). Exposure to elevated temperatures has no deleterious effect on the lycopene-synthesizing system, because fruit held at a high temperature (above 30°) rapidly begins to synthesize this pigment when transferred to a lower temperature (Went *et al.*, 1942). These observations explain why tomatoes exposed on the vine to wide temperature fluctuations ripen normally as long as the nycto-temperature falls below 30° (Sayre *et al.*, 1953).

(e) *Inhibitors*. Streptomycin, guanidine hydrochloride, isonicotinic acid hydrazide, maleic hydrazide, tetronic acid and terramycin all inhibit carotenogenesis in seedlings, whilst penicillin is without effect (Schopfer *et al.*, 1952a, b; Netien and Lacharme, 1955). Tetronic acid is 60 times more effective than streptomycin and isonicotinic acid hydrazide is unique in inhibiting carotenogenesis specifically.

(ii) *Protista*

(a) *Carbon sources*. In the mould *Phycomyces blakesleeanus* maltose and glucose are equally carotenogenic; xylose and fructose, on the other hand, are much less effective, although they support growth as well as maltose and glucose (Garton *et al.*, 1951). Replacement of glucose by acetate markedly reduces carotenogenesis (Friend *et al.*, 1955). In *Rhodotorula rubra*, glycerol is the most effective single carbon source (Nakayama *et al.*, 1954) and this is also true of *My-cobact. phlei* and *Mycobact. rhodochrous* (Goodwin and Jamikorn, 1956).

There is one reported instance when variation in the carbon source of a medium alters qualitatively the carotenoids synthesized. *Mycobact. lacticola* produces carotenes and neutral xanthophylls when cultured on agar; on mineral oils, on the other hand, carotenes and acidic carotenoids (astaxanthin) are synthesized (Haas and Bushnell, 1944).

(b) *Nitrogen sources.* Replacement of asparagine in the basal culture medium by leucine (or valine) greatly stimulates carotenogenesis in *Phycomyces blakesleeanus* (Goodwin and Lijinsky, 1952; Chichester *et al.*, 1955). These reason for this has already been discussed (p. 280). The failure of leucine to stimulate carotenogenesis in, for example, *Rhodospirillum rubrum* (Goodwin and Osman, 1953) *Sarcina lutea* (Arnaki and Stary, 1952) and *Corynebact. poinsettiae* (Starr and Saperstein, 1953), is probably due either to the failure to metabolize leucine to HMG-CoA, or to the fact that although leucine is metabolized to HMG-CoA, this compound is not the rate-limiting factor in carotenogenesis.

When asparagine in the basal medium is replaced by NH_4NO_3, growth and carotenogenesis are equally inhibited in *Phycomyces blakesleeanus*. Addition of any single member of the tricarboxylic acid cycle restores normal growth, but the effect on carotenogenesis varies with the acid used; this is a pH effect (see p. 297) (Friend *et al.*, 1955; Goodwin *et al.*, 1956b).

(c) *Light. Photosynthetic organisms.* Complete exclusion of light has no effect on the carotenoid levels of *Chlorella vulgaris* grown heterotrophically (Goodwin, 1954b); on the other hand, under the same conditions *Euglena gracilis* var. *bacillaris* produces only one fifth the amount of carotenoids in the dark compared with the light (Goodwin and Jamikorn, 1954).

The optimum light intensity for carotenogenesis in the blue-green algae, *Anacystis nidulans* and *Anabaena* spp. is 400–800 ft c. (Handke, 1954). In the green mutant of *Rhodopseudomonas spheroides* the situation is quite different; maximum carotenoid levels were found at the lowest light intensity examined (50 ft c.) and they were five times greater than in cells cultured under an intensity of 5000 ft c. (Cohen-Bazire *et al.*, 1957).

Non-photosynthetic organisms. Light stimulates carotenogenesis in a number of fungi including *Phycomyces blakesleeanus* (Garton *et al.*, 1951; Chichester *et al.*, 1954), *Penicillium sclerotiorum* (Mase *et al.*, 1957), *Rhodotorula gracilis* (Praus, 1952), *Neurospora crassa* (Haxo, 1956) and *Fusarium oxysporum* (Carlile, 1956). In the case of *Phycomyces blakesleeanus* and *Penicillium sclerotiorum* the effect is quantitative. However, in *N. crassa* the colourless polyenes, phytoene and phytofluene, are increased at the expense of the coloured carotenoids (Sheng and Sheng, 1952; Zalokar, 1954) and in *R. gracilis* the ratio α - + β-carotene: torulene changes from 1·67:1 in the dark to 2·29:1 in the light (Praus, 1952).

Light exerts a triggering effect on carotenogenesis in *N. crassa* (Zalokar, 1955), *P. blakesleeanus* (Chichester *et al.*, 1954) and *F. oxysporum* (Carlile, 1956). In *N. crassa*, for example, exposures of dark-grown cultures to light and oxygen for as short a period as one minute, stimulates such cultures, when returned to darkness and incubated aerobically, to synthesize carotenoids almost to the same extent as that obtained under permanent illumination. Oxygen is essential for both photo-activation and for dark synthesis of pigments after activation. The photo-activation is not temperature-dependent.

(d) *Oxygen.* The only anaerobes which synthesize carotenoids are the photosynthetic bacteria (see p. 274). Carotenoid levels are greatly reduced when *Rhodospirillum rubrum* is grown under semi-aerobic conditions (Goodwin and Osman, 1953) and synthesis is almost completely inhibited in *Rsp. rubrum* and *Rhodopseudomonas spheroides* growing under strongly aerobic conditions (Cohen-Bazire *et al.*, 1957).

(e) *Temperature.* The carotenoids produced by many carotenogenic fungi, e.g. *Rhodotorula rubra* and *R. penaus* (Nakayama *et al.*, 1954) and *Phycomyces blakesleeanus* (Friend and Goodwin, 1954) remain qualitatively the same over a wide temperature range, but, in general, the amounts synthesized are less the lower the temperature. However, in one case marked qualitative changes are associated with variation in temperature of cultivation (Skoda, 1951; Nakayama *et al.*, 1954). The yellow mycelia characteristic of low temperature (8°) cultural conditions contain predominantly (90%) α- and β-carotenes, whilst the red mycelia produced at 25° contain torulene and torularhodin as the major pigments. If 5° cultures are transferred to 28° then torulene and torularhodin are rapidly synthesized.

In the bacteria so far examined *Sarcina aurantiaca* (Reader, 1925), *Mycobact. phlei* (Goodwin and Jamikorn, 1956) and certain marine *Corynebact.* spp (Hodgkiss *et al.*, 1954) the situation is the opposite to that in fungi, low temperatures being more conducive to carotenogenesis than high temperatures. Furthermore, *Corynebact* spp. cultured at high temperatures (37°) do not resume pigment synthesis when transferred to low temperatures. High temperatures favour xanthophyll synthesis in *Mycobact. phlei* (Turian, 1953) but the effect is much less marked than in *R. gracilis*.

(f) *pH*. When *Phycomyces blakesleeanus* is cultivated on a standard glucose-asparagine medium, the pH of the culture drops from an initial value of 6·2 to around 2·6–3·0. If this change is prevented by buffering the medium, then although growth is normal, β-carotene synthesis is almost completely inhibited. Similarly if *P. blakesleeanus* is grown originally on a medium low in glucose, it will, when washed and resuspended in a glucose solution, synthesize β-carotene only if the medium is unbuffered (Goodwin and Willmer, 1952).

It has already been noted that on a glucose-NH_4NO_3 medium growth is stimulated by addition of small amounts (final concentration 0·02M) of any member of the tricarboxylic acid cycle (p. 295); stimulation of carotenogenesis, however, varies with the acid used. This variation is due to differences in the final pH of the medium in the presence of different acids. For example, if the citrate concentration is reduced from 0·02M to 0·01M the final pH is also lower and there is a corresponding increase in carotonegenesis (Friend *et al.*, 1955).

(g) *Growth factors*. Low thiamine levels tend to reduced carotenogenesis somewhat in *Phycomyces blakesleeanus* (Friend and Goodwin, 1954) and in *Bacillus lombardopelligrini* and *B. boquet* (Lutz, 1947). In *Corynebact. poinsettiae*, however, thiamine appears to play a much more important role; on a medium containing 0·1µg/ml thiamine, the colonies are pink and contain mainly lycoxanthin (? rhodopin) and spirilloxanthin; when the medium contains 100 µg/ml thiamine, orange colonies form in which the spirilloxanthin level is greatly reduced and cryptoxanthin, absent from the pink cultures, appears in relatively large amounts (a pink mutant of *Corynebact. poinsettiae* and *Corynebact. michiganese* behaves similarly) (Starr and Saperstein, 1953).

(h) *Inhibitors*. Various compounds have been shown to inhibit carotenogenesis in a number of organisms (see Goodwin, 1959a), but they have provided little information leading to a further understanding of the mechanism of carotenogenesis. Diphenylamine on the other hand, has proved a most useful compound in this connection. Its action has been discussed on p. 285; here it will be sufficient to indicate its effect on various organisms (Table 4). Other

TABLE 4. Organisms in which Diphenylamine inhibits Carotenogenesis
and Stimulates Synthesis of Colourless Polyenes

Organism	Reference
Non-photosynthetic bacteria	
Mycobact. phlei	Turian (1950), Turian and Haxo (1952), Goodwin and Jamikorn (1956)
Mycobact. spp.	Kühlwein (1953)
Neisseria spp.	Ellinghauser and Pelczar (1957)
Photosynthetic bacteria	
Rhodospirillum rubrum	Goodwin and Osman (1953, 1954), Cohen-Bazire and Stanier (1958)
Chromatium spp.	Goodwin and Land (1956)
Chlorobium spp.	Goodwin and Land (1956)
Fungi	
Allomyces spp.	Turian (1957), Turian and Haxo (1954)
Neurospora crassa	Turian (1957)
Phycomyces blakesleeanus	Goodwin (1952b)
Rhodotorula gracilis	Praus and Dyr (1957); Slechta *et al.* (1958)
Rhodotorula mucilaginosa	Villoutreix (1957, 1960)
Rhodotorula rubra	Wittman (1956)

compounds tested which have an effect similar to diphenylamine
are not numerous, they include methylheptenone (Mackinney *et al.*,
1952, 1953a,b) and 2-hydroxydiphenyl (Villoutreix, 1960), although
the latter does not cause the accumulation of large amounts of
colourless polyenes.

The effect of diphenylamine is not universal, for example, it
has no specific effect on any alga so far examined (Goodwin, 1954b;
Goodwin and Jamikorn, 1954) or on *Rhodopseudomonas* spp. (Goodwin, 1955) or seedlings of higher plants (Goodwin, 1958).

(i) *Stimulators.* One of the most interesting recent general observations in this field of carotenoids studies was that made by Barnett *et al.* (1956) who found that the amount of β-carotene produced separately by two mating types, ($+$) and ($-$) strains, of the
mould *Choanephora cucurbitarum* was stimulated more than ten
times when the two strains were grown in mixed culture. Stimulation also occurred if the two strains were separated by cellophane
during incubation. These observations have been confirmed by
Plempel (1957) and by Hesseltine and Anderson (1957) in a number

of the family *Choanephoraceae.* Under suitable conditions 38 mg of carotene (at least 75% of which is the β-isomer) is produced per 100 ml. of culture medium (Anderson *et al.*, 1958; Ciegler *et al.*, 1959). Table 5 summarizes the results obtained and also shows that a combination of vegetable oil, detergent and β-ionone are necessary for maximum yields. β-Ionone is particularly interesting in this respect, because Mackinney *et al.* (1952, 1953a,b) found that when it was added at an activator rather than a substrate level it stimulated carotenogenesis in *Phycomyces blakesleeanus.* However, neither [6-^{14}C]-nor [9-^{14}C]-β-ionone gave rise to labelled β-carotene

TABLE 5. Effect of various Medium Adjuncts on Carotene Production by *Blakslea trispora* (Anderson *et al.*, 1958)

Addition	Organisms		
	NRRL 2456(+)	NRRL 2457 (—)	2456x2547
	(Carotene production μg/100 ml medium)		
A. O*	420	470	1980
B. 4% Vegetable oil	560	400	4000
C. Ionone (0·1%)+	300	320	1760
D. Detergent	40	390	640
(Triton X-100, 0·12%)			
E. B+C	390	420	11000
F. B+D	1550	1080	6500
G. C+D	24	75	280
H. B+C+D	820	1490	12960

* Basal medium (g./l.). Acid-hydrolyzed maize, 75; acid-hydrolysed casein, 2; corn steep liquor, 5; KH_2PO_4, 0·5; thiamine HCl, 1·0 (mg.) pH 6·2. Shake cultures. Incubation time, 6 days.
+ Added aseptically to 2-day cultures.

(Engel *et al.*, 1953; Mackinney *et al.*, 1953b) and the addition of β-ionone did not dilute out the incorporation of [^{14}C]glucose into β-carotene (Chichester *et al.*, 1954). However, in heterothallic cultures of *Blakslea trispora* the effect of β-ionone appears to be at the substrate level (Ciegler *et al.*, 1959).

Resorcinol increases carotenoid production in *Penicillium sclerotiorum* (Motonaga and Miyanoue, 1961).

III. FORMATION OF VITAMIN A FROM CAROTENOIDS

A. *Structural Requirements*

Early investigators on carotenoid vitamin A interrelationships soon discovered that not all carotenoids were active as vitamin A precursors in animals, and before the mechanism of formation of vitamin A is considered it will be appropriate to summarize the structural criteria necessary for biological activity.

(i) *Structure of the ring.*

Table 6 lists the naturally occurring carotenoids which are active, and where known, their activity relative to β-carotene, which has the highest biological potency of all carotenoids. As α- and γ-carotenes are only one half as active as β-carotene

TABLE 6. Naturally Occurring Carotenoids with Vitamin A Activity

Name	Structure	Biological potency (β-carotene $=$ 100%)
α-Carotene	(III)	53
β-Carotene	(I)	100
γ-Carotene	(IV)	43
β-Zeacarotene	(XXIX)	40
Cryptoxanthin	(IX)	57
Echinenone	4-oxo-β-carotene (XXXIV)	44
β-Apo-8'-carotenal	(see Table 8)	40
Mutatochrome	5,8-epoxy-β-carotene (XXXV)	50

and as lycopene is biologically inactive, it follows that one β-ionone residue is a first essential for activity. The bio-

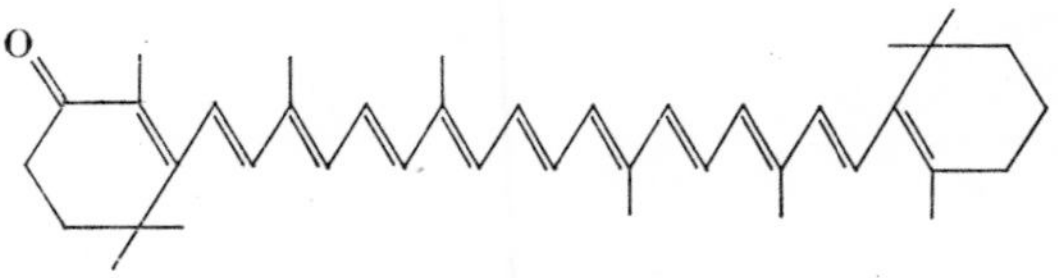

(XXXIV)

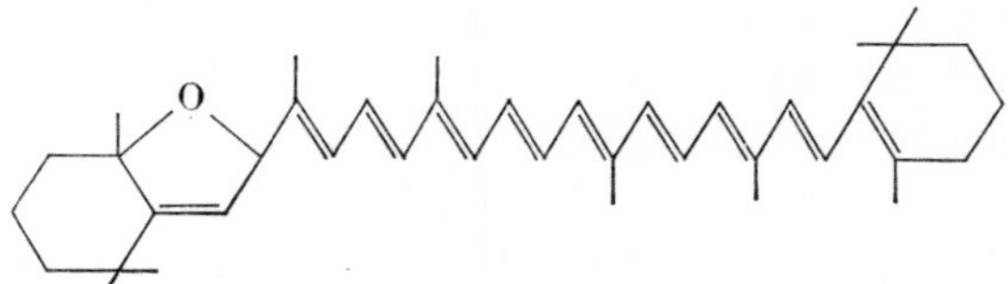

(XXXV)

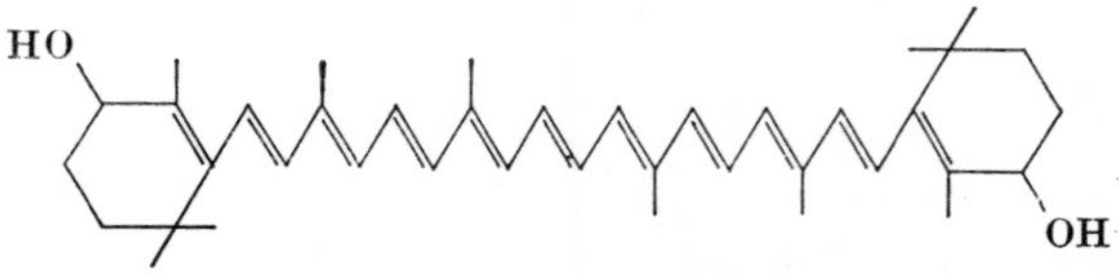

(XXXVI)

logical inactivity of lutein (VI), zeaxanthin (X) and isozeaxanthin (XXXVI) indicates that the β-ionone ring must not be hydroxylated (Isler and Zeller, 1957). 5,6-Epoxy derivatives with the remainder of the β-ionone ring unsubstituted, e.g. β-carotene 5,6,5',6'-diepoxide (XXXVII), have slight activity (Karrer *et al.*, 1945; Isler and Zeller, 1957); presumably the animal can to some extent remove the oxygen and convert the compound back into a β-carotene derivative in the body. On the other hand, 5,8-epoxides, e.g. aurochrome (XXXVIII) are biologically inactive (von Euler and

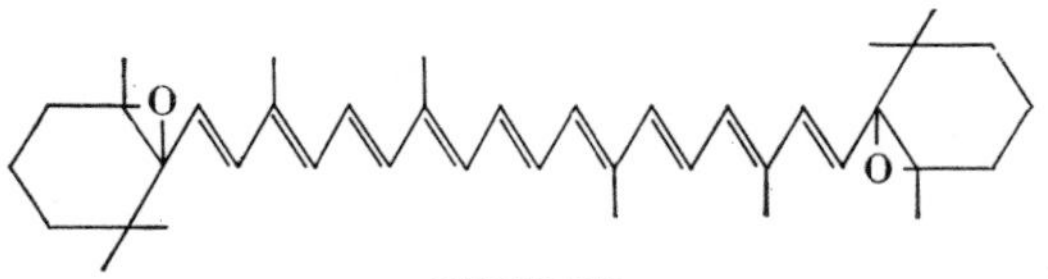

(XXXVII)

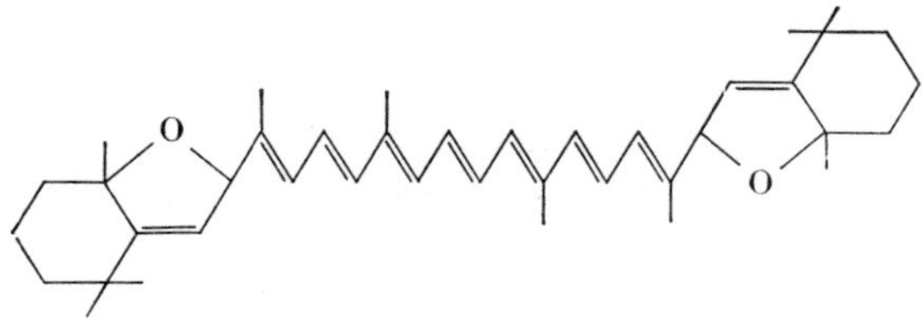

(XXXVIII)

Karrer, 1950). Variations in the structure of the β-ionone residue of the carotenoid molecule by organic chemists (see Isler and Zeller, 1957) have produced some compounds which still, somewhat surprisingly, retain activity (Table 7). Of particular interest is bis-dehydro-β-carotene (XXXIX) which theoretically would give rise vitamin A_2 (XLV). Its low activity is consistent with this (vitamin A_2 has only about 40% the activity of vitamin A), but no report has been published as to which vitamin appears in the liver on feeding this compound.

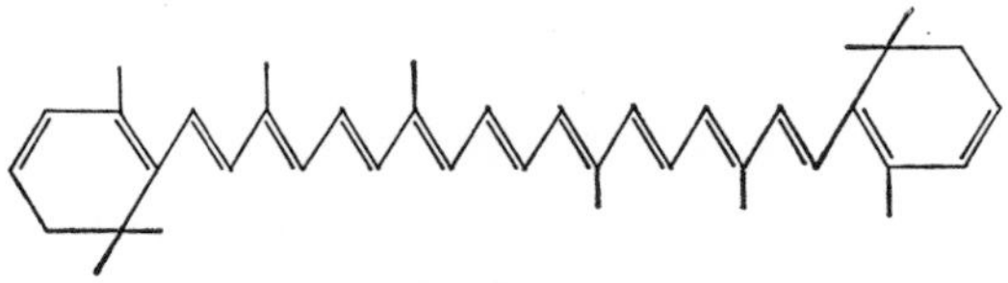

(XXXIX)

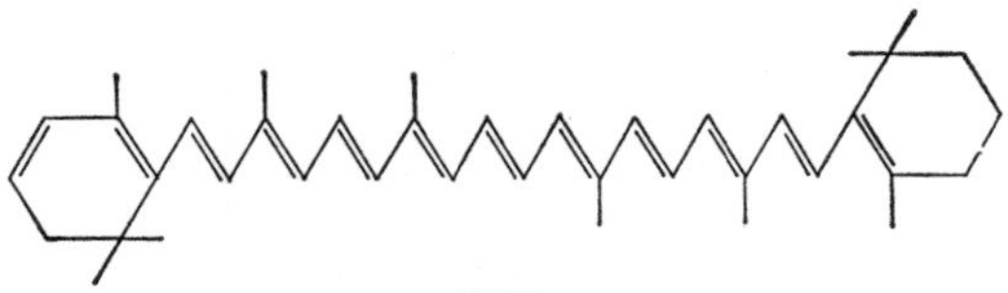

(XL)

TABLE 7. Synthetic Carotenoids with Vitamin A Activity (Isler and Zeller, 1957)

Name	Structure	Biological activity (β-carotene = 100%)
Bisdehydro-β-carotene	3, 4, 3', 4'-dehydro-β-carotene (**XXXIX**)	38
Monodehydro-β-carotene	3,4-dehydro-β-carotene (**XL**)	75
Isocryptoxanthin	4-hydoxy-β-carotene (**XLI**)	48
2,2'-Dimethyl-β-carotene	(**XLII**)	50
1-Desmethyl-1-ethyl-β-carotene	(**XLIII**)	53
1,1'-Bisdesmethyl-1,1'-diethyl-β-carotene	(**XLIV**)	38
β-Carotene diepoxide	5,6,5',6'-diepoxy-β-carotene (**XXXVII**)	15

The interesting report that astaxanthin (**XLVI**) maintains normal growth (Grangaud *et al.*, 1961) and vision but not reproduction

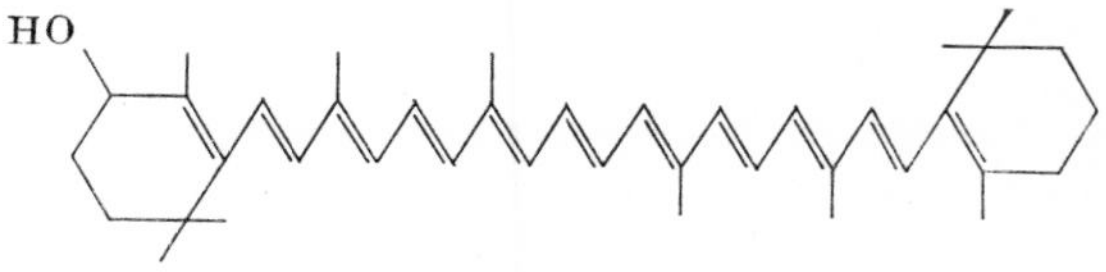

(XLI)

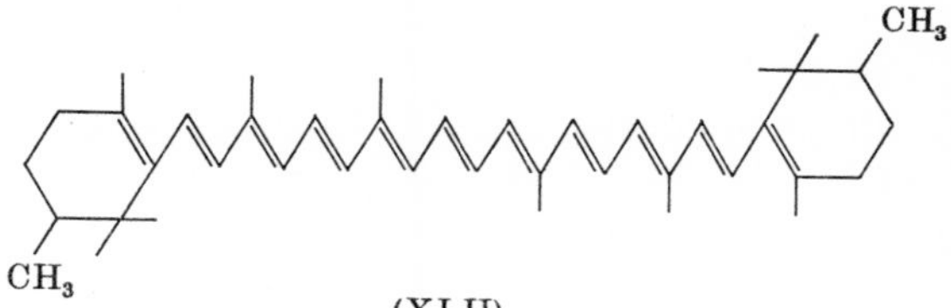

(XLII)

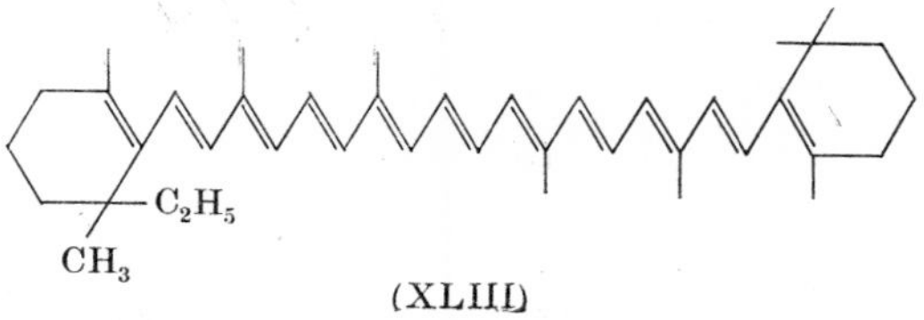

(XLIII)

in the albino rat (Massonet, 1957) appears to be an exception to the general rules just discussed. Astaxanthin is apparently far more effective in curing xerophthalmia than in stimulating growth (Grangaud *et al.*, 1961). It is also apparently a pro-vitamin A in the fish *Gambusia holbrookii* (Grangaud and Massonet, 1955; Grangaud *et al.*, 1956).

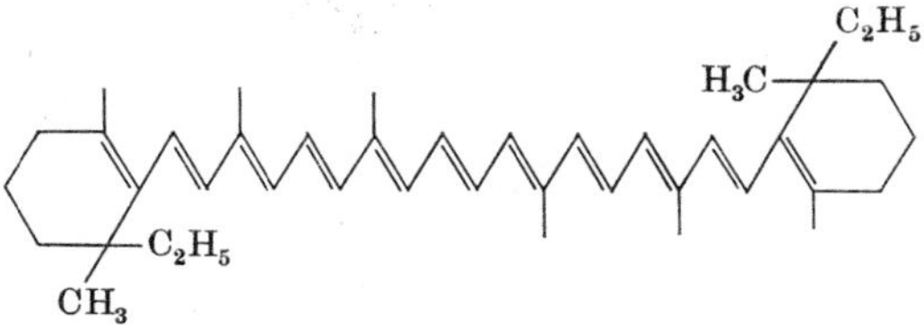

(XLIV)

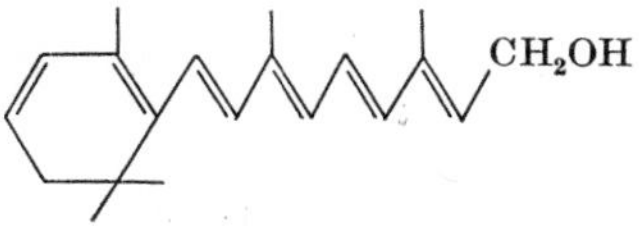

(XLV)

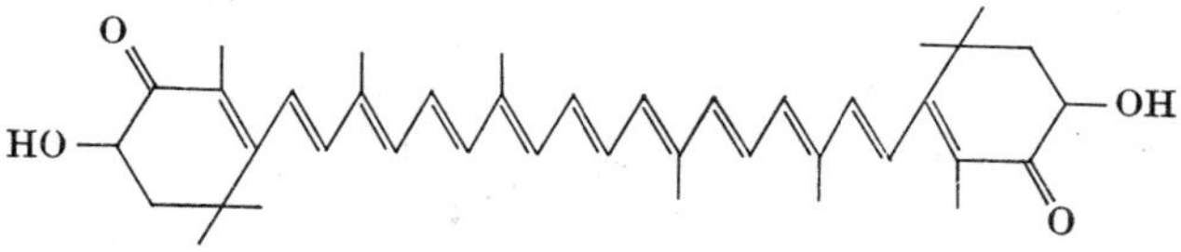

(XLVI)

(ii) *Structure of the chain.*

Unilateral degradation of the side chain of β-carotene yields a series of apocarotenoids, many of which have now been synthesized (see Glover, 1960a). All those which retain the vitamin A side chain intact are biologically active (Table 8). The quantitative variations observed in the activity of the apocarotenoid series will be considered later in relation to views on the mechanism of conversion of β-carotene into vitamin A. From the view of biological activity it matters little whether the terminal grouping of the apocarotenoid is an aldehyde, carboxyl or carbonyl grouping.

If the complete molecule of β-carotene is shortened as in Isler's "C_{30} model substance" (XLVII) or lengthened as in decapreno-β-carotene (XLVIII), biological activity is lost (Isler and Zeller, 1957). This would be expected in the case of (XLVII) because vitamin A cannot be obtained from it; however, it could theoretically be obtained from (XLVIII), but presumably this compound cannot fit on to the appropriate enzyme surface. On the other hand, 16,16'-

TABLE 8. Synthetic β-Apocarotenoids with Vitamin A Activity (Glover, 1960)

Name	Structure
β-Apo-8'-carotenal*	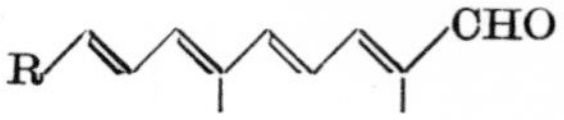
β-Apo-10'-carotenal	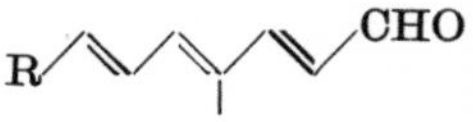
β-Apo-12'-carotenal	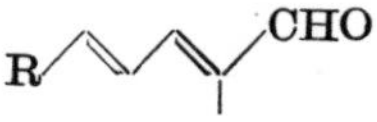
β-Apo-12'-carotenoic acid methyl ester	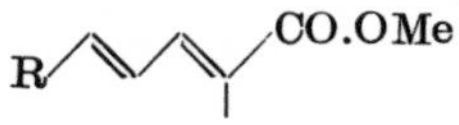
γ-(15-Hydroxyretinyl) tiglic acid methyl ester	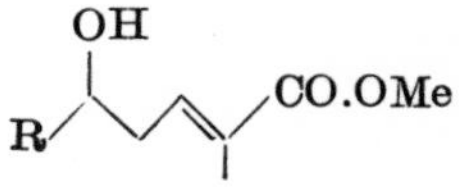
β-Apo-14'-carotenol	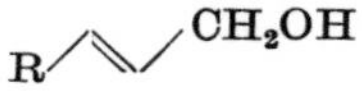
β-Apo-14'-carotenoic acid methyl ester	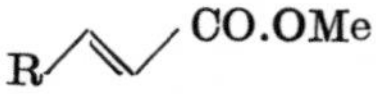
2-(15-Hydroxyretinyl) acetic acid methyl ester	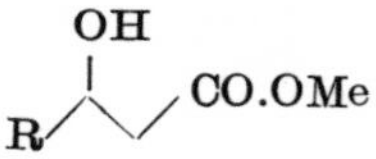

* R =

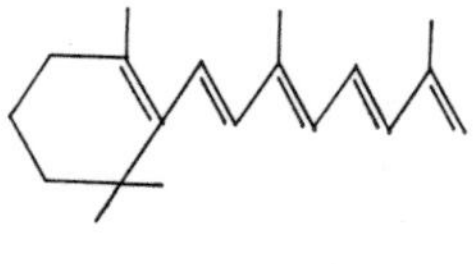

bishomo-β-carotene (XLIX) has biological activity (20% as active as all *trans* β-carotene) (Deuel *et al.*, 1952).

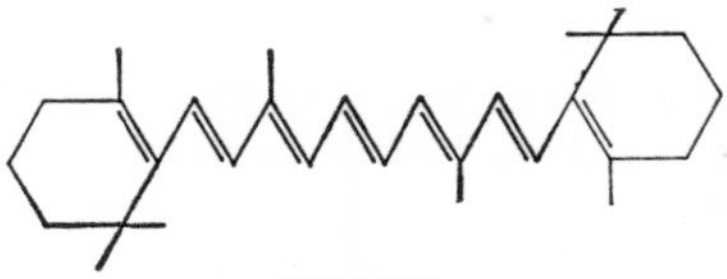

(XLVII)

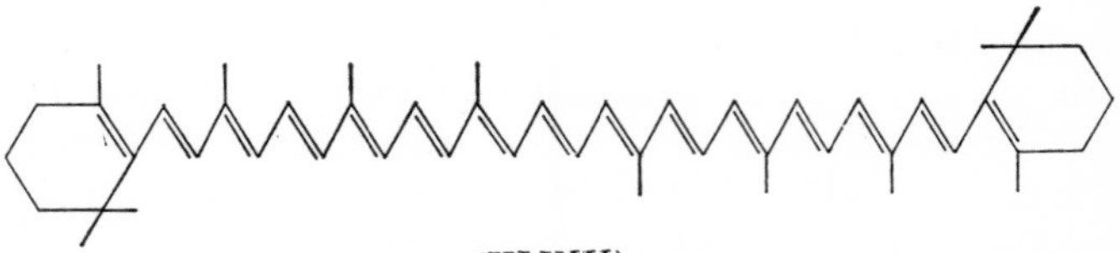

(XLVIII)

Any alteration in the isoprenoid nature of the chain of β-carotene, for example, removal of the methyl group at C-13 and C-13', removing two hydrogens as in dehydro-β-carotene (retro-β-carotene) (L) or addition of two hydrogens (7,7'-dihydro-β-carotene) (LI), completely destroys biological activity (Isler and Zeller, 1957).

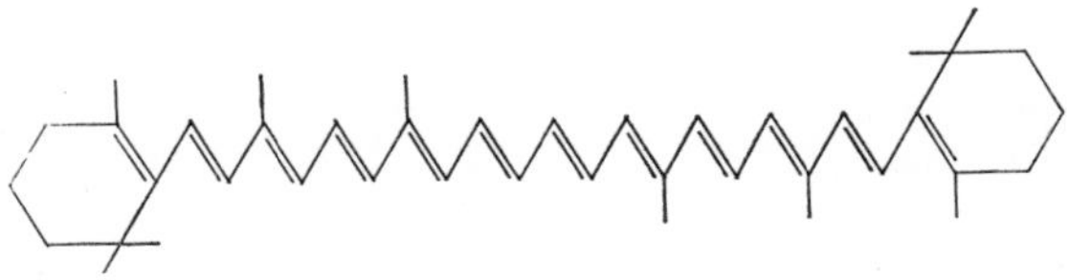

(XLIX)

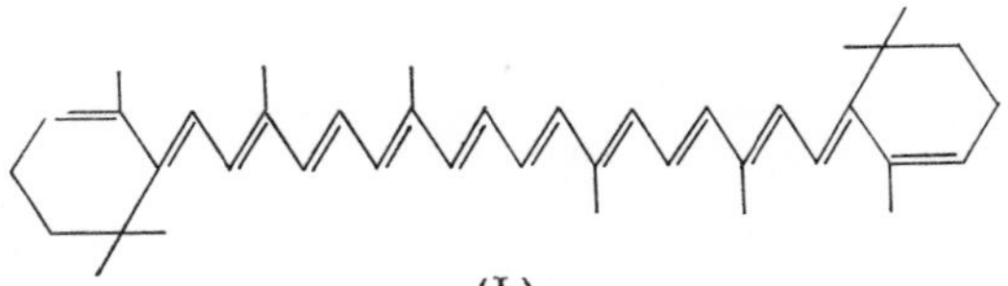

(L)

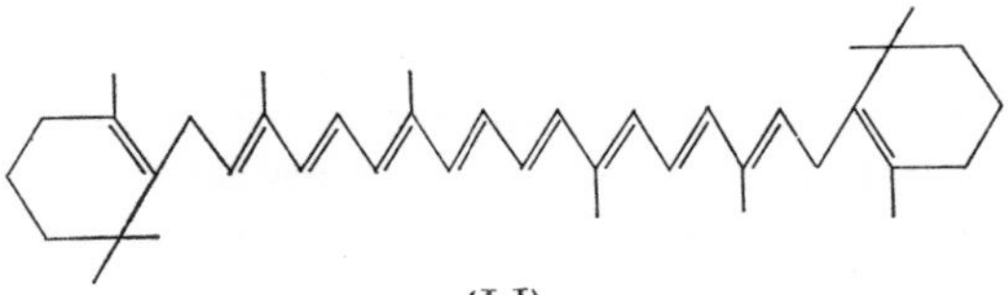

(LI)

(iii) *Stereoisomerization*

The effect of variation in the shape of the β-carotene molecule caused by *cis-trans* isomerization on the biopotency of the compound has been studied in detail by Zechmeister and Deuel and their colleagues (see e.g. Zechmeister, 1949). Table 9 shows how marked are the differences encountered in the activity of different isomers. The exact mechanism accounting for these variations has not yet been elucidated; the simplest possibility is that only the all *trans* form is active and that *cis* isomers are active only in so far as they can be isomerized back to the all *trans* form in the digestive tract. However, Zechmeister (1960) believes that the most important aspect of the problem is whether an isomer has the right shape to fit on to the enzyme surface. In support of this he quoted the observation that all *trans*-γ-carotene and pro-γ-carotene (a poly*cis* isomer of similar shape to the all *trans* molecule) have equal biological activity in the rat, and that in the chick pro-γ-carotene is, in fact, 25% more effective than the all *trans* isomer (Greenberg *et al.*, 1949).

TABLE 9. The Vitamin A Activity of *cis*-Isomers
of β-Carotene and γ-Carotene (Zechmeister, 1960)

Compound	Structure	Biological activity (β-carotene = 100)
β-Carotene isomers		
Central mono *cis*	15-*cis*	30-50
Neo-β-carotene U	9-*cis*	38
Neo-β-carotene B	9,13-di*cis*	53
11,11-di*cis**	—	30
γ-Carotene isomers		
All *trans*		43
Neo-γ-carotene P	—	19
Pro-γ-carotene*		43

* These compounds contain "hindered" *cis* configurations.

B. *Biochemistry of Conversion*

(i) *Site of conversion*

As β-carotene is the most important precursor of vitamin A, it has been the compound almost exclusively used in studies designed to elucidate the mechanism of the conversion of biologically active carotenoids into vitamin A.

Moore in 1929 first demonstrated the conversion of carotene into vitamin A and as the vitamin A formed accumulated in the liver, it was natural to assume that the conversion took place in that metabolically active organ. However, many experiments suggested that injected β-carotene was much less effective than ingested β-carotene (see Goodwin, 1952a), and eventually Sexton *et al.* (1946) in a thorough investigation showed that carotene administered parenterally by the intraperitoneal, intravenous, intrasplenic or intracardiac route, was ineffective in curing vitamin A deficiency. They pointed out that these investigations tended to implicate the intestine as the site of conversion and this was soon demonstrated in three different laboratories using goats and rats as experimental animals (Glover *et al.*, 1947, 1948; Goodwin and Gregory, 1948; Wiese *et al.*, 1947; Thompson *et al.*, 1947, 1949). All these conclusions were based on the observation that the feeding of β-carotene resulted in an increase in the vitamin A present in the thoracic lymph drawn off by a cannula set in the thoracic duct. Since these original experiments the intestinal conversion has been demonstrated in many other animal species (see Goodwin, 1952a). The possibility that the conversion was being carried out by the intestinal flora was ruled out by experiments with animals with sterile intestinal lumina (produced by treatment with sulphasuccidine) (Patel *et al.*, 1951). Later investigations have indicated that tissues other than the intestine can carry out the conversion of carotene into vitamin A (Bieri and Pollard, 1954; McGillivray *et al.*, 1956; Worker, 1956, 1959), but they are much less effective than the intestine. McGillivrary (1961) found that when carotene is injected intravenously it undergoes non-specific reactions which are initiated in the blood immediately after injection. Some of the products of these reactions are converted into vitamin A.

(ii) In vitro *conversion*

A great deal of effort has been expended without complete success in attempts to obtain a satisfactory *in vitro* system which will effectively convert β-carotene into vitamin A (Glover, 1960a,b; Worker, 1959). Such a preparation would materially help in working out the mechanism involved. Recently Olson (1960, 1961a,b, 1962) has reported that intestinal loops will carry out the reaction (about 2·5% conversion) provided bile salts are present to enhance the absorption of the substrates. The conversion requires oxygen, takes place in either a bicarbonate or phosphate buffer and does not require the presence of a divalent ion. The isolated intestines of the fish *Gambusia holbrooki* are reported to convert β-carotene and as taxanthin into vitamin A (Grangaud *et al*, 1961).

(iii) *Mechanism of conversion.*

Two possibilities exist (Fig. 4); (i) central fission at (a) (Fig. 4) to yield vitamin A aldehyde (retinene) (11, Fig. 4) which is reduced to vitamin A; (ii) the pathway of "attrition" by which β-carotene, following oxidation at (b) (Fig. 4), undergoes stepwise β-oxidation until vitamin A aldehyde is reached which, because of the methyl group on its β-carbon atom, cannot undergo further oxidation. One of the attractions of the attrition theory is that it would explain why β-carotene is twice as active as α-carotene or γ-carotene without having to invoke indeterminate factors such as "efficiency of conversion". A great deal of careful work by Glover and his colleagues (see Glover, 1960a, b) on the metabolism and biological activity of various β-apocarotenoids which could reasonably be expected to be intermediates in the stepwise degradation of β-carotene has forced them to the following conclusions: (a) that the attrition pathway is not the main metabolic route from β-carotene to vitamin A, and (b) that when vitamin A is formed from β-apocarotenoids, the degradation is not necessarily β-oxidative. They further found that after feeding [15,15′-^{14}C] -β-carotene to rats, the specific activity of the isolated [1-^{14}C]vitamin A was much higher than those of the isolated β-apocarotenoids; this confirms their previous conclusions from feeding experiments with non-isotopic material. The natural occurrence of β-apo-8′-carotenal supports the conclusion that stepwise degradation of β-carotene can take place in Nature to some extent (Brubacher *et al.*, 1960).

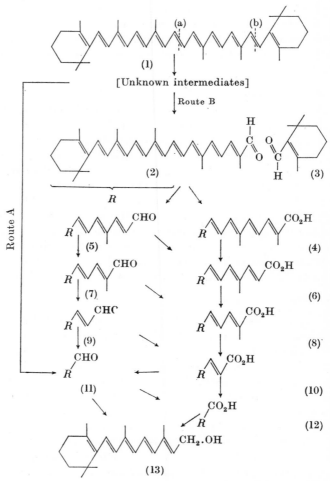

Fig. 4. Possible mechanisms for the conversion of β-carotene into vitamin A (Glover, 1960a).

One therefore returns to the central fission theory as being the most probable, and the main support for this is nutritional. It has been claimed that under optimal conditions one molecule of β-carotene is converted into two molecules of vitamin A (Koehn, 1948; Burns *et al.*, 1951). However, there are many earlier reports which indicate that the conversion is much less efficient (see Goodwin, 1952a; Glover, 1960b). The mechanism of the conversion is still undecided, but the attack is probably oxidative, because Olson, as indicated above, states that O_2 is required, and because retinene a potential product of oxidative fission, is very rapidly reduced to vitamin A in the intestinal mucosae (Glover *et al.*, 1948).

C. *Interconversion of Vitamin A and Retinene*

(i) *General*.

Retinene, vitamin A aldehyde (LII) is the prosthetic group of rhodopsin, the photosensitive pigment for scotopic or dimlight vision (Wald, 1943). It also exists in a bound form in eggs of many animals (Plack *et al.*, 1957, 1959). Obviously retinene must be formed *in vivo* from vitamin A and Wald and Hubbard (1948–1949) and Bliss (1949) demonstrated that the enzyme *alcohol dehydrogenase* [alcohol: NAD oxidoreductase] is present in the retina and, in the presence of NAD as co-factor, carries out the reversible reaction (7). As already noted retinene is rapidly converted into vitamin A in

$$\text{Vitamin A} + \text{NAD}^+ \quad \rightleftarrows \quad \text{retinene} + \text{NADH} + \text{H}^+$$

$$\text{C}_{19}\text{H}_{27}\text{CH}_2\text{OH} \qquad\qquad \text{C}_{19}\text{H}_{27}\text{CHO} \tag{7}$$

the intestinal mucosae which suggests that the equilibrium of reaction is far over to the left. This was shown to be so in the retina (Bliss, 1951). Retinene of the right spatial configuration (see below) combines with the specific retinal protein, opsin, spontaneously (Wald and Brown, 1950); the removal of retinene in this way stimulates its continued production from vitamin A, in spite of the unfavourable equilibrium.

(ii) *Stereoisomers of Vitamin A and Retinene*.

In 1953 Hubbard and Wald found that all-*trans*-retinene (LII), synthesized from all-*trans* vitamin A, would not combine *in vitro* with opsin; on the other hand, if the retinene were first isomerized by exposure to light, then part of the isomerized material reacted readily with opsin. Eventually after numerous painstaking investigations (see Morton and Pitt, 1957), it was discovered that only one *cis*-isomer, the 11-*cis*-isomer (LIII), would combine with opsin to form rhodopsin. However, the product liberated during the bleaching by light of rhodopsin synthesized *in vitro* from 11-*cis*-retinene is all-*trans*-retinene (Wald and Brown, 1956). So, in order to complete the visual cycle (Fig. 5) and regenerate rhodopsin, all-*trans*-retinene must be isomerized to 11-*cis*-retinene. Non-enzymatic photo-isomerization is ruled out because, (a) in this case a mixture of isomers would be obtained; (b) free retinene is not present in the eye in significant amounts

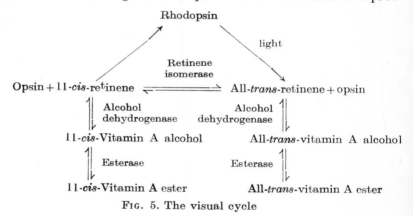

(Krinsky, 1958), and (c) the activating wavelengths are mainly in the violet and ultraviolet region of the spectrum and little of radiations of these wavelengths would penetrate to the retina. The prob-

FIG. 5. The visual cycle

lem was resolved when Hubbard (1955–1956) discovered an enzyme, *retinene isomerase* [all-*trans*-retinene 11-*cis-trans*-isomerase], in the retina which isomerize all-*trans*-retinene specifically to 11-*cis*-retinene. In the dark the equilibrium mixture contains 95% all-*trans*-retinene, and in *in vitro* experiments the enzyme does not appear to work fast enough to account for the rate of regeneration of rhodopsin in the living eye. Either (a) the enzyme functions more efficiently *in vivo* or (b) 11-*cis*-retinene can also be formed from 11-*cis*-vitamin

A, by the action of alcohol dehydrogenase. This implies the isomerization of vitamin A itself, but an enzyme for this reaction has not yet been described. However, the process must occur and be very effective in some invertebrates; in the euphausiid crustacean *Meganyctiphanes norvegica*, for example, at least 90% of the vitamin A in the eye is in the 11-*cis* configuration (Wald and Burg, 1956–7; Wald and Brown, 1956–7).

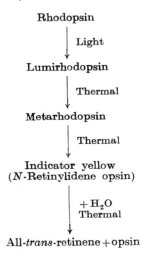

FIG. 6. The action of light on rhodopsin.

It is interesting to find that much smaller doses of 11-*cis*-vitamin A than of all-*trans*-vitamin A are required for maintaining normal vision in rats whereas the reverse is true with respect to growth-promoting activity (Chatzinoff *et al.*, 1958).

It is not appropriate here to discuss in detail the action of light on rhodopsin. This has recently been dealt with authoritatively by Wald (1960) and by Pitt and Morton (1960). The overall effect is indicated in Fig. 6 but this clearly remains incomplete (see Hubbard and Kropf, 1960).

D. *Vitamin A_2*

Vitamin A_2 (XLV) occurs mainly in fresh water fish, but it is also present in small amounts in marine fish; it occurs together with vitamin A in marine amphibia (Morton, 1960). In fresh water fish, retinene₂ (LIV) effectively replaces retinene as the visual pigment, giving rise to porphyropsin; furthermore, in some species which do not produce any vitamin A (Balasundaran *et al.*, 1956) vitamin A_2 must also function in all the systemic activities of vitamin A. However, in rats it has only about 30–40% of the biological activity of vitamin A.

(LIV)   (LV)

Little is known about the formation of vitamin A_2; in 1939 Morton and Creed fed β-carotene to dace and perch and noted an accumulation of vitamin A_2 in the liver oils. The dehydrogenation of the β-ionone ring could occur at the carotene level, or vitamin A could be first formed and then converted into vitamin A_2. The latter appears to be the pathway which occurs in the liver of the fresh water fish *Gambusia holbrookii* (Grangaud and Moatti, 1958), but confirmatory reports have not yet appeared.

Vitamin A_2 cannot be reduced to vitamin A in mammalian livers (Shantz *et al.*, 1946), but this change does appear to take place in amphibia. Wald (1946) showed that the tadpoles of *Rana catesbiana* have retinene$_2$ as the prosthetic group of their visual pigment; this is replaced by retinene during metamorphosis. This was confirmed by Wilt (1959) who showed that the change also occurred *without feeding*, when metamorphosis was induced by thyroxine.

However, in other amphibia this situation is not so clear cut; for example, retinene$_2$ is found in adult newts *Triturus cristatus* and *T. carnifex* (Collins *et al.*, 1953) and retinene in the larvae of *Bufo marinus* (Peskin, 1957).

E. *Vitamin A Acid*

This substance (LV), which was first synthesized by Arens and Van Dorp (1946) is as potent as vitamin A in the growth bioassay if it is injected as the sodium salt (Arens and Van Dorp, 1946); on the other hand, its activity when given orally is much less than vitamin A [10% according to Arens and Van Dorp (1946) and 42% according to Kofler and Rubin (1960)]. The fascinating aspect of the biochemistry of vitamin A acid is that it appears to function without being converted into vitamin A. This observation suggested that it was the metabolically active form of vitamin A, and would explain away the fact that in many tissues where vitamin A appears to be functional e.g. in epithelial tissues, vitamin A itself cannot be detected (Sharman, 1949). Recent work indicates that although more than one form of active vitamin A exists, all forms can be produced from vitamin A, but some cannot be formed from vitamin A acid; for example, vitamin A acid cannot be converted into visual pigments (Dowling and Ward, 1960) and will not function in the activities of the reproductive cycle which are dependent on vitamin A (Thompson *et. al.*, 1961); furthermore, it will not cure external eye lesions in the chick (Krishnamurthy and Bieri, 1962).

At present there is no evidence that vitamin A acid is a natural product. Varandani *et al.* (1961) for example, injected labelled vitamin A intraperitoneally into rats and vitamin A acid could not be detected amongst the labelled metabolites isolated 16 hours later. However, the oxidation of retinene to vitamin A acid is reported to be brought about in the rat jejunum (Dmitrovskii, 1961) and by liver *aldehyde dehydrogenase* [aldehyde: NAD oxidoreductase], *liver aldehyde oxidase* [aldehyde: O_2 oxidoreductase] and milk *xanthine oxidase* [xanthine: O_2 oxidoreductase] (Weissbach *et al.*, 1961; Futterman, 1962; Futterman and Richardson, 1962). Furthermore, Krishnamurthy and Bieri (1962) have recent reported that studies with [6,7-^{14}C]vitamin A acid injected into chicks indicate that most of the dose is firmly bound to protein and that a significant amount of activity is not extracted by ethanol-ether even after acidification of the homogenate.

REFERENCES

Anderson, D. G., Norgard, D. W., and Porter, J. W. (1960). *Arch. Biochem. Biophys.* 88, 68.

Anderson, D. G., and Porter, J. W. (1961). *Fed. Proc.* 20, 350; *Plant Physiol.* 36, XIV; *Comm. 5th Int. Cong. Biochem. Moscow*, Pergamon Press London, p. 45.

Anderson, D. G., and Porter, J. W. (1962). *Arch. Biochem. Biophys.* 94, 509.

Anderson, I. C. and Robertson, D. S. (1960). *Plant Physiol.* 35, 531.

Anderson, R. F., Arnold, M., Nelson, G. E. N., and Ciegler, A. (1957). *Abst.* 132nd *Meeting Amer. Chem. Soc.*, p. 17A.

Anderson, R. F., Arnold, M., Nelson, G. E. N., and Ciegler, A. (1958). *Agric. Food Chem.* 6., 543.

Arens, J. F., and Van Dorp, D. A. (1946). *Nature, Lond.* 157, 1960; 158, 60, 622.

Arnaki, M., and Stary, Z. (1952). *Biochem. Z.* 323, 376.

Balasundaran, S., Cama, H. R., Sunderasan, P. R., and Varma, T. N. R. (1956). *Biochem. J.* 64, 150.

Bandurski, R. S. (1949). *Botan. Gaz.* 111, 95.

Bandurski, R. S., Scott, F. M., Pflug, M., and Went, F. W. (1953). *Amer. J. Bot.* 40, 41.

Barlow, G. B., and Patrick, A. D. (1958). *Nature, Lond.* 182, 662.

Beeler, D., and Porter, J. W. (1962). *Biochem. biophys. Res. Comm.* 8, 367

Barnett, H. L., Lilly, V. G., and Krause, R. F. (1956). *Science* 123, 141.

314 THE BIOSYNTHESIS OF VITAMINS AND RELATED COMPOUNDS

Benedict, C. R., Fuller, R. C., and Bergeron, J. A. (1961). *Biochim. biophys. Acta*, **54**, 525.
Bieri, J. G., and Pollard, C. J. (1954). *Brit. J. Nutrit.* **8**, 32.
Blass, U., Anderson, J. M., and Calvin, M. (1959). *Plant Physiol.* **34**, 329.
Bliss, A. F. (1949). *Biol. Bull.* **97**, 221.
Bliss, A. F. (1951). *Arch. Biochem. Biophys.* **31**, 197.
Braithwaite, G. D., and Goodwin, T. W. (1957). *Biochem. J.* **67**, 13P.
Braithwaite, G. D., and Goodwin, T. W. (1958). *Nature, Lond.* **182**, 1304.
Braithwaite, G. D., and Goodwin, T. W. (1960). *Biochem. J.* **76**, 1, 5, 194.
Brubacher, G., Gloor, U., and Wiss, O. (1960). *Chimia*, **14**, 19.
Burns, M. J., Hauge, S. M., and Quackenbush, F. W. (1951). *Arch. Biochem. Biophys.* **30**, 341, 347.
Carlile, M. J. (1956). *J. gen. Microbiol.* **14**, 643.
Chatzinoff, A., Millman, N., Oroshnik, W., and Rosen, F. (1958). *Amer. J. Ophthal.* **46**, 205.
Chichester, C. O., Wong, P. S., and Mackinney, C. (1954). *Plant Physiol.* **29**, 238.
Chichester, C. O., Nakayama, T., Mackinney, G., and Goodwin, T. W. (1955). *J. biol. Chem.* **214**, 575.
Chichester, C. O., Yokoyama, H., Nakayama, T. O. M., Lukton, A. and Mackinney, G. (1959). *J. biol. Chem.*, **234**, 598.
Ciegler, A., Arnold, M., and Anderson, R. F. (1959) *Appl. Microbiol.*, **7**, 94, 98
Claes, H. (1954). *Z. Naturforsch.* **9b**, 461.
Claes, H. (1956). *Z. Naturforsch.* **11b**, 260.
Claes, H. (1957). *Z. Naturforsch.* **12b**, 401.
Claes, H. (1958). *Z. Naturforsch.* **13b**, 222.
Claes, H. (1959). *Z. Naturforsch.* **14b**, 4.
Cohen, R. Z., and Goodwin, T. W. (1962). *Phytochemistry* **1**, 67.
Cohen-Bazire, G., Sistrom, W. R., and Stainer, R. Y. (1957). *J. cell. comp. Physiol.* **49**, 25.
Cohen-Bazire, G., and Stanier, R. Y. (1958). *Nature, Lond.* **181**, 250.
Collins, F. D., Love, R. M., and Morton, R. A. (1953). *Biochem. J.* **53**, 629, 632.
Davies, B. H. (1961). *Phytochem.* **1**, 25; *Biochem. J.* **80**, 48P.
Davies, B. H., and Goodwin, T. W. (1959). *Biochem. J.* **73**, 10P.
Davies, B. H., Goodwin, T. W., and Mercer, E. I. (1961) *Biochem. J.* **81**, 40P.
Davies, B. H., Jones, D., and Goodwin, T. W. (1963) *Biochem. J.* **87**, 326.
Davis, J. B., Jackman, L. M., Siddons, P. T., and Weedon, B. C. L. (1961). *Proc. chem. Soc.* p. 261.
Decker, K., and Uehleke, H. (1961). *Hoppe-Seyl. Z.* **323**, 61.
Deuel, H. J. Jr., Inhoffen, H. H., Ganguly, J., Wallcave, L., and Zechmeister, L. (1952). *Arch. Biochem. Biophys.* **40**, 352.
Dituri, F., Rabinowitz, J. L., Hullin, R. P., and Gurin, S. (1957). *J. biol. Chem.* **229**, 825.
Dmitrovskii, A. A. (1961). *Biokhimiya*, **26**, 126.
Dowling, J. E., and Wald, G. (1960). *Vitam. and Horm.* **18**, 515.
Ellinghauser, H. C., and Pelczar, M. J. (1957). *J. Bact.* **73**, 130.
Engel, B. G., Würsch, J., and Zimmermann, M. (1953). *Helv. chim. Acta* **36**, 1771.
Friend, J., and Goodwin, T. W. (1954). *Biochem. J.* **57**, 434.
Friend, J., Goodwin, T. W., and Griffiths, L. A. (1955). *Biochem. J.* **60**, 649.
Futterman, S. (1962). *J. biol. Chem.* **237**, 677.
Futterman, S., and Richardson, D. C. (1962). *Fed. Proc.* **21**, 473.
Garton, G. A., Goodwin, T. W., and Lijinsky, W. (1961). *Biochem. J.* **48**, 154.
Glover, J. (1960a). *Ann. Reps. Chem. Soc.* **56**, 331.
Glover, J. (1960b). *Vitam. & Horm.*, **18**, 371.
Glover, J., Goodwin, T. W., and Morton, R. A. (1947). *Biochem. J.* **41**, xiv.

Glover, J, Goodwin, T. W., and Morton, R. A. (1948). *Biochem. J.* **43**, 109, 512.
Glover, J., and Redfearn, E. R. (1953). *Biochem. J.* **54**, viii.
Goodwin, T. W. (1952a). "The Comparative Biochemistry of the Carotenoids", Chapman and Hall, London.
Goodwin, T. W. (1952b). *Biochem. J.* **50**, 550.
Goodwin, T. W. (1954a). *Biochem. J.* **58**, 90.
Goodwin, T. W. (1954b). *Experientia*, **10**, 213.
Goodwin, T. W. (1955). *Souvenir Soc. Biol. Chem. Ind.* p. 271.
Goodwin, T. W. (1956). *Arch. Mikrobiol.* **24**, 313.
Goodwin, T. W. (1958). *Biochem. J.* **70**, 503, 612.
Goodwin, T. W. (1959a). *Advances in Enzymol.* **21**, 295.
Goodwin, T. W. (1959b). *In* "Biosynthesis of Terpenes and Sterols" (Wolstenholme G. E. W., and O'Connor, M., eds.) Churchill, London.
Goodwin, T. W. (1960). "Recent Advances in Biochemistry". Churchill, London.
Goodwin, T. W. (1962a). *In* "Comparative Biochemistry" (M. Florkin and H. S. Mason, eds.) Vol. 4, Academic Press, New York.
Goodwin, T. W. (1962b). "Proceedings of the 5th International Congress of Biochemistry, Moscow.", Pergamon Press, London **7,** 294.
Goodwin, T. W. (1962c). *Wiss., Veroff. des Dtsch. Gesell. für Ernahrung*, **9**, 1
Goodwin, T. W., and Gregory, R. A. (1948) *Biochem. J.* **43**, 505.
Goodwin, T. W., Griffiths, L. A., and Modi, V. V. (1956b). *Biochem. J.* **62**, 259.
Goodwin, T. W., and Henshall, J. D. (1962). Unpublished observations.
Goodwin, T. W., and Jamikorn, M. (1952). *Nature, Lond.* **170**, 104.
Goodwin, T. W., and Jamikorn, M. (1954). *J. Protozool.* **1**, 216.
Goodwin, T. W., and Jamikorn, M. (1956). *Biochem. J.* **62**, 269, 275.
Goodwin, T. W., Jamikorn, M., and Willmer, J. S. (1953). *Biochem. J.* **53**, 51.
Goodwin, T. W., and Land, D. G. (1956). *Arch. Mikrobiol.* **24**, 305.
Goodwin, T. W., and Land, D. G. (1956). *Biochem. J.* **62**, 553.
Goodwin, T. W., Land, D. G., and Osman, H. G. (1955). *Biochem. J.* **59**, 491.
Goodwin, T. W., Land, D. G., and Sissins, M. E. (1956a). *Biochem. J.* **64**, 486.
Goodwin, T. W., and Lijinsky, W. (1952). *Biochem. J.* **50**, 268.
Goodwin, T. W., and Osman, H. G. (1953). *Biochem. J.* **53**, 541.
Goodwin, T. W., and Osman, H. G. (1954). *Biochem. J.* **56**, 222.
Goodwin, T. W., and Phagpolngarm, S. (1960). *Biochem. J.* **76**, 197.
Goodwin, T. W., and Willmer, J. S. (1952). *Biochem. J.*, **51,** 323.
Grangaud, R., and Massonet, R. (1955). *C. R. Acad. Sci., Paris* **241**, 1087.
Grangaud, R., Vignais, P., Massonet, R., and Moatti, J. P. (1956). *C.R. Acad. Sci., Paris* **243**, 170.
Gragaud, R., and Moatti, J. (1958). *C. R. Soc. Biol., Paris*, **152,** 1245.
Grangaud, R., Massonet, R., Conquy, J., and Ridolfo, J. (1961) *C. R. Acad. Sci., Paris* **252**, 1854; **253**, 336.
Greenberg, S. M., Calbert, C. E., Pinckard, J. H., Deuel, H. J. Jr., and Zechmeister, L. (1949). *Arch. Biochem.* **24**, 31.
Griffiths, M., Sistrom, W. R., Cohen-Bazire, G., and Stanier, R. Y. (1955) *Nature, Lond.* **176**, 1211.
Griffiths, W. T., Goodwin, T. W., Mercer, E. I., and Treharne, K. J. (1962). (Unpublished)
Grob, E. C. (1959). *In* "Biosynthesis of Terpenes and Sterols". G. E. W., Wolstenholme, and M. O'Connor (ed.) Churchill, London
Grob, E. C., and Boschetti, A. (1962). *Chimia*, **16,** 15.
Grob, E. C., and Bütler, R. (1954). *Helv. chim. Acta* **37**, 1908.
Grob, E. C., and Bütler, R. (1955). *Helv. chim. Acta* **38**, 1313.
Grob, E. C., and Bütler, R. (1956). *Helv. chim. Acta* **39**, 1975.
Grob, E. C., Kirschner, K., and Lynen, F. (1961). *Chimia* **15**, 308.

Haas, H. F., and Bushnell, L. D. (1944). *J. Bact.* **48**, 219.
Handke, M. H. (1954). *Wiss. nat. Z. Martin Luther Univ. Halle-Wittenberg* **4**, 89.
Haxo, F. (1952). *Biol. Bull.* **103**, 286.
Haxo, F. (1956). *Fortschr. Chem. org. Naturst.* **12**, 169.
Haxo, F. T., and Clendenning, K. A. (1953). *Biol. Bull.* **105**, 103.
Heilbron, I. M. (1942). *J. chem. Soc.*, p. 79.
Hendricks, S. B., and Borthwick, H. A. (1959). *Proc. Nat. Acad. Sci., Wash.*, **45**, 344.
Hesseltine, C. W., and Anderson, R. F. (1957). *Mycologia*, **49**, 449.
Hodgkiss, W., Liston, J., Goodwin, T. W., and Jamikorn, M. (1954). *J. gen. Microbiol.* **11**, 438.
Hopkins, F. G. (1912). *J. Physiol.* **44**, 425.
Hubbard, R. (1955–1956). *J. gen. Physiol.* **39**, 935.
Hubbard, R., and Kropf, A. (1960). *Nature, Lond.* **188**, 68.
Hubbard, R., and Wald, G. (1953). *J. gen. Physiol.* **36**, 415.
Hutner, S., and Provasoli, L. (1951). *In* "Protozoa", (A. Lwoff ed.) Academic Press, New York.
Isler, O., and Zeller, P. (1957). *Vitam. & Horm.* **15**, 31.
Jackman, L. M., and Jensen, S. L. (1961). *Acta chem. scand.* **15**, 2058.
Jensen, S. L. (1959). *Acta chem. scand.* **13**, 842, 2142, 2143.
Jensen, S. L. (1960). *Acta chem. scand.* **14**, 953.
Jensen, S. L. (1961). *Acta chem. scand.* **15**, xl.
Jensen, S. L. (1963). *Acta chem. scand.* **17**, 500.
Jensen, S. L. Cohen-Bazire, G., and Stanier, R. Y. (1961). *Nature, Lond.* 192, 1168.
Jensen, S. L., Cohen-Bazire, G., Nakayama, T. O. M., and Stanier, R. Y. (1958). *Biochim. biophys. Acta.* **29**, 477.
Karrer, P., Jucker, E., Rutschmann, J., and Steinlin, K. (1945). *Helv. chim. Acta* **28**, 1150.
Karrer, P., and Jucker, E. (1950). "Carotenoids" (trs. E. A. Braude). Elsevier, Amsterdam.
Kay, R. E., and Phinney, B. (1956). *Plant Physiol.* **31**, 226.
Koehn, C. J. (1948). *Arch. Biochem. Biophys.* **17**, 337.
Kofler, M., and Rubin, S. H. (1960). *Vitamins & Hormones*, 18, 315.
Krezeminski, L. F., and Quackenbush, F. W. (1960). *Arch. Biochem. Biophys.* **88**, 267.
Krinsky, N. I. (1962). *Fed. Proc.* **21**, 92.
Krinsky, N. I. (1958). *J. biol. Chem.* **232**, 881.
Krishnamurthi, S., and Bieri, J. G. (1962). *Fed. Proc.* **21**, 475.
Kuhlwein, H. (1953). *Arch. Mikrobiol.* **19**, 363.
Lincoln, R. E., and Porter, J. W. (1950). *Genetics*, **35**, 206.
Lotspeich, F. J., Krauss, R. F., Lilly, V. G., and Barnett, H. L. (1959). *J. biol. Chem.*, **234**, 3109.
Lotspeich, F. J., Krause, R. F., Lilly, V. G., and Barnett, H. L. (1961), *Fed. Proc.* **20**, 269.
Lutz, A. (1947). *Ann. Inst. Pasteur*, **73**, 1089.
McCollum, S. P. (1954). *Food Res.* **19**, 182.
McCollum, E. V., and Davis, M. (1913). *J. biol. Chem.* **15**, 167.
McCollum, E. V., and Davis, M. (1914). *J. biol. Chem.* **19**, 245.
McCollum, E. V., Simmonds, N., Becker, J. E., and Shipley, P. G. (1922). *J. biol. Chem.*, **53**, 293.
McGillivray, W. A. (1961). *Brit. J. Nutrit.* **15**, 313.
McGillivray, W. A., Thompson, S. Y., and Worker, N. A. (1956). *Brit. J. Nutrit.* **10**, 126.

Mackinney, G., Chandler, B. V., and Lukton, A. (1958). *Comm. 4th Int. Cong. Biochem.* Vienna, p. 130.

Mackinney, G., Nakayama, T., Buss, C. D., and Chichester, C. O. (1952). *J. Amer. chem. Soc.* **74**, 3456.

Mackinney, G., Chichester, C. O., and Wong, P. S. (1953a). *J. Amer. chem. Soc.* **75**, 5428.

Mackinney, G., Nakayama, T., Chichester, C. O., and Buss, C. D. (1953b). *J. Amer. chem. Soc.* **75**, 236.

Mackinney, G., Rick, C. M., and Jenkins, J. A. (1956). *Proc. nat. Acad. Sci., Wash.* **42**, 404.

Mapson, L. W., and Cruickshank, E. M. (1947). *Biochem. J.* **41**, 197.

Mase, Y., Rabourn, W. J., and Quackenbush, F. W. (1957). *Arch. Biochem. Biophys.* **68**, 150.

Massonet, R. (1957). *Arch. sci. Physiol.* **11**, 223.

Mathews, M. M., and Sistrom, W. R. (1959). *J. Bact.* **78**, 778.

Mego, J. L., and Jagendorf, A. T. (1963). *Biochim. biophys. Acta* **53**, 237.

Mercer, E. I., Davies, B. H., and Goodwin, T. W. (1963). *Biochem. J.* **87**, 317.

Modi, V. V., and Patwa, D. K. (1961). *Enzymol.* **23**, 27.

Moore, T. (1929). *Lancet* i, 490; *Biochem. J.* **23**, 803.

Moore, T. (1957). "Vitamin A." Elsevier, New York.

Morton, R. A. (1960). *Vitam., & Horm.* **18**, 543.

Morton, R. A., and Creed, R. H. (1939). *Biochem. J.* **33**, 318.

Morton, R. A., and Pitt, G. A. J. (1957). *Fortschr. Chem. org. Naturst.* **14**, 244.

Moster, J. B. and Quackenbush, F. W. (1952). *Arch. Biochem. Biophys.* **38**, 297.

Nakayama, T. (1958). *Arch. Biochem. Biophys.* **75**, 352, 356.

Motonaga, K., and Miyanoue, T. (1961). *Takamine Kenkyusho Nempo*, **13**, 106.

Nakayama, T., Mackinney, G., and Phaff, H. J. (1954). *Leeuwenhoekned. Tijdschr.* **20**, 217.

Netien, G., and. La Charme, J. (1955). *Bull. Soc. Chim. biol., Paris* **37**, 634.

Olson, E. M., Harvey, J. D., Hill, D. C. and Branion, H. D. (1959). *Poultry Sci.* **38**, 950.

Olson, J. A. (1960). *Biochim. Biophys. Acta* **37**, 166.

Olson, J. A. (1961a). *Comm. 5th Int. Cong. Biochem.* p. 238.

Olson, J. A. (1961b). *J. biol. Chem.* **236**, 349.

Olson, J. A. (1962). *Fed. Proc.* **21**, 473.

Osborne, T. B., and Mendel, L. B. (1914). *J. biol. Chem.*, **17**, 401.

Pardee, A. B., Schachman, H. K., and Stanier, R. Y. (1952). *Nature, Lond.* **169**, 282.

Patel, S. M., Mehl, J. W., and Deuel, H. J. (1951). *Arch. Biochem.* **30**, 103.

Pennock, J. F., Hemming, F. W., and Morton, R. A. (1962). *Biochem. J.* **82**, 11P.

Peskin, J. G. (1957). *Anat. Record.* **128**, 600.

Pitt, G. A. J., and Morton, R. A. (1960). *Symp. Biochem. Soc.* **19**, 67.

Plack, P. A., Kon, S. K., and Thompson, S. Y. (1959). *Biochem. J.* **464**.

Plack, P. A., Thompson, S. Y., and Kon, S. K. (1957). *Biochem. J.* **68**, 2P.

Plempel, M. (1957). *Arch. Microbiol.* **26**, 151.

Porter, J. W., and Anderson, D. G. (1962). *Arch. Biochem. Biophys.* **91**, 520.

Porter, J. W., and Lincoln, R. E. (1950). *Arch. Biochem.* **27**, 390.

Praus, R. (1952). *Chem. Listy*, **46**, 643.

Praus, R., and Dyr, J. (1957). *Chem. Listy*, **51**, 1559, 1939.

Purcell, A. E., Thompson, G. A., and Bonner, J. (1959). *J. biol. Chem.* **234**, 1081.

Rabourn, W. J., and Quackenbush, F. W. (1959). *Arch. Biochem. Biophys.* **44**, 159.

Reader, V. (1925). *Biochem. J.* **19**, 1039.

Roux, E., and Husson, C. (1952). *C. R. Acad. Sci., Paris* **234**, 1573.

Rudney, H. (1959). In "Biosynthesis of Terpenes and Sterols" (G. E. W. Wolstenholme and M. O'Connor, eds.). Churchill, London.

Rüegg, R., Schwieter, U., Ryer, G., Schudel, P., and Isler, O. (1961). *Helv. chim. Acta* **44**, 985.

Saperstein, S., Starr, M. P., and Filfus, J. A. (1954). *J. gen. Microbiol.* **10**, 85.

Sapozhnikov, D. I. I., Maerskaya, A. N., Krasovskaya-Antropova, T. A. Prialgruskaite, L. L. and Turchino, U. S. (1959). *Biokhimiya* **24**, 34.

Sayre, C. B., Robinson, W. B., and Wishnetzky, T. (1953). *Proc. Amer. Soc. hort Sci.* **61**, 381.

Schlegel, H. G. (1958). *Arch. Mikrobiol.* **31**, 231.

Schlegel, H. G. (1959). *J. Bact.* **77**, 310.

Schopfer, W. H., Grob, E. C., and Besson, G. (1952a). *Arch. Sci. (Genève)* **5**, 5.

Schopfer, W. H., Grob, E. C., Besson, G. and Keller, V. (1952b). *Arch. Sci. (Genève)*, **5**, 1.

Sexton, E. F., Mehl, J. W., and Deuel, H. J. (1946). *J. Nutrit.* **31**, 299.

Seybold, A., and Egle, K. (1938). *Planta*, **28**, 87.

Shantz, E. M., Embree, N. D., Hodge, H. C., and Wills, J. H Jr. (1946). *J. biol. Chem.* **763**, 455.

Sharman, I. M. (1949). *Brit. J. Nutrit.* **3**, viii.

Sheng, T. C., and Sheng, G. (1952). *Genetics* **37**, 264.

Shneour, E. A., and Zabin, I. (1958). *J. biol. Chem.* **234**, 770.

Shneour, E. A. (1962). *Biochim. biophys. Acta* **62**, 534.

Sissins, M. E. (1956). Ph. D. Thesis, University of Liverpool.

Skoda, J. (1951). *Chem. Listy* **41**, 413.

Slechta, L., Gabriel, O., and Hoffman-Ostenhof, O. (1958). *Nature, Lond.* **181**, 268.

Starr, M. P., and Saperstein, S. (1953). *Arch. Biochem. Biophys.* **43**, 157.

Steele, W. J., and Gurin, S. (1960). *J. biol. Chem.* **235**, 2778.

Steenbock, H. (1919). *Science* **50**, 352.

Steenbock, H., and Boutwell, P. W. (1920). *J. biol. Chem.* **41**, 81.

Steenbock, H., Snell, M. T., and Boutwell, P. W. (1921). *J. biol. Chem.* **47**, 303.

Stephenson, M. (1920). *Biochem. J.* **14**, 715.

Suzue, G. (1960). *Arch. Biochem. Biophys.* **88**, 180; *Biochim. biophys. Acta* **45**, 616.

Suzue, G. (1961). *Biochim. biophys. Acta* **50**, 593.

Tavormina, P. A., Gibbs, M. H., and Huff, J. W. (1956). *J. Amer. chem. Soc.* **78**, 4498.

Thompson, S. Y., Ganguly, J., and Kon, S. K. (1947). *Brit. J. Nutrit.* **1**, V.

Thompson, S. Y., Ganguly, J., and Kon, S. K. (1949). *Brit. J. Nutrit.* **3**, 50.

Thompson, J. N., Howell, J. Mc., and Pitt, G. A. J. (1961). *Biochem. J.* **80**, 16P, 25P.

Tomes, M., L., Quackenbush, F. W., and Kargl, T. E. (1956). *Botan. Gaz.* **117**, 248.

Tomes, M. L., Quackenbush, F. W., and McQuistan, M. (1954). *Genetics* **39**, 810.

Turian, G. (1950). *Helv. chim. Acta* **33**, 1988.

Turian, G. (1953). *Helv. chim. Acta* **36**, 937.

Turian, G. (1957). *Physiol. Plantarum* **10**, 667.

Turian, G., and Haxo, F. (1952). *J. Bact.* **63**, 690.

Turian, G., and Haxo, F. (1954). *Botan. Gaz.* **115**, 254.

Van Niel, C. B. (1947). *Leeuwenhoek ned. Tijdschr.* **12**, 156.

Van Niel, C. B., Goodwin, T. W., and Sissins, M. E. (1956). *Biochem. J.* **63**, 408.
Varandani, P. T., Wright, G. J., Wolf, G., and Johnson, B. C. (1961). *Fed. Proc.* **20**, 452.
Varma, T. N. R., and Chichester, C. O. (1962). *Arch. Biochem. Biophys.*, **96**, 265.
Varma, T. N. R., Chichester, C. O., Nakayama, T., Lukton, A., and Mackinney, G. (1959). *Nature, Lond.* **183**, 188.
Villoutreix, J. (1957). *Bull. Soc. pharm. Nancy*, **33**, 8.
Villoutreix, J. (1960). *Biochim. biophys. Acta* **40**, 434, 442.
Von Euler, H., and Karrer, P. (1950). *Helv. chim. Acta* **33**, 1481.
Wald, G. (1943). *Vitam. & Horm.* **1**, 195.
Wald, G. (1946). *Harvey Lectures* **41**, 148.
Wald, G. (1960). *Vitam. & Horm.* **18**, 417.
Wald, G., and Brown, P. K. (1950). *Proc. nat. Acad. Sci., Wash.* **36**, 84.
Wald, G., and Brown, P. K. (1956). *Nature, Lond.* **177**, 174.
Wald, G., and Brown, P. K. (1956–7). *J. gen. Physiol.* **40**, 627.
Wald, G., and Burg, S. P. (1956–7). *J. gen. Physiol.* **40**, 609.
Wald, G., and Hubbard, R. (1948–9) *J. gen. Physiol.* **32**, 367
Weissbach, H., Goodwin, F., and Maxwell, E. S. (1961) *Biochim. biophys. Acta,* **49**, 384.
Wald, G., and Hubbard, R. (1958–9). *J. gen. Physiol.* **32**, 367.
Yamamoto, H. Y., Chichester, C. O., and Nakayama, T. O. M. (1962) *Photochem. Photobiol.* **1**, 53.
Went, F. W., Le Rosen, A., and Zechmeister, L. (1942). *Plant. Physiol.* **17**, 91.
Wiese, C. F., Mehl, J. W., and Deuel, H. J. (1947). *Arch. Biochem.* **17**, 75.
Wilt, F. H. (1959). *Developmental Biol.* **1**, 199.
Withrow, R. B., Klein, W. H., Price, L., and Elstrad, V. (1953). *Plant Physiol.* **28**, 1.
Wittman, H. (1956). *Arch. Mikrobiol.* **25**, 373.
Wolf, G., and Johnson, B. C. (1960). *Vitam. & Horm.* **18**, 403.
Worker, N. A. (1956). *Brit. J. Nutrit.* **10**, 126.
Worker, N. A. (1959). *Brit. J. Nutrit.* **13**, 400.
Wurhmann, J. J., Yokoyama, H., and Chichester, C. O. (1957). *J. Amer. chem. Soc.* **79**, 4569.
Yamamoto, H., Yokoyama, H., Simpson, K., Nakayama, T. O. M., and Chichester, C. O. (1961). *Nature, Lond.* **191**, 1299.
Yamamoto, H., Nakayama, T. O. M., and Chichester, C. O. (1962a). *Arch. Biochem. Biophys.* **97**, 168.
Yamamoto, H., Chichester, C. O., and Nakayama, T. O. M. (1962b) *Arch. Biochem. Biophys.* **96**, 645.
Yokoyama, H., Chichester, C. O., Nakayama, T., Lukton, A., and Mackinney, G. (1957). *J. Amer. chem. Soc.* **79**, 2029.
Yokoyama, H., Chichester, C. O., and Mackinney, G. (1960). *Nature, Lond.* **186**, 235.
Yokoyama, H., Nakayama, T. O. M., and Chichester, C. O. (1962). *J. biol. Chem.* **237**, 681.
Zalokar, M. (1954). *Arch. Biochem. Biophys.* **50**, 71.
Zalokar, M. (1955). *Arch. Biochem. Biophys.* **56**, 318.
Zechmeister, L. (1949). *Vitam. & Horm.* **7**, 59.
Zechmeister, L. (1960). *Fortschr. Chem. org. Naturst.* **18**, 223.

CHAPTER 15

THE VITAMINS E (TOCOPHEROLS) AND VITAMINS K

I. INTRODUCTION

The aim of this very short chapter is mainly to draw the attention of workers interested in problems of biosynthesis to the existence of these two groups of compounds. No detailed investigations on either set have been reported, but the structures pose fascinating biosynthetic questions.

II. VITAMINS E (TOCOPHEROLS)

A. *Introduction*

Mattill and Conklin (1920) first indicated from nutrition experiments that a lipid-soluble factor was specifically concerned with fertility. This was confirmed by Evans and Bishop (1922) and the factor eventually became known as vitamin E. Evans *et al.* (1936) subsequently isolated three closely related compounds from wheat germ oil, and gave the name α-tocopherol to the compound with the greatest activity in preventing death and resorption of the foetus in female rats, the characteristic lesion in vitamin E deficiency. In 1938 Fernholz elucidated the structure of α-tocopherol and Karrer *et al.* (1938) synthesized it. Examination of the two other factors showed that they and α-tocopherol were all methylated derivatives of toco

(I)

(I). The use of refined techniques in dealing with small amounts of tocopherols has resulted in the identification of 8 naturally occurring tocopherols (Table 1). The best sources of all these compounds are the higher plants, in particular vegetable oils.

TABLE 1. The Structures of the Naturally
Occurring Tocopherols

Compound	Structure
α-Tocopherol	5,7,8-trimethyltocol
β-Tocopherol	5,8-dimethyltocol
γ-Tocopherol	7,8-dimethyltocol
ζ-Tocopherol (palm oil, wheat bran)	α-tocopherol with 3 double bonds in the C-2 side chain*
$\zeta(\zeta_2)$-Tocopherol (rice)	5,7-dimethyltocol
ε-Tocopherol	α-tocopherol with 3 double bonds in the C-2 side chain*
η-Tocopherol	7-methyltocol
δ-Tocopherol	8-methyltocol

* Complete proof of these structures is still awaited (see e.g. Green *et al.*, 1959, 1960).

Apart from the well-known sterility effect, vitamin E deficiency results in a number of other pathological states, e.g. nutritional muscular dystrophy and exudative diathesis. Because of this and because of the recent implication of vitamin A in reproduction (Thompson and Pitt, 1961), it is wise not to persist in calling vitamin E the anti-sterility vitamin.

B. *Biosynthesis*

(i) *General factors controlling synthesis in higher plants*

The most thorough study on the pattern of tocopherol synthesis in germinating seeds and developing seeds is that of Green (1958) who separated the tocopherols chomatographically before assaying them. In laboratory experiments the total tocopherol level in seedlings germinated in the dark remained essentially constant for wheat (14 days) and pea (8 days) seedlings. On the other hand, the levels in germinating sweet corn increases considerably between 9 and 16 days after the onset of germination. The same general pattern was observed if the seeds were germinated in the light; Baszynsky (1959) similary found that the synthesis of tocopherols by maize seedlings was the same in light and darkness. So the conclusions must be that the pattern of synthesis can vary from plant to plant but different plants behave differently and that light has no effect in any species.

A further interesting aspect of Green's work is that the ungerminated seeds contain a mixture of tocopherols, but as barley and pea seeds germinate, the α-tocopherol levels increase, whilst the remainder decrease by a corresponding amount (Table 2). As the

TABLE 2. The Tocopherol Levels in Wheat Seedlings Germinated in Darkness (Green, 1958)

Time of germination (days)	Tocopherols (μg/plant)				
	α	β	ε	ξ	(Total)
4	0·49	0·22	0·26	0·18	1·15
5	0·60	0·26	0·29	0·00	1·15
6	0·63	0·19	0·21	0·12	1·15
8	1·14	0·00	0·00	0·00	1·14
14	1·20	0·00	0·00	0·00	1·20

plants continue to grow, α-tocopherol continues to be essentially the only vitamer synthesized. However, as soon as seed formation and, particulary, seed maturation begins the other tocopherols begin to appear. Some typical values for barley ears are given in Table 3.

TABLE 3. The Tocopherol Levels in Barley Ears (Green, 1958)

Age of Plant (days)	Condition	Tocopherols (μg./ear)						
		α	β	γ	ε	ξ	η	Total
93	Unripe	4·9	0	0	0	0	0	4·9
106	Unripe	13·5	2·9	Trace	8·9	14·5	Trace	39·7
122	Ripe	15·2	9·6	Trace	18·0	25·1	Trace	67·9

The significance of these changes in relation to a biosynthetic pathway is not yet clear, but the results with young wheat and pea seedlings strongly suggest that α-tocopherol is being formed from the other compounds. The general increase in total tocopherols during seed maturation noted by Green (1958) has also been reported in pistachio seeds (*Pistacia vera* L.) by Giovannini and Condorell (1958).

Booth and Hobson-Frohock (1961) have found that the α-tocopherol levels in leaves are highest in old, dormant and dying leaves, and lowest in young and actively growing leaves. Once again the significance of this to the problem of biosynthesis of tocopherols is difficult to evaluate. Sironval and Tannir-Lomba (1960) reported that the vitamin E content of mature leaves of *Fragaria vesca* L. var. *semperflorens* grown under long day conditions (16 hr) and beginning to flower was about twice that of leaves from plants grown under short day conditions and which remained vegetative.

(ii) *Mechanism of synthesis*

It would appear fatuous to discuss the mechanism of synthesis of the tocopherols when it has become apparent in the preceding section that virtually nothing is known about the details of the reaction. It is only raised here in order to point out the basic similarity between the ubiquinones (II) and more particularly their isomers, the ubichromenols (III) and the tocopherols (I). The terpenoid side chains

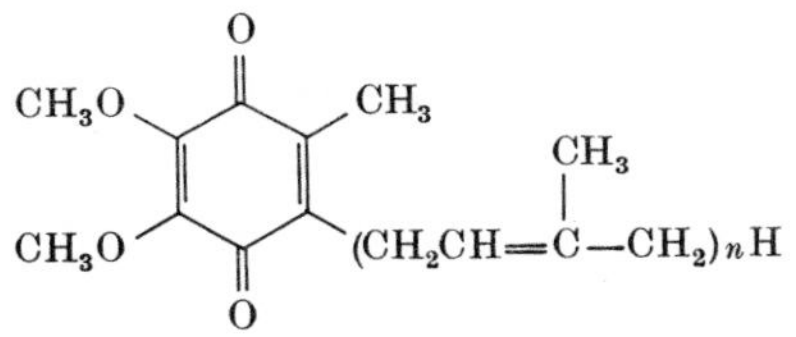

(II)

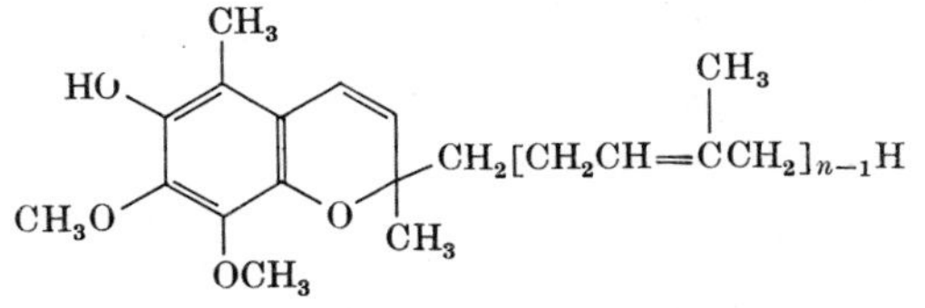

(III)

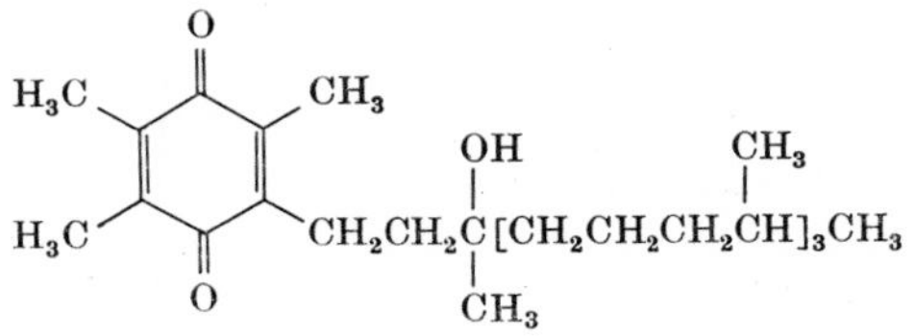

(IV)

of the ubiquinones arise from mevalonate (Gloor and Wiss, 1959; 1960; Glover *et al.* 1961; Lawson *et al.*, 1961) and the aromatic ring probably from phenylalanine, via shikimic acid (Olson *et al.*, 1960, 1961, 1962). The tocopherols could arise from similar precursors via a compound related to α-tocopherylquinone (IV). However, the recent work of Slaters' group (Slater, 1960) indicates that this compound is not present in animal tissues; it does not appear to have been looked for in plant tissues. It should further be emphasized that structurally obscure benzoquinone metabolites of tocopherols have been obtained from animals (Martius and Costelli, 1957; Simon *et al.*, 1956).

III. Vitamins K

A. *Introduction*

Dam (1929) first reported that chicks reared on a synthetic ration developed a pathological condition characterized by an increased blood clotting time. He named the factor present in various foodstuffs which would cure this condition vitamin K (Koagulations vitamin) (Dam, 1935). Two compounds with vitamin K activity were eventually isolated by Binkley *et al.* (1939), Dam *et al.* (1939) and Karrer and Geiger (1939). Vitamin K_1 (2-methyl-3-phytyl-1,4-naphthoquinone (V) was obtained from lucerne (alfalfa); it occurs in all leafy tissues but after a period when it was consistently reported to be absent from chloroplasts, its position there has been reaffirmed (Kegel *et al.*, 1962). It is important not to confuse it with Kofler's quinone (plastoquinone) (VI) which is specifically associated with chloroplasts (Kofler *et al.*, 1959; Trenner *et al.*, 1959). Vitamin K_2 was obtained from putrefied fish meal by Doisy's group (Binkley *et al.*, 1939) and considered to have a 30-C side chain consisting of 6 isoprenoid residues. However, Isler *et al.* (1958a,b) have shown that the side chain actually contains 7 isoprenoid residues and that Doisy's vitamin K_2 is 2-methyl 3-(all-*trans*-farnesylgeranylgeranyl)-1,4-naphthoquinone (VII). As Isler's group also isolated from their fish meal extract small amounts of 2-methyl-3-farnesylfarnesyl-1,4-naphthoquinone (VIII), a compound with the structure originally assigned to vitamin K_2, they propose that (VII) be termed vitamin K_2 (35) and (VIII) vitamin K_2 (30). All the three vitamins K mentioned have been synthesized by Isler's group (see Isler and Wiss, 1959). Two other vitamins K_2 have been reported, that from *Mycobacterium tuberculosis* has a 45-C side chain (Noll, 1958), and that from rat tissues fed 2-methyl-1,4-naphthoquinone has an unsaturated 20-C side chain

(Martius, 1958); a third vitamin K-active naphthoquinone has been isolated from *Mycobact. phlei* but has not been fully identified (Brodie *et al.*, 1958). Vitamin K is also present in the photosynthetic bacteri-

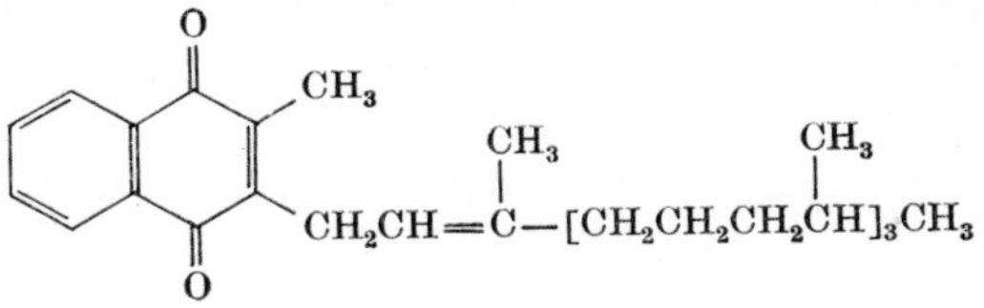

(V)

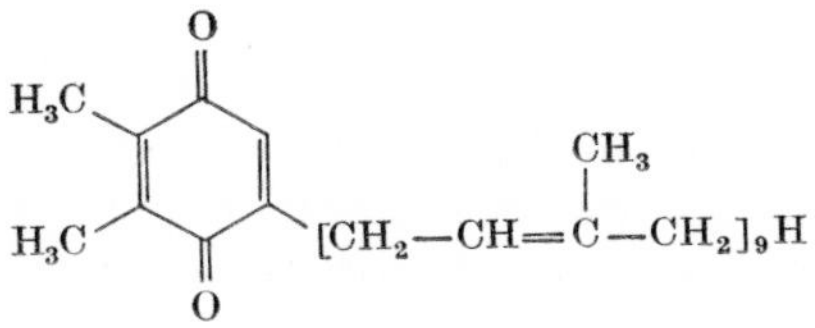

(VI)

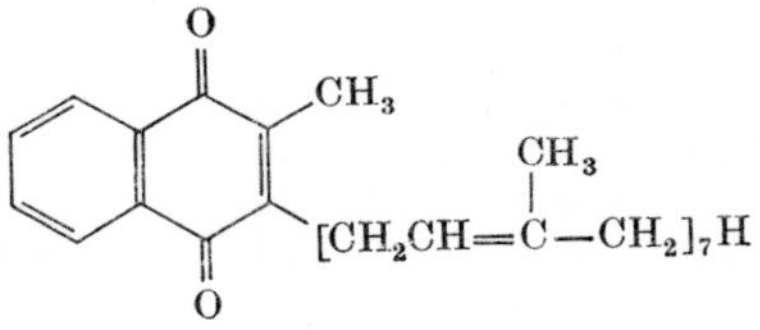

(VII)

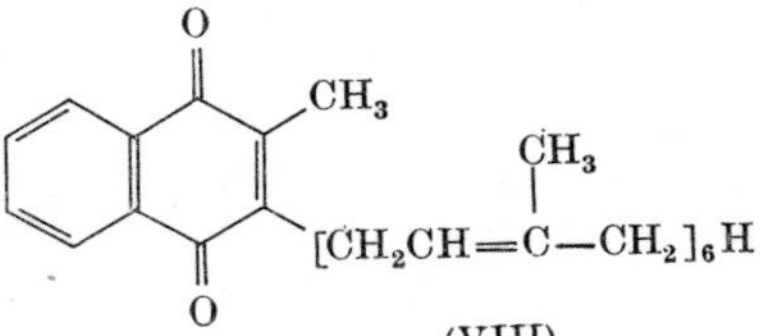

(VIII)

um *Chromatium* (Green *et al.*, 1959; Fuller *et al.*, 1961) and a survey of the occurrence of vitamins K in bacteria has recently been published (Bishop *et al.*, 1962).

B. *Biosynthesis*

Very little is known about the biosynthesis of vitamin K. Dam and his colleagues (Dam and Glavind, 1938; Dam *et al.*, 1940, 1947) found that vitamin K was synthesized by seedlings of *Picea canadensis* germinated in the dark but not by dark-germinated *Pisum sativum*;

synthesis was, however, greater in seedlings of *Picea canadensis* germinated in the light. More recent experiments using modern analytical methods have confirmed the vitamin K is synthesized by leaves only in the light (Lichtenthaler, 1962).

With regard to bacterial synthesis of vitamin K_2, Isler and Wiss (1959) state that it "varies within wide limits and appears to be very dependent on the composition of the bacterial flora. Vitamin K_2 can also be produced on artificial media containing aspartic acid, ammonium citrate and glucose".

Martius and Esser (1958) administered [^{14}C]-2-methyl-1,4-naphthoquinone (menadione) to chicks and rats and isolated a radioactive vitamin K which appeared to have an unsaturated 20-C side chain. They suggested that all vitamins K administered to animals are degraded to menadione and then built up to vitamin K_2 (20) by the animals. The more recent work of Billeter and Martius (1960) confirms this view; these investigators report the conversion of vitamin K_1 into vitamin K_2 (20) by the chick and the rat.

REFERENCES

Baszynski, T. (1959). *Acta Soc. Bot. Polon.* **28,** 621.
Billeter, M., and Martius, C. (1960). *Biochem. Z.* **333,** 430.
Binkley, S. B., Cheney, L. C., Holcomb, W. F., McKee, R. W., Thayer, S. A., MacCorquadale, D. W., and Doisy, E. A. (1939). *J. Amer. chem. Soc.* **61,** 2558.
Bishop, D. H. L., Pandya, K. P., and King, H. K. (1962). *Biochem. J.* **83** 606.
Booth, V. H., and Hobson-Frohock, A. (1961). *J. Sci. Fod Agric.* **12,** 251.
Brodie, A. F., Davis, B. R., and Fieser, L. F. (1958). *J. Amer. chem. Soc.* **86,** 6454.
Dam, H. (1929). *Biochem. Z.* **215,** 475.
Dam, H. (1935). *Biochem. J.* **29,** 1273.
Dam, H., and Glavind, J. (1938). *Biochem. J.* **485.**
Dam, H., Geiger, A., Glavind, J., Karrer, P., Karrer, W., Rotschild, E., and Salomon, H. (1939). *Helv. chim. Acta* **22,** 310.
Dam, H., Glavind, J., and Nielson, R. (1940). *Hoppe-Seyl. Z.* **265,** 80.
Dam, H., Glavind, J., and Gabrielson, E. K. (1947). *Acta physiol. scand.* **13,** 9.
Evans, H. M., and Bishop, K. S. (1922). *Science* **55,** 650.
Evans, H. M., Emerson, O. H., and Emerson, G. A. (1936). *J. biol. Chem.* **113,** 319.
Fuller, R. C., Smillie, R. M., Rigopoulos, N., and Yount, V. (1961). *Arch. Biochem. Biophys.* **95,** 197.
Fernholz, E. (1938). *J. Amer. chem. Soc.* **60,** 700.
Giovannini, E., and Condorelli, G. (1958). *Ric. Sci.* **78,** 1863.
Gloor, U., and Wiss, O. (1959). *Arch. Biochem. Biophys.* **83,** 216.
Gloor, U., and Wiss, O. (1960). *Biochem. biophys. Res. Comm.* **2,** 222.
Glover, J., Lawson, D. E. M., Morton, R. A., and Threlfall, D. R. (1961). "Proceedings of the 5th International Congress of Biochemistry," (in press). Pergamon Press, London.

Green, J. (1958). *J. Sci. Fd Agric.* **9,** 801.

Green, J., McHale, D., Marcinkiewicz, S., Mamalis, P., and Watt, P. R. (1959). *J. chem. Soc.*, p. 3362.

Green, J., Mamalis, P., Marcinkiewicz, S., and McHale, D. (1960). *Chem. Ind. London* **79,** 73.

Green, J., Price, S. A., and Gare, L. (1959). *Nature, Lond.* **184,** 1339.

Isler, O., Rüegg, R., Chopard-dit-Jean, L. H., Winterstein, A., and Wiss, O. (1958a). *Chimia (Switz.)* **12,** 69.

Isler, O., Rüegg, R., Chopard-dit-Jean, L. H., Winterstein, A., and Wiss, O. (1958b). *Helv. chim. Acta* **41,** 786.

Isler, O., and Wiss, O. (1959). *Vitam. & Horm.* **17,** 53.

Karrer, P., Fritsche, H., Ringier, B. H., and Salomon, H. (1938). *Helv. chim. Acta* **21,** 520, 820.

Karrer, P. and Geiger, A. (1939). *Helv. chim. Acta* **22,** 945.

Kegel, L. P., Henninger, M. D., and Crane, F. L. (1962). *Biochem. biophys. Res. Comm.* **8,** 294.

Kofler, M., Langemann, A., Rüegg, R., Chopard-dit-Jean, L. H., Rayroud, A., and Isler, O. (1959). *Helv. chim. Acta* **42,** 1283.

Lawson, D. E. M., Threlfall, D. R., Glover, J., and Morton, R. A. (1961). *Biochem. J.* **79,** 201.

Lichtenthaler, H. K. (1962). *Planta* **54,** 431.

Martius, C. (1958). *Dtsch. med. Wschr.* **83,** 1701.

Martius, C., and Costelli, J. (1957). *Biochem. Z.* **329,** 449.

Martius, C., and Esser, H. O. (1958). *Biochem. Z.* **331,** 1.

Mattill, H. A., and Conklin, R. E. (1920). *J. biol. Chem.* **44,** 137.

Noll, H. (1958). *J. biol. Chem.* **232,** 919.

Olson, R. E., Dialameh, G. H., and Bentley, R. (1960). *Fed. Proc.* **19,** 20.

Olson, R. E., Bentley, R., Dialameh, G. H., and Gold, P. (1962). *Biochem. J.* **82,** 14P.

Olson, R. E., Bentley, R., Dialameh, G. H., Gold, P. H., Ramsey, V., and Springer, C. (1961). "Comm. 5th International Congress of Biochemistry" p. 469.

Simon, E. J., Ersengart, A., Sundheim, L., and Milhorat, A. T. (1956). *J. biol. Chem.* **221,** 807.

Sironval, C., and El Tannir-Lomba (1960). *Nature, Lond.* **185,** 855.

Slater, E. C. (1960). "Proceedings of the 4th International Congress of Biochemistry, Vienna" **11,** 316. Pergamon Press, London.

Thompson, J. N., and Pitt, G. A. J. (1961). *Biochem. J.* **80,** 16P, L5P.

Trenner, N. R., Arison, B. H., Erickson, R. E., Shunk, C. H., Wolf, D. E., and Folkers, K. (1959). *J. Amer. chem. Soc.* **81,** 2026.

AUTHOR INDEX

(Numbers in italics refer to pages on which reference is listed.)

M

Ma, R., 150, *157*
Maas, W. K., 133, 134, 138, *143*
McCalla, A. G., 40, *66*
McCann, P., 110, *130*
McCay, P. B., 219, 220, *228*, *230*
McClary, J. E., 5, *22*
McClung, L. S., 28, *67*
McCollum, E. V., 240, *268*, 270, *316*
McCollum J. P., 224, *230*
McCollum, S, P., 287, *316*
McConnell, W. B., 92, *94*
McCormick, D. B., 58, 59, *65, 66*, 161, 162, *165*, 218, *231*
McCormick, M. H., 205, *209*
Maccorquadale, D. W., 324, *326*
McCoy, E., 148, *156, 157*
McCoy, R. H., 154, *157*
McCullough, W. G., 262, *267*
McDougall, B. M., 115, 116, *127*
McElroy, L. W., 30, 40, *66*
McEvoy, D., 35, 37, 38, 42, 43, 45, 46, 49, 50, *63, 64, 66*
McGillivray, W. A., 307, *316*
McGlohon, V. M., 132, *144*
McHale, D., 321, 325, *327*
McIntosh, E. N., 134, *143*
Mack, P. B., 39, *68*
McKee, R. W., 324, *326*
McKibben, J. R., 154, *157*
Mackinney, G., 253, *266*, 279, 280, 281, 283, 295, 296, 298, 299, *314*, *317, 319*
Maclaren, J. A., 34, 35, 42, 46, *65*
McMillan, F. H., 257, *268*
McNutt, W. S., 34, 42, 43, 46, 55, *64, 66*, 106, *128*
McQuistan, M., 286, *319*
Macrae, T. F., 159, *165*
McVeigh, I., 12, 14, *21*, 30, 39, *63*, *81, 95*, 160, *165*
Madden, R. J., 69, 79, *95, 99*
Maeuskaya, A. N., 292, *317*
Magasanik, B., 105, 121, *128*, *129*

Mainil, J., 26, *63*
Maizel, B., 16, *22*
Major, R. T., 131, *144*
Makino, K., 60, *65*
Maley, G. F., 51, 52, 54, 55, *65*, 106, 108, *128, 129*
Malkin, A., 86, *97*
Mamalis, P., 321, 325, *327*
Mann, T., 204, *209*
Mannering, G. J., 30, *65*
Mand, Y., 18, *22, 23*, 214, *230, 231*
Mantrova, G. V., 178, *185*
Mapson, L. W., 212, 215, 219, 221, 223, 224, 225, 226, *228*, *229, 230*, 293, *317*
Marcinkiewicz, S., 321, 325, *327*
Mardeshev, S. R., 137, *143*
Marion, L., 90, 93, *95, 96*
Marnati, M. P., 180, *184*
Martin, J. B., 195, *201*
Martius, C., 324, 325, 326, *326*, *327*
Mase, Y., 295, *317*
Mason, H. S., 71, 74, *97*, 247, *268*
Massonet, R., 302, 303, 307, *315*, *317*
Masuda, T., 49, 50, 51, 52, 53, 55, 57, 58, *63, 65*
Mathew, C. K., 115, *128*
Mathews, M. M., 278, *317*
Mathias, A. P., 56, *63*
Matsuo, Y., 192, *201*
Matsuura, K., 59, 61, *65*
Matsuyama, A., 135, *143*
Mattern, C. F. T., 183, *186*
Mattill, H. A., 320, *327*
Mattson, F. H., 195, *201*
Maudgal, R. K., 243, 247, 248, *268*
Maxwell, E. S., 213, *229, 230, 319*
May, F. L., 76, *97*
Mayberry, R. H., 218, *231*
Maynard, L., 224, *229*
Mead, J. F., 236, *238, 239*
Meade, R. E., 28, 29, *66, 67*
Medairy, G. C., 30, *66*
Mego, J. L., 294, *317*
Mehl, J. W., 306, 307, *317, 318*, *319*

SUBJECT INDEX

A

Acetal phosphatides, see Plasmalogens

Acetic acid,
    incorporation into anabasine, 90
    incorporation into carotenoids, 279
    incorporation into cholesterol, 242
    incorporation into fatty acids, 235—237
    incorporation into nicotinic acid, 90
    incorporation into riboflavin, 50
    incorporation into squalene, 242

Acetoin, in riboflavin biosynthesis, 49—50, 53

Acetolactate, 136

Acetyl-CoA carboxylase, 146

Acetyl-CoA: CO_2 ligase (ADP), see Acetyl-CoA carboxylase

Active acetaldehyde, 20

Active acetate, 2, 132

Active formaldehyde, 101, 119

Active formate, 101

Active glycine in riboflavin synthesis, 45

Active isoprene, 251

Active methylene, 101

Active pyruvate, see α-Lactyl-2-thiamine pyrophosphate

Active sulphate, 199

Acyl-CoA: acetyl-CoA acyltransferase, see β-Ketothiolase

N-Acylsphingosine, see Ceramide

Adenine, in riboflavin biosynthesis, 42, 49
    incorporation into pteroyltriglutamic acid, 107

Adenosine 3'-phosphate 5'-sulphatophosphate, see Active sulphate

S-Adenosylmethionine, 190

S-Adenosylmethionine: nicotinamide methyltransferase, see Nicotinamide methyltransferase

α-Adenylcobamide, 173

Agnosterol, 143

β-Alanine,
    formation of, 137—138
    in nicotinic acid synthesis, 90
    in pantothenic acid synthesis, 133

Alcohol dehydrogenase, 309

Alcohol: NAD oxidoreductase, see Alcohol dehydrogenase

Aldehyde dehydrogenase (liver), 313

Aldehyde: NAD oxidoreductase, see Aldehyde dehydrogenase (liver)

Aldehyde: O_2 oxidoreductase, see Aldehyde oxidase (liver)

Aldehyde oxidase (liver), 313

Aldonolactonase, 214

Alkaloids, 90—94

Alloxan, 41, 57

All-*trans*-retinene: 11-*cis*-*trans*-isomerase, see retinene isomerase

p-Aminobenzoic acid, in folic acid synthesis, 111

p-Aminobenzoylglutamate, 111

1-Amino-4-formylbutadiene-2-carboxylic acid, 75